Cross-cultural Rehabilitation

For W B Saunders

Editorial Director: Mary Law
Design Direction: Judith Wright

Cross-cultural Rehabilitation

An International Perspective

Edited by

Ronnie Linda Leavitt PhD MPH PT

Associate Professor, University of Connecticut, USA

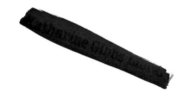

 W.B. SAUNDERS

London • Edinburgh • Philadelphia • Toronto • Sydney • Tokyo

W B SAUNDERS
An imprint of Harcourt Publishers Limited

First published 1999
  Reprinted 2001

ISBN 0 702 022454

British Library Cataloguing in Publication Data
A catalogue record for this book is available from the British
Library.

Library of Congress Cataloging in Publication Data
A catalog record for this book is available from the Library
of Congress

Note
Medical knowledge is constantly changing. As new information becomes available, changes in treatment, procedures,
equipment and the use of drugs become necessary. The
authors and the publishers have, as far as it is possible,
taken care to ensure that the information given in this text is
accurate and up to date. However, readers are strongly
advised to confirm that the information, especially with
regard to drug usage, complies with the latest legislation
and standards of practice.

The authors and publishers have made every effort to trace
the copyright holders for borrowed material. If they have
inadvertently over-looked any, they will be pleased to make
the necessary arrangements at the first opportunity.

The
publisher's
policy is to use
**paper manufactured
from sustainable forests**

Printed in China

Contents

Contributors

Alejandro Brice PhD CCC-SLP
Department of Communicative Disorders,
College of Health and Public Affairs, University
of Central Florida, FL, USA

Lynda R. Campbell CCC-SLP
Department of Communication Disorders, Saint
Louis University, Saint Louis, MO, USA

Nguyen Thi Minh Chau BS PT
Project Assistant, Health Volunteers Overseas,
Hanoi, Vietnam

Huib Cornielje MPH MSc(Med) DipPhys
Department of Public Health, Hogeschool,
Leiden, The Netherlands

Valerie Lesley Dawson PhD MSc
Chairperson, Department of Rehabilitation
Studies, West Bank

Paulo de Lyz Girov Martins Ferrinho
PhD MSc(Med) MMed(Com)
Instituto de Higiene e Medicina Tropical and
Centro de Malaria e de Outras Doencas
Tropicais of the Universidade Nova de Lisboa,
Lisboa, Portugal

Harry Finkenflügel MEdM MSc BSc
Faculty of Human Movement Sciences, Vrije
Universiteit, Amsterdam, the Netherlands

Lawrence Daniel Golin BSc MDiv PT
Formerly at Memorial Christian Hospital, Cox's
Bazar, Bangladesh. Presently International
Director for Ministries to Disabled Persons,
Association of Baptists, Harrisburg, PA, USA

Nora Ellen Groce PhD
International Health Division, Yale School of
Public Health, Yale University, New Haven, CT,
USA

Gale Haradon PhD OTR
Chair and Associate Professor, Department of
Occupational Therapy, University of Texas
Health Science Center at San Antonio, San
Antonio, TX, USA

Nguyen Thi Huong BS PT
Head, Rehabilitation Department, Central
Medical Technology School, Ho Chi Minh City,
Vietnam

Kevin Hylton
Department of Sociology and Anthropology,
Howard University, Washington, DC, USA

Benedicte Ingstaad
Section for Medical Anthropology, Institute of
General Practice and Community Medicine,
University of Oslo, Oslo, Norway

Jennifer Jelsma MPhil BSc(Phys) DipTertEd
Senior Lecturer in Physiotherapy, Department
of Rehabilitation, University of Zimbabwe,
Harare, Zimbabwe

Sharon Johnson
Director of Rehabilitation Services, Government
Services Center, Duluth, MN, USA

Elizabeth Kay PhD PT
Physical Therapy Program, Northern Illinois
University, DeKalb, IL, USA

Richard Ladyshewsky MHSc BMR (PT)
School of Physiotherapy, Curtin University of
Technology, Shenton Park, Australia

Ronnie L. Leavitt PhD MPH PT
Associate Professor, Department of Physical
Therapy, University of Connecticut, Storrs, CT,
USA

Sophie Levitt BSc(Physiotherapy) Rand. FCSP
Consultant Physiotherapist and Tutor,
Developmental Paediatrics and Neurology,
London, UK

Christine A. Loveland PhD
Professor of Anthropology, Sociology-
Anthropology Department, Shippensburg
University, Shippensburg, PA, USA

Catherine Marshall PhD
Director of Research, American Indian
Rehabilitation Research and Training Center,
Northern Arizona University, Flagstaff, AZ,
USA

Helen L. Masin PhD PT
Graduate Programs in Physical Therapy,
University of Miami, Coral Gables, FL, USA

M. Miles
Birmingham, UK

Christine A. Nelson PhD OTR FAOTA
Morelos, Mexico

Aldred H. Neufeldt PhD
Professor, Community Rehabilitation Studies
Program, The University of Calgary, Calgary,
Canada

Brian O'Toole
CBR Consultant, Georgetown, Guyana, South
America

Tomlin J. Paul MB BS MPH
Department of Community Health & Psychiatry,
University of the West Indies, Kingston, Jamaica

Rebecca Reviere PhD
Professor, Department of Sociology and
Anthropology, Howard University, Washington
DC, USA

Martha Elena Rubi OT
Morelos, Mexico

Patty Ruppelt PT
Physical Therapist, Oakland, CA, USA

Estelle Schneider MS PT
Physical Therapist, San Francisco, CA, USA

Karin Schumacher PT MPH
Independent Consultant, Denver, CO, USA

Hector Segovia
Executive Director and Founder, Centre for the
Promotion of Integral Rehabilitation (CEPRI),
Managua, Nicaragua

Jo Simister
Post-graduate student, University of Ulster, UK

Joseph W. Smey EdD PT
Professor and Dean, School of Allied Health,
University of Connecticut, Storrs, CT, USA

Shoma Stout
UCB-UCSF Joint Medical Program, Health and
Medical Sciences, University of California,
Berkeley, CA, USA

Marigold J. Thorburn MD
Consultant, 3D Projects, Spanish Town;
Associate Lecturer, Faculty of Medical Sciences,
University of the West Indies, Mona, Jamaica

Ahmed Younis DPhil BSc TDip
Physiotherapy Lecturer, School of Health
Sciences, Robert Gordon University, Aberdeen,
UK

Maude Zhanje BSc(Hons)(Physio)
Physical Therapist, Children's Rehabilitation
Unit, Harare, Zimbabwe

Jean Anne Zollars MA PT
Physical Therapist, Albuquerque, NM, USA

Preface

As we anticipate a new millennium, the world is in a state of transformation. Many countries are experiencing considerable demographic shifts along with an increasingly wide range of ethnic identification, religion, material reality, beliefs and behaviors – all leading to rich diversity and cultural complexity. At the same time, health professionals are becoming much more aware of the need to become culturally competent in order to be most effective in their interaction with patients. Rehabilitation professionals have yet to address the issue of cultural competence adequately. The time is ripe for an emerging subspecialty within the fields of rehabilitation medicine and medical anthropology; that is, the field of cross-cultural and international rehabilitation.

As my professional career has expanded to include physical therapy, public health and medical anthropology, I have been frustrated by the way medical and rehabilitation professionals generally focus solely on their area of clinical expertise and rarely pay adequate attention to the socio-cultural context in which our clients live. This frustration has been exacerbated by the dearth of accessible literature and resources in the newly emerging specialty of cross-cultural rehabilitation. For those of us wanting to develop our clinical or academic expertise in this arena, there have been few people or places to turn to for tangible learning tools. To begin to fill the gap, I had thought about editing a book such as this for many years. However, it wasn't until the 1995 meeting of the World Con-

federation of Physical Therapy (WCPT) in Washington DC that I committed myself to such a project. The cross-cultural and international atmosphere was exhilarating. Many people from around the world gave presentations about disability and rehabilitation in their community or country. They gathered for informal conversations about the need for innovative models of rehabilitation specific to a particular environment. The 'buzz words' of the 90s were everywhere – diversity, multi-culturalism, cultural sensitivity, and more. In essence, it was, and remains, apparent that rehabilitation professionals have a moral and pragmatic imperative to become culturally competent.

Because there is so little published material on cross-cultural and international rehabilitation, I faced the challenge of how to be broad minded and expansive, yet focused and specific. I found this to be no easy task. This book is not meant to be merely an academic exercise; my intent is for the reader to gain practical information. I hope the information herein will help to bring together the art and science of rehabilitation with applied medical anthropology. I look forward to the time when a new generation of professionals will offer contributions to expand this field of study by publishing other related, yet more specialized materials.

As we enter the next century, we must genuinely collaborate with our clients and colleagues, including those trained in other disciplines and community level workers, in order to obtain the best possible functional outcome for the client. In teaching my physical therapy students, I have tried, not always successfully, to impress upon them that it may be less important to teach a patient exercises than it is to understand what having an impairment or disability means to the patient. Only with a full appreciation of the patient's life ways and sociocultural context can we best facilitate the rehabilitation process.

I challenge myself and my colleagues to travel the path of intercultural learning toward cultural competence and cultural proficiency. We must move away from ethnocentrism and cultural incapacity toward acceptance and respect for difference, continuing self-assessment, vigilance towards the dynamics of differences, ongoing expansion of cultural knowledge and resources, and adaptations to services. This challenge shall remain with us throughout our lifetimes.

It is truly a privilege to make a contribution to a profession which has given me so much.

Ronnie Leavitt

Connecticut, USA 1999

Acknowledgments

I would like to express my deep appreciation to the many people whose participation and support were critical to the publication of *Cross-cultural Rehabilitation: An International Perspective.*

- to my professional colleagues who encouraged me to undertake this endeavor and often had to suffer the consequences during periods of stress. Special appreciation goes to Inge Reaviel and Mary Gannotti for their kind words and deeds.

- to the contributing authors, truly a diverse and dedicated group from a wide variety of disciplines and nations. They are clinicians and researchers on the cutting edge who will hold a unique place in the development of the emerging specialty of cross-cultural rehabilitation. Each has helped to improve the lives of persons with disabilities.

- to my many friends and family members who have given me their friendship, love and support over the years. Through my personal and professional good times and bad, you have been there. Special thanks and acknowledgment must go to my parents, David and Frieda Lawrence, my sister, Leslie Lawrence and my children, Alan and Kenny Leavitt.

1

Introduction to *Cross-cultural Rehabilitation: An International Perspective*

Ronnie Leavitt

INTRODUCTION

Persons with disabilities (PWD) and their rehabilitation have yet to attract the attention they deserve from the global health care community. Even though the World Health Organization (WHO) sponsored the International Year of Disabled Persons in 1981, and the United Nations Decade of Disabled Persons (1982–1992) focused some attention on the issues, particularly in the developing world, the need for further discussion remains great, especially on how attitudes and responses to disability differ from culture to culture. Disability exists in all societies, yet how individual cultures have defined what constitutes a disability and its significance depends upon each society's values. Attitudes toward individuals with a disability, concepts of rehabilitation, the sociocultural, biological and economic implications of disability, and policy affecting individuals with a disability also vary.

Despite a range of estimates and some disagreement, it is generally thought that there are about 450 million PWD in the world, or around 10% of the population (Helander et al 1989, PAHO 1994). The incidence and prevalence of many health and disability conditions vary within and between countries and are affected by such variables as ethnicity, race, socioeconomic status, geography, migration history, armed conflict, and health beliefs and behaviors. The prevalence of moderate and severe disability – that is, people who are more likely to need rehabilitation – is estimated at 5.2% (Helander 1993). Without improved programs in disability prevention, both the absolute numbers and relative proportions of PWD will grow in the coming decades as the world's population increases and as medical advances allow for the survival of more children under the age of 5 and more elderly people over 65.

It is projected that by the year 2000 more than 80% of the world's population with a disability will live in the Third World (Marfo & Walker 1986). The WHO and the Pan American Health Organization (PAHO) estimate that rehabilitation services for individuals with disabilities in the Third World serve a minute fraction (1–3%) of the total number of those in need (WHO 1981, Helander et al 1989, PAHO/WHO 1994). However, the situation for PWD can be improved upon in the 21st century. New models of care – known as community based rehabilitation (CBR) – are developing: they will undoubtedly be a useful addition to the more traditional models of rehabilitation services. CBR could prove more successful in reaching large numbers of people and allowing individuals with a disability to lead a more satisfying life.

Population and professional demographics

The world contains a kaleidoscope of individuals and cultures: people have a wide range of ethnic identification, religion, material reality, beliefs and behaviors that lead to rich diversity and cultural complexity. In the global context, however, Caucasian people, though the minority, generally speaking have far greater economic resources and political power. Hence, they have more access to rehabilitation services and are more likely to be the ones providing services to others in a multi-cultural environment.

Changing demographics within the USA provides a good example of the pragmatic reasons why rehabilitation professionals need to pay more attention to culture. Between 1980 and 1990, the total US population increased by 9.8%. The rate of growth, however, varied widely: the Asian/Pacific Island population rate of growth was 107.8%, the Hispanic/Latino 53%, the

Native American 37.9%, the black 13.2% and white 6% (US Bureau of the Census 1990). During the last 2 decades, there has been a tremendous influx of immigrants into the USA from South and Central America and from Asia; this trend is expected to continue. By the year 2050, it is projected that white, non-Hispanic Americans will represent 52.8% of the total population (down from the current rate of approximately 70–75%). Hispanic Americans will account for 24.5%, African Americans 13.6%, Asian/Pacific Island Americans 8.2% (US Department of Commerce 1996) and Native Americans 0.19%. People of color (a term used in the USA to include people of African-American, Hispanic-American, Asian-American or Native-American descent) will increase in numbers and therefore require more rehabilitation services.

In addition, again using the USA as an example, there is considerable disparity between the number of individuals from particular ethnic groups enrolled in health professional schools and their representation in the society as a whole. Although people of color make up approximately 25–30% of the US population, they comprise only 7.9% of all health profession degree recipients in the 1990s (Carter & Wilson 1993) and the same proportion of the American Physical Therapy Association in 1996 (APTA 1996).

Within a more global context, the shortage of rehabilitation professionals is dramatic, no matter what their ethnicity or country of origin. For example, the World Confederation for Physical Therapy (WCPT) is an international body for physical therapy and physical therapists from 67 countries, with a reported membership in 1996 of national organizations representing about 215 000 individual members. Although not all physical therapists join WCPT, particularly in the Western world, a review of the membership easily demonstrates the problem of inadequate numbers and distribution of physical therapists. The largest number of therapists (44 000) are from the USA, followed by Germany (31 000). In contrast, the whole of Africa has 2800 members, over 2000 of whom are in South Africa, leaving only 800 to serve the rest of the continent. Some 30 000 physical therapists serve all of Asia, with over 12 000 of these from Japan. In South America, there are only 2600 members coming from six countries (WCPT 1996).

Not only are the absolute numbers of trained personnel insufficient, but in many cases rehabilitation professionals will be from a different cultural background than the person they are treating, whether in their own country, in increasingly multi-cultural settings, or whether they work in another country. The groups included in a discussion of cross-cultural themes generally have limited economic or political power to influence the systems around them, including those for health care and rehabilitation. This can result in a cultural clash and conflicting expectations. Typically, the majority population (or, in some countries, those with political and economic power, even if they are in the minority) rarely concerns itself with the clients in a clinical encounter or considers the under-representation of people of color or the lack of diversity within their professions.

Can professionals work effectively with people from other backgrounds? If the answer is yes, it is logical that increased knowledge about the sociocultural context of the other person can only improve the relationship. It would seem imperative to be aware of the impact of culture on each individual – the patient and the professional – and thus on patient–therapist interactions. With more insight – and fewer preconceived stereotypes – the ability to develop a mutually advantageous relationship is bound to be enhanced.

CULTURAL COMPETENCE

Today, and in the foreseeable future, rehabilitation practitioners, organizations, and systems need to be *culturally competent.* Cultural competence acknowledges and incorporates – at all levels – the importance of culture, the assessment of cross-cultural relations, vigilance towards the dynamics that result from cultural differences, the expansion of cultural knowledge, and the adaptation of services to meet culturally unique needs (Cross et al 1989).

A culturally competent practitioner:

• Has the capacity for cultural self-assessment. Practitioners must recognize the immense influence of culture and be able to assess the effect it has on their own and other people's life views and actions. It is not merely the 'other' who has a unique culture, but each one of us. Understanding our own values, attitudes, beliefs and behaviors is a prerequisite to successful interventions.

• Values diversity, with an awareness, acceptance, and even celebration of differences in life view, health systems, communication styles, and other life-sustaining elements. Individuals share common basic needs and cultural universals such as a family unit, parental roles, educational system, health care system, forms of work, and forms of self-expression. Yet they have different ways of going about meeting those needs: values, attitudes and behaviors are variable and unique to each individual. Not only is there great inter-cultural diversity in the world, but also within cultures there is a wide range of intra-cultural diversity. Patients and their families, as well as health professionals within a particular group, each exemplify a range of health beliefs and behaviors and are again influenced by a huge array of cultural variables.

• Is conscious of the dynamics of difference. With cultural interaction comes the possibility of misjudging the other's intentions and actions. Each party to an interaction brings to the encounter a specific set of experiences and styles. One must be vigilant to minimize misperception, misinterpretation, and misjudgement.

• Institutionalizes cultural knowledge. Cultural knowledge must be accessed and incorporated into the delivery of services. It is impossible, and not necessary, to learn all there is to know about all cultural sub-groups, but clinicians must be aware of the ethnographic information related to the community and relevant beliefs and behaviors of their clients and their clients' families.

• Adapts to diversity. A system is adapted to create a better fit between the needs of the people requiring services and those facilitating the process by which the needs can be met. Interventionists must develop culturally sensitive models as well as help people unfamiliar with more mainstream models to interpret and negotiate them. No one model or approach is universally applicable (Cross et al 1989, Lynch & Hanson 1992).

Cross et al (1989) describe at least six possibilities along a continuum of cultural competence, starting with the least competent:

• Cultural *destructiveness* may involve the extreme of cultural genocide but is more commonly seen when people are actively denied services or treated in a dehumanizing manner.
• Cultural *incapacity* occurs when systems lack the capacity to work effectively with individuals from another culture. The system maintains bias, supports stereotypes, and assumes a paternal stance.
• Cultural *blindness* presumes an unbiased philosophy and that all people are the same. Policy and practices do not recognize the need for culturally specific approaches to solve problems. Services are inherently ethnocentric, ignore cultural strengths, encourage assimilation, and blame victims for their problems.
• Cultural *pre-competence* moves toward the more positive end of the continuum. The system recognizes its weaknesses and explores alternatives. There is a commitment to responding appropriately to differences.
• Cultural *competence* is characterized by acceptance and respect for difference, continuing self-assessment regarding culture, vigilance toward the dynamics of differences, ongoing expansion of cultural knowledge and resources, and adaptations to services.
• Cultural *proficiency* occurs when culture is held in high regard. The need to conduct research, disseminate the results, and develop new approaches that might increase culturally competent practice is recognized.

Rehabilitation professionals have an ethical responsibility to strive for cultural competence and cultural proficiency.

CROSS-CULTURAL REHABILITATION: AN INTERNATIONAL PERSPECTIVE

Philosophy

The information in *Cross-cultural Rehabilitation: An International Perspective* represents an effort to facilitate the development of cultural competence and cultural proficiency. It is intended to broaden the horizons of the many individuals concerned with rehabilitation who traditionally work within their own sociocultural contexts and national boundaries. Rehabilitation clinicians are not likely to appreciate the great differences in the lives of PWD or their rehabilitation care when faced with less familiar multi-cultural or cross-cultural settings within their own country or in the international arena. Nor would they be likely to know the best ways to alleviate obstacles thwarting care. Yet, in the next millennium, world and national population patterns will continue to shift, and practitioners will increasingly be required to share and practice their knowledge and skills in diverse settings within their own country and abroad. The challenges to delivering effective and humanistic care will become even greater than they are today. It is essential that attention be paid to the macro- and microlevel culture in which the rehabilitation worker and the client live.

The traditional rehabilitation paradigm assumes a very biomedical, clinical orientation. This book hopes to convince rehabilitation professionals to be more oriented to sociocultural domains, areas that are typically found within the social science and public policy arena. This includes a greater appreciation of the importance of material conditions and social relations: That is, culture, ethnicity, economic status, political environment, religion, gender, and other such variables that clinicians often ignore. With greater insight into the social, cultural, and economic conditions that others experience, attempts to improve the life situation of PWD are likely to be more successful. There is a presumed goal of increased access and improved quality of services for those who might not otherwise receive ideal, or even any, rehabilitation services.

An essential point is that the information presented here can be extrapolated to other cultures. *Cross-cultural Rehabilitation* is based on the premise that it is possible to usefully generalize or learn from one context (specific geographic location or population group) and apply the lesson to another context. This is true even though each culture has specific culturally defined ways to physically and emotionally support PWD, and each situation must be looked at within its unique context. A description of beliefs and behaviors regarding disability and rehabilitation in Miami, Florida, for example, has relevance to providing service in London, England, Harare, Zimbabwe, or Chittagong, Bangladesh. There must be a greater understanding of how or why people think or behave in a particular manner. There needs to be an increased appreciation of the sociocultural, political, and economic context affecting people's lives. And in a world where no answers are set in stone, it is necessary to learn from the experience of others. What makes a rehabilitation program effective or not in an African nation might provide some insight into the effectiveness of a program in Europe – and vice versa. The details of a specific model or approach may differ, but the principle of paying strict attention to the culture applies.

Cultural pluralism is the underlying philosophy within this book. That is, cultures are different but not inherently better or worse than one another: each has cultural strengths and weaknesses. When differences occur, it is necessary to know how to deal with these in the most constructive manner to facilitate the desired outcome.

Organization and content

Cross-cultural Rehabilitation: An International Perspective covers theory, practice, and professional development areas of study that are,

more often than not, omitted from the curriculum for rehabilitation professionals. Although culture and its importance, particularly as it relates to PWD, has begun to receive attention, many professionals still do not consider it relevant to their professional practice. This domain is beyond the scope of what rehabilitation students and clinicians usually study, and thus they rarely access the texts and journals in medical anthropology and medical sociology that do look to define the meaning of disability and rehabilitation within cross-cultural settings. Even these texts, however, are not specific to rehabilitation professionals and do not use profession-specific examples. Some rehabilitation professional texts (for example those on pediatrics or geriatrics) have a chapter on cultural issues, but their coverage of the topic is limited in both breadth and depth. In addition, the didactic and clinical educational materials are generally presented from a Eurocentric point of view with regard to disability, health, and illness. This contributes to a less-than-ideal delivery of professional service to people from diverse backgrounds. In this book, the goal is to present theoretical and practical examples from a wide variety of cultures that specifically relate to the disciplines associated with the rehabilitative process. It cites cross-cultural within nation examples as well as international experiences.

Rehabilitation includes all measures to reduce the impact of disabling and handicapping conditions and may enable PWD to maintain themselves in their environment. Optimally, it allows individuals with a disability to achieve full social integration into society. Key characteristics of rehabilitation include an attempt to meet the physical, psychological, and social needs of a person with an impairment. Hence, this book is written for a range of practitioners who may be involved with the process of rehabilitation.

In order for this book to be as multi-cultural as possible, it includes contributors from a wide variety of rehabilitation disciplines practicing throughout the world. Most are physical therapists, but occupational therapists, rehabilitation counselors, speech and language pathologists, physicians and special educators appear as well, as do medical anthropologists and sociologists. The authors live and work in a variety of countries and in a wide range of settings. Although it is impossible to include all countries and sub-groups, readers should benefit from this broad representation. There is no one viewpoint expressed, although all of the authors appreciate the need to encourage the aforementioned paradigm shift.

Except for asking all authors to use 'person first language' regarding persons with a disability (as opposed to a 'disabled person'), the terminology preserves each author's preferences. The resulting language inconsistencies – for example, less developed countries, developing countries, Third World countries, the South, all representing a particular group of nations – reflect actual variations in the real world. The cultural perspective of each author has been maintained.

Also regarding terminology, it must be recognized that broad categories fail to represent sub-groups and the presence of intra-cultural diversity. For example, the category 'Asian' encompasses at least 18 subgroups and 'Hispanic' or 'Latino' encompasses over 20 subgroups. Also, people increasingly prefer to identify themselves by using a multi-racial category, a trend that should continue to grow as the frequency of inter-ethnic relationships increases (Knutson et al 1995).

An additional word of caution is in order. Broad categories can perpetuate culturally biased racial or ethnic stereotyping and prejudices. Clearly, this is not the intent. Rather, the intent is to incorporate knowledge about the people one is working with, considering the broad cultural landscape in which they live as well as their individual characteristics in order to recognize inter- and intra-ethnic diversity. It is necessary to take into account all the variables that might influence the professional–patient interaction.

Section 1, 'The Theoretical Basis for Developing Cultural Competence', provides a general overview of several salient domains, the most important of which is culture. Other major topics include attitudes toward PWD, health beliefs and behaviors as they relate to disability and rehabilitation, cross-cultural communication, and the influence of socioeconomic status and race and ethnicity on one's life. Baseline knowledge of these critical domains is necessary to appreciate the need to explore alternative ways to approach people from different cultures and alternative models of care. These themes are carried through the entire book and certainly enhance one's ability to gain the most from the case examples and research chapters.

Section 2, 'Professional Issues', focuses on more general information relevant to the development of the rehabilitation professions in cross-cultural settings. For example, a history of the development of rehabilitation, and specifically community based rehabilitation, begins this section. Other topics include those associated with the development of uniform terminology to ease communication, epidemiological characteristics in the assessment of disability, teaching methods suited for a cross-cultural encounter and the development of functional assistive devices that are culturally appropriate.

Section 3, 'The Practice of Rehabilitation in Cross-cultural and International Environments: Case Examples', reflects extensive personal experience and, in some cases, more formal descriptive research and study. These chapters are mostly ethnographic in nature. An ethnography is 'the work of describing a culture . . . it aims to understand another way of life from the native point of view' (Spradley 1979, p. 3). Although these chapters are not full-scale ethnographies, each attempts, as far as possible, to describe cultural behaviors in terms of the actors' definition. That is, the authors present both the emic (insider's) view and etic (outsider's) view in order to understand the cultural context and cognitive processes of the people studied, rather than impose them from cross-cultural (hence ethnocentric) perspectives. In particular, this section examines disability and rehabilitation in specific cultural contexts. The ethnographer observes, asks questions, and listens in order to understand beliefs, attitudes, values, morals, and other environmental factors that encompass and influence people's lives.

Community based rehabilitation (CBR) programs are the focus of many of the chapters. These programs represent the newest philosophy and models that are considered a logical alternative to the more prevalent biomedical Western model typically found in the developed world and in the major cities of the developing world. This is useful to new students in the field as well as to those who take a more serious and academic interest in this topic. Generally, more information on CBR is becoming available, but much of it is not easily accessible to the mainstream student of cross-cultural and international rehabilitation. Hence, there is an urgent need to share information and ideas concerning CBR so that the most effective and efficient models may develop.

Section 4, 'Cross-cultural Research', also includes ethnographic studies but these chapters focus on answering specific questions. Cross-cultural research examples provide the reader with actual qualitative and quantitative data supporting the presence of diversity of beliefs and behaviors. This will stimulate reha-bilitation professionals to further study the notions of disability and rehabilitation in cross-cultural contexts. Despite progress in this arena, many questions are yet to be asked and answered.

Section 5 'The Practice of Cultural Competence in the 21st Century', summarizes the most salient points presented in the preceding sections. Prominent is the theme that all human experiences, including the experience of disability, are grounded in culture. Rehabilitationists must make an effort to understand the specific explanatory models of PWD and develop culture-specific rehabilitation models. The authors propose that rehabilitation be part of a broader commitment to collaboration with the client, community development, and public health. Section 5 also provides specific suggestions to help prepare for immersion in a cross-cultural setting and recommendations to facilitate cultural competence.

Taken as a whole, this book is intended to have practical application as well as theoretical and descriptive interest and value.

REFERENCES

American Physical Therapy Association Office of Minority and International Affairs, APTA, Washington, DC

Carter D J, Wilson (1993) Minorities in higher education: 1992 eleventh annual status report. American Council on Education, Washington, DC

Cross T L, Bazron B J, Dennis K W, Isaacs M R 1989 Towards a culturally competent system of care, Vol. 1. National Technical Assistance Center for Children's Mental Health, Georgetown University, Washington, DC

Helander E 1993 Prejudice and dignity: an introduction to CBR. United Nations Development Fund publication no. E93-111-B.3, UN, Washington, DC

Helander E, Mendes P, Nelson G, Goerdt A 1989 Training in the community for persons with disabilities. World Health Organization, Geneva

Knutson L, Leavitt R, Sarton B 1995 Race, ethnicity and other factors influencing children's health and disability: implications for pediatric physical therapists. Pediatric Physical Therapy 7: 175–183

Lynch E, Hanson M 1992 Developing cross-cultural competence. Paul H Brookes, Baltimore

Marfo K S, Walker B 1986 Childhood disability in develop-ing countries: issues in habilation and special education. Praeger, New York

Pan American Health Organization 1994 Health conditions in the Americas. World Health Organization, Washington, DC

Pan American Health Organization/World Health Organiz-ation 1994 Situational analysis of disabilities and rehabili-tation in the English speaking Caribbean. World Health Organization, Washington, DC

Spradley J 1979 The ethnographic interview. Holt, Rinehart and Winston, New York

United States Bureau of the Census 1990 Current population reports. US Bureau of the Census, Washington, DC

United States Department of Commerce 1996 Population projections of the United States by age, sex, race and Hispanic origin, 1995 to 2050. US Bureau of the Census, Washington, DC

World Confederation for Physical Therapy 1996 Annual report. WCPT, London, UK

World Health Organization 1981 World health: international year of disabled persons. World Health Organization, Geneva

The theoretical basis for developing cultural competence

This first section introduces some theoretical concepts that are often ignored by rehabilitation professionals. The most important of these are the notion of cultural variability with regard to disability and rehabilitation and the unequivocal need for consideration of social and cultural variables such as income, ethnicity, race, and language when addressing issues associated with disability and rehabilitation. Section 1 is the first step towards facilitating the development of 'cultural competence'. Practical application of these concepts is found in Section 3 and Section 4.

Chapter 2, 'The concept of culture', by Christine Loveland, a cultural and medical anthropologist, introduces the basic terminology and theory related to the concept of culture, and the relationship of disability and rehabilitation to culture. It describes principles that are relevant to practice, such as the need to be aware of cultural universals as well as different cultural value systems, and the notions of ethnocentrism and cultural relativism.

Loveland also introduces the specific topic of culture and disability – a theme that is evident throughout this book. Loveland notes (as do other contributors to this book) that the concept of disability is not a cultural universal. That is, disability is not a concept found in all known cultures. If disability does exist as a recognized category, there is variation in its meaning. Also, having a disability is a necessary but not necessarily sufficient condition for membership in a subculture of people with a disability (PWD).

Loveland describes three approaches within the field of medical anthropology: applied medical anthropology, bioculturalism, and critical anthropology. Although each, to a certain extent, is represented within this book, the most commonly represented approach is applied medical anthropology whereby there is an effort to use data and theories 'in the real world'. That is, there is an attempt to use anthropological findings to improve the effectiveness of health care programs. This field is closely allied with the international public health movement.

Loveland also introduces the subject of medical sociology. A thread that runs throughout most of the chapters, emanating from this domain, is the idea that PWD are often seen as 'deviant' and are marginalized, so that they lack political and economic power.

The study of culture and medical anthropology is a massive subject. Chapter 2 is an introduction and is not intended to provide an in-depth analysis or critique of alternative anthropologic theories, philosophical points of view, or methodologies of ethnographic research. Loveland suggests further reading for practitioners who wish to delve more deeply into these domains.

In Chapter 3, ' "Appearances" of disability, discrimination and the transformation of rehabilitation service practices', Aldred Neufeldt draws on medical sociology and anthropology to introduce the social dimensions of disability. Neufeldt begins by emphasizing how important it is to recognize our tendency to see the world from our own perspective. This perspective is often quite limited, based on superficial appearances of other cultures or individuals rather than well-founded knowledge. When exploring the reality of disablement, Neufeldt suggests that the lived experiences of PWD most likely approximate reality. He urges rehabilitation practitioners to have 'more than a passing familiarity with prevalent "appearances" of disability' in order to appreciate the reality of disability.

Neufeldt provides a sampling of attitudes toward disability, historically and today. He suggests that there has been strong evidence of a consistent negative bias and cultural intolerance toward PWD. Neufeldt argues that the 'continuing reality is that the presence of disablement contributes to discriminatory practices'. He examines the kinds and extent of discriminatory practices toward PWD.

Only in recent years has a paradigm shift begun to occur with regard to shaping rehabilitation services. It is now recognized that both consumers of services and providers need to be co-participants in the process. Neufeldt describes three approaches that are plausible: a consumer-directed model, a professional-directed model, and a conjointly-directed model. Each approach proposes an active alliance of providers with consumers to increase the likelihood of appropriate service interventions. Finally, he suggests guidelines for user-sensitive rehabilitation services that are not culture bound.

Neufeldt also comments on the debate concerning the most appropriate language to use when discussing disability. As noted in Chapter 1, in this book 'person first' language is the norm; in order to emphasize the person first and the disability second, it is appropriate to say 'person with a disability'. Neufeldt offers some alternative thoughts: based on the World Health Organization (WHO) definitions of 'impairment', 'disability', and 'handicap' (see Ch. 10), a disability results when a person with an impairment encounters an inaccessible environment. Hence, it is the environment which disables the person and 'person with a disability' would therefore be incorrect.

Neufeldt also links Loveland's introduction to culture with medical anthropologist Nora Groce's description of culture-specific, disability-related beliefs and behaviors. In Chapter 4, 'Health beliefs and behavior towards individuals with disability cross-culturally', Groce focuses on ideas about disability that are intimately tied to a larger culturally based system of health beliefs and health behaviors. Groce elaborates on Loveland's brief introduction to the concepts of health beliefs and behaviors, discussing the non-material culture of a group of individuals. This information is much more difficult to access and to assess from one's own cultural context.

Groce, like Loveland, proposes that few concepts of disability are universally applicable. In fact, individuals and societies conceptualize and treat individuals with disabilities in different ways. These cultural interpretations vary depending upon how a society attaches value and meaning to a particular type of disability. According to Groce, three major categories of social beliefs seem to exist cross-culturally and tend to predict how well an individual will fare in a particular community. These are:

- *causality*: the cultural explanations for why a disability occurs
- *valued and devalued attributes*: specific physical or intellectual attributes that are valued or devalued in a particular society
- *anticipated role*: the role an individual with a disability is expected to play as an adult in a community.

Groce provides many practical illustrations that complement Neufeldt's theoretical perspective, although she offers some examples in which PWD are viewed as having more positive attributes and experiences than does Neufeldt. She describes an array of individual and societal models of belief, often referred to as explanatory models (explanatory models and cultural practices of particular sub-cultures are also described by Leavitt, Thorburn, Jelsma and Zhanje, Simister and Younis, and others in the case example and research sections of *Cross-cultural Rehabilitation*).

'Some influences of religions on attitudes towards disabilities and people with disabilities', Chapter 5, by M. Miles, offers a look at one particular cultural variable, that of religion. Despite a great range of variation, religion often reflects social organization and reinforces social structure, and it can encourage the oppression or empowerment of PWD. Miles offers examples from Christian, Jewish, Buddhist, Islamic and Hindu texts that focus on the social construction of disability in particular cultures. Arguably the most important sociocultural variable affecting the status of PWD in the world today, including the accessibility and quality of rehabilitation, is economic conditions.

Poverty, without doubt the most prevalent economic condition throughout much of the world, and heavily represented within particular ethnic enclaves, is highly associated with poor health in general, and specifically an increase in disability and a decrease in rehabilitation services. In Chapter 6, 'Poverty and health: an international overview', medical sociologists Rebecca Reviere and Kevin Hylton explore these relationships using examples from a wide variety of nations throughout the world.

Every chapter in *Cross-cultural Rehabilitation* describing the practice of rehabilitation within a particular context notes the effect of socioeconomic conditions on the everyday lives of PWD. Although it is difficult to directly compare the 'absolute' poverty of, for example, people in Bangladesh or Vietnam to the 'relative' poverty of children in Miami, Florida, or Romania, poverty has direct and indirect consequences.

Some of the themes that emerge in later chapters have a direct relationship to the information presented by Reviere and Hylton. For example, the lack of rehabilitation facilities, personnel, and technology is better understood by realizing that access to all health care services may be limited at best. The 'feminization of poverty' is also a reality; thus, an even greater burden is placed on women and their children, who are more likely to suffer economically. This is especially relevant because it is apparent that most PWD are cared for by women (usually the mother) or live in a female-headed household.

Practitioners most often do not come from impoverished backgrounds themselves. Yet, the overarching consideration of socioeconomic status profoundly influences the everyday existence of PWD and the ability of both the practitioner and the client to develop and implement a rehabilitation plan at the individual, community, or national level. No practitioner can become culturally competent in a cross-cultural setting without taking into account the reality of the client's economic status.

In Chapter 7, 'Understanding racial prejudice, discrimination and racism, and their influence on health care delivery', Joseph Smey explores the theoretical concepts of prejudice, stereotyping, discrimination, and racism. He details their effects on health care equity and the ability to develop effective interpersonal relations, particularly with those of another racial or ethnic group. Although it is widely acknowledged that there are many 'isms' in the world, and in fact much of this book focuses, directly and indirectly, on 'handicappism', or discrimination against PWD, racism is singled out because of its prominence as a topic of ongoing national dialogue in the USA. This should not be interpreted as a denial of the presence of other insidious 'isms' in the global society.

Smey proposes that changing demographics in the USA and throughout the world have important implications for rehabilitationists. As noted in Chapter 1, there is an increasing likelihood that clinicians will not reflect the diversity of the communities they serve and that clinicians will work with PWD who are from a different ethnic group than themselves. Thus, racism is more likely to play a role in the interaction. This chapter is addressed primarily to the practitioners who are in the white majority in the industrialized nations. These individuals are more likely to unconsciously perpetuate rather than be the target of racism. Still, in many middle-income and lower-income nations power is typically held by either the white minority, or people of color who are of a particular ethnic or tribal group, and the influences of prejudice, discrimination and racism on the majority population remain all too present. Therefore, these theoretical domains are pertinent to many patient–therapist interactions.

Discussions of the influence of race and racism tend to be extremely controversial. Debates on whether race is a useful categorization and on the biological and sociological implications of race and ethnicity have been going on for decades. Once again, this is a very broad and complex topic. Smey presents a perspective that supports the notion that race and ethnicity often negatively influence the health status of and health care received by individuals (including PWD) and the ability of individuals from different racial and ethnic groups to

develop the most effective personal and/or working relationships possible. He enumerates several themes crucial to the efforts of any individual or group to reduce the impact of racism. Of critical importance is a need for introspective examination of one's self and personal value systems with regard to beliefs, attitudes, and behaviors toward people from other racial or ethnic groups. Also critical is an understanding of the costs of racism to us as individuals and the society that we live in, as well as the benefits of changing the present system.

In the last chapter in Section 1, 'Cross-cultural communication', speech and language pathologists Alejandro Brice and Lynda Campbell combine the theoretical basis for cross-cultural communication with the practical application of these principles. The notion that communication, which is both a cultural and a language phenomenon, is vital to any health-related intervention by a practitioner is obvious. Less obvious is the relationship of communication style to the prevailing cultural value systems. Typically, when we communicate with people from a different culture we base our interpretation of the encounter on our own world view. A world view based on our own culture and language may include the tendency to stereotype or show bias. This can lead to ineffective communication or miscommunication, along with conflict.

Brice and Campbell reinforce and expand upon many of the points introduced by Loveland, most importantly the typology of comparative value systems. They examine the interrelationships between culture and communication and suggest strategies to minimize barriers to communication. In cross-cultural encounters there is, by definition, cultural difference between the participants. In industrialized countries, many of the rehabilitationists come from 'individualistic' and 'vertical' societies that tend to have 'low-context' communication styles; the sub-groups that they work with or study belong to 'collectivist', 'horizontal' societies with 'high-context' communication patterns.

Possibly the most difficult variable or set of

cultural differences frustrating many professionals from Western cultures who work with people from non-Western cultures is that based on views concerning time. Brice and Campbell, by describing monochronic versus polychronic time views as one of the prominent cultural variables, help us to better understand the differences in viewpoint and style. In addition, Brice and Campbell present information that is useful for practitioners to consider when working with the families of PWD, offering examples of specific differences in communication styles between Latino-Hispanic people and African-American people. They also explore aspects of family relationships and note that families have varying degrees of cohesion (enmeshed vs. disengaged) and adaptability (chaos vs. rigidity). These characteristics are likely to affect the cross-cultural communication process. Lastly, Brice and Campbell note three elements in building trust – caring, consistency, and credibility – in order to minimize conflict and maximize the involvement of families in the rehabilitation process.

In sum, Section 1 lays the foundation for understanding the themes and practices that underlie the notion of cultural competence. In each cross-cultural encounter, the relevance of the local material and non-material culture must be paid attention to. Of special significance are the importance of local socioeconomic conditions and health beliefs and behaviors regarding disability and rehabilitation. At the practical level, these chapters stress the need for a greater understanding of the meaning of disability in a particular cultural context and the necessity of designing culturally appropriate models of rehabilitation. Understanding this material brings the clinician a step closer to cultural competence.

2

The concept of culture

Christine Loveland

CULTURE

At birth humans must begin to adjust to a natural environment in which oxygen sustains life and to a social environment in which culture sustains life. Only when deprived of oxygen or of the usual cultural supports do people realize how crucial both are to existence. In the case of culture, this can occur when people leave their home culture or when they interact with others from different cultural backgrounds. Both scenarios have become increasingly common as global travel and population movements result in frequent cross-cultural interaction. This interaction contains the potential for enhanced communication and understanding but it also contains the possibility of miscommunication and misunderstanding. This is very evident in all areas of clinical medicine; for example in rehabilitation settings the therapist and the patient may come from different cultural backgrounds and view the entire situation in very different ways. People in the patient's culture may see disability as something to be hidden, while the therapist's goal is to reintegrate the patient into society. The patient and her family may be very resistant to the rehabilitation professionals' efforts since they cannot imagine a culture in which people with disabilities (PWDs) assume public roles. If all of the people involved in this situation – patient, family, medical personnel – understand each other's cultural perspectives, it is more likely that the therapeutic outcome will be successful.

Cultural relativism

Ethnocentrism is the belief that one's own culture is superior to others and is the standard by which other cultures should be judged. In the example above, it would be important for the therapist to understand why PWDs are isolated and stigmatized in the patient's culture. With this understanding, even though the therapist might disagree both with the belief and the behavior, he would be able to consider them in any proposed rehabilitation regimen. The therapist would be practicing cultural relativism, the belief that the customs and behavior of people in other cultures should be understood within their own cultural contexts. Cultural relativism does not mean that everyone has the same set of values or that everyone agrees on everything; it may, in fact, mean that people in a cross-cultural interaction 'agree to disagree'.

It is easier to achieve an attitude of cultural relativism when it is remembered that people do not biologically inherit a culture, they learn it, and any normal human infant can learn any culture – its values, its customs, its beliefs. Cultures, like people, develop and change in response to the environment and conditions present in a particular time and place; they adapt if it is necessary and possible to do so. Cultures are not static or unchangeable and all of the elements of a culture – the economic system, the political organization, the religion, the family structure – are interconnected. They are woven together into an intricate tapestry; pull one thread, change one color of the tapestry and the composition of the entire picture may be altered. That is why it is unrealistic to ask a person to change her beliefs about illness and disability without recognizing the possibility that this may challenge or alter other learned values and behaviors.

The importance of nonmaterial culture in rehabilitation

People usually learn their core values, beliefs and attitudes early in life and change them only with great difficulty. They may resist discussion of them, considering them personal, private, or even sacred. These elements of culture make up what is called nonmaterial culture, which is abstract and often difficult for those outside the culture to understand. Frequently the nonmaterial culture can be learned by outsiders only through lengthy and careful observation. On the other hand, the material culture encompasses all of the more easily seen parts of culture – architecture, clothing, food, technology – and similarities and differences between cultures in this area are readily visible. In a rehabilitation context, beliefs about the cause(s) of disability, including religious beliefs and beliefs about the roles (appropriate behavior) of the person with a disability, the family, and the therapist would belong to the nonmaterial culture. The available facilities, technology, and rehabilitation equipment would be a part of the material culture. Sometimes similarities in the material cultures obscure profound differences in the nonmaterial cultures and people in a cross-cultural interaction are surprised and shocked when misunderstanding develops. For example, just because a patient and therapist live in similar houses, wear similar clothing, and even speak the same language does not mean that they share the same religion, the same attitudes about disability, or the same beliefs about the appropriate behavior for women and men.

Religious beliefs

Religious beliefs provide one of the best examples of the importance of nonmaterial culture in rehabilitation. People in many cultures believe that illness, accidents, disability, and even death are supernatural punishments for the misbehavior of either the patient or a member of the patient's family. Sometimes powerful emotions such as jealousy and anger are blamed for such misfortunes; these emotions may have been unleashed in the past, even before the patient was born. If that is the case, taking a patient's history entails more than recording relevant medical information; it means an examination of the psychosocial background of the patient's relatives and ancestors. In fact, outside of biomedicine, most medical systems consider the causes of illness and disability to lie within the souls and minds of those involved, not under a microscope or on an X-ray film. While biomedicine treats and alleviates the symptoms, only a truly holistic treatment which includes the emotional or psychological causes can effect a cure (for specific examples see Anderson 1996, Gropper 1996, Galanti 1991, Knutson et al 1995). Rehabilitation professionals must respect such beliefs and be aware that patients and families may not discuss them with medical personnel, especially if these personnel do not appear to share these beliefs (see Chs. 4 and 5).

Two excellent examples of a lack of cross-cultural respect and understanding in a medical setting are documented in the films *Peace has not been made* (Vang & Finck 1983) and *A Choice for K'aila* (Morrison 1990). The first film is about an immigrant Hmong (a Laotian highland people) family's unfortunate experience with an urban American hospital after their young son severely cut his hand. Although the hospital staff used translators and assumed that the family understood the medical situation and need for treatment, the Hmong, who had retained the beliefs learned in Laos, saw their son's injury and surgery from a very different perspective. Especially important was their belief that the soul leaves the body when a person is unconscious and their subsequent opposition to general anesthesia and surgery. As a result, they took their son home before the nerve damage in his hand was repaired, renamed the hospital 'the experimentation house', and vowed never to use the hospital again. In this case, cultural differences resulted in a very poor outcome for everyone involved and left a young boy with permanent loss of function in his hand.

The second film details the opposition of a Canadian Native American family to a liver transplant for their critically ill son. They believed that the soul of the organ donor would enter their son's body and that his quality of life after a transplant would be poor. Canadian social service agencies and the medical staff of the hospital did not share these beliefs and this resulted in a bitter argument with the family.

Ultimately the family prevailed and their son died in his mother's arms at home. In both of these examples elements of culture, particularly the linking of illness and medical treatment to religious beliefs, were crucial in the rejection of biomedical procedures. In both cases, people outside of the patients' cultures had limited understanding of them.

Euro-American values

Beliefs about the supernatural and its relationship to illness and disability are just one part of nonmaterial culture, and many other values and norms can be important in cross-cultural interaction. Although it can be risky to generalize about cultures because of the danger of stereotyping, many observers have identified recurrent themes and patterns in cultures (see, for example, Locke 1992, Lynch & Hanson 1992). These patterns can provide overall structure to cross-cultural interaction as long as it is remembered that they are guidelines and that there will be great individual variation within each culture. Ferraro (1998) has contrasted many of the world's cultures (Latin America, the Middle East, Africa, Asia) with those cultures that have Euro-American values (Canada, Northern and Western Europe, Australia, New Zealand). His typology (Ferraro 1998, p. 109) is given in Table 2.1.

Table 2.1 Comparative value orientations (Ferraro, G P The cultural dimension of international business, 1998. Reproduced by permission of Prentice-Hall, Inc., Upper Saddle River, NJ.)

Euro-American	Cross-cultural comparison
Individualism	Collectivism
Precise time reckoning	Loose time reckoning
Future oriented	Past oriented
Doing (working, achieving)	Being (personal qualities)
People controlling nature	Nature controlling people
Youthfulness	Old age
Informality	Formality
Competition	Cooperation
Relative equality of sexes	Relative inequality of sexes

In general, those cultures which have been most heavily influenced by Euro-American values will match those cultural characteristics listed in the left column of Table 2.1, while those least influenced by these values will fit the characteristics listed in the right column. Euro-American values emphasize the importance of the individual and the ability of each person to affect her future through hard work. In this type of cultural orientation, both time and nature are commodities to be used profitably and the success (or lack of success) of each person is credited to that individual. If the medical personnel in a rehabilitation setting have this type of cultural value system they will emphasize the autonomy and personal responsibility of their patients, expect their patients to be on time for appointments and to work hard while they are there. In contrast, if their patients have a cultural value system that emphasizes the importance of the group over the individual, a casual approach to punctuality, and acceptance of fate, they may arrive after their scheduled appointment time with several family members and feel that there is little point in working too hard since much of what happens to people (including disability) is predetermined. In this situation, effective rehabilitation can be derailed by cross-cultural misunderstanding and personal conflicts. In order to achieve the best possible therapeutic outcome, it therefore is imperative for rehabilitation personnel to understand not only their own culture(s) but also that of their patients. This, potentially, is just as important as their knowledge of anatomy, physiology, or manual skills.

Summary

In summary, culture refers to the learned behaviors, values, norms, and symbols that are passed from generation to generation within a society. People learn what is appropriate and acceptable within their own culture and may come to view their way of doing things as the only correct way. This attitude is called ethnocentrism, and it is common in all of the world's cultures. Successful cross-cultural communication and interaction

benefit from cultural relativism, which rejects ethnocentrism, stresses the variability of culture, and emphasizes the need to try and understand other cultures in their own context. We may be better able to do this by recognizing that culture has two major components: material culture and nonmaterial culture. People often are more willing to change elements of their material culture than their nonmaterial culture, contributing to cultural lag, in which the physical aspects of culture (such as styles of dress and new technology) change much more rapidly than the nonphysical aspects (such as attitudes toward new styles of dress, and appropriate uses of new technology). This lag is common in biomedicine as technology (e.g. life-support systems) and research results (e.g. those in genetics) present clinicians and patients with challenging religious and ethical dilemmas. People may reject or be ambivalent toward elements of the material culture, such as a proposed medical treatment, because of the values in their nonmaterial culture. This means that rehabilitation professionals should be aware of the importance of culture (their own as well as that of their patients) and of the interconnectedness of the different parts of the material and nonmaterial culture. Such awareness is a necessity for those whose work environments include people from different cultural backgrounds. In today's world, that describes almost everyone.

SUBCULTURES

Subcultures are smaller units within a culture that share many of the cultural traits of the majority of people in the larger culture but are in some way(s) distinct from them. By definition a person who belongs to a subculture also belongs to the larger culture, and a subculture is always a part of a greater cultural entity. Complex societies typically encompass many different subcultures and people in these societies frequently engage in cross-cultural interaction without ever leaving the geographical boundaries of their home country. The two films mentioned earlier in this chapter provide excellent examples of this. In the first film, the

Hmong family belonged to a subculture in their homeland, since the majority of Laotians are not Hmong, and the Hmong share a distinct cultural heritage and language. They also belong to a subculture (Hmong-American) in their new country, the USA, since they retain elements of their traditional culture that differ from the culture of the majority of Americans. However, now the Hmong also belong to larger subcultures in the United States, including Laotian-Americans and Asian-Americans. In the second film, the family also belonged to a subculture within Canada since they were Native Americans, but they further refined this by identifying themselves as members of specific Native American (or First Nation) cultures. The fact that the family members in both films differed in physical appearance from the majority of people in their cultures must also be considered since this is often important in the development of subcultures.

Acculturation and assimilation

Acculturation is a process through which people in subcultures adopt traits from the larger culture. Perhaps the first generation of immigrants finds it difficult to learn a new language and way of life, but their children succeed in doing so. This second generation may be bilingual and perhaps even bicultural, able to function effectively in two cultural settings. However, the children in the third generation may know little about their grandparents' language and culture and be almost fully assimilated. Assimilation involves the loss of cultural traits and their replacement by cultural traits from another culture. Assimilation is often most complete for populations that are not physically distinct from the majority, do not retain contact with their original culture, and do not maintain residential and educational segregation. Both the Hmong and Native Americans have physical traits that differ from the majority group and some Native Americans also live on reservations that physically separate them from the majority group. Both of these situations make assimilation more difficult.

Ethnicity and racial categorization

Subcultures such as Native Americans, Asian-Americans, and the Hmong (both in Laos and the USA) are frequently called racial or ethnic groups. What does this mean? Ethnicity is based on an element or elements of culture and an ethnic group has a religion, language, place of origin, and/or way of life that distinguishes it from other people in a particular culture. There may be dozens of ethnic groups in a pluralistic society (as in many African countries, for example). In a more homogeneous society (such as Japan) there may be very few. The worldwide trend is toward more heterogeneity, however, because of immigration and the movement of refugee populations. Defining race or racial group is much more problematic than defining ethnicity or ethnic group. Typically, racial categorization is done on the basis of appearance or phenotype, and the physical trait that is given most importance is skin color. This is so arbitrary and the variation within so-called races is so extensive that many scientists no longer use the term race (see Harrison et al 1988 and Lieberman and Jackson 1995 for discussions of this topic from an anthropological perspective). Scientists also point out that only about four of more than 100 000 genes in human beings code for skin color (Scupin 1995, p. 30) and that this is a very minor physical characteristic by which to categorize huge groups of people.

The association of specific physical traits with ethnic and racial groups is arbitrary (for example, what if height or eye color were used to define races rather than skin color?), is not based on science, and should not be used to stereotype people in any cultural setting, including a rehabilitation setting. Both race and ethnicity are cultural categories. If people in a particular subculture tend to speak and behave in a distinct and consistent way, it is because they learned the behavior, not because it is innate or genetically based.

Occupation, sexual orientation, religion, language, place of ancestral origin – all potentially are foundations for the development of a subculture because in each case the people involved differ in some way from other people in a culture. What about disability? If able-bodied people are in the majority, do PWDs belong to a distinct subculture? Do they consider themselves to be part of a (sub)culture of disability? Do other people see them in this way? As is often the case in cross-cultural inquiry, we can ask the same questions in every culture, but we will not receive the same answers.

CULTURE AND DISABILITY

Cultural universals are concepts or customs found in all known cultures. The concept of disability is not a cultural universal. As Ingstad & Reynolds (1995, p. 7) point out:

the concept of disability itself must not be taken for granted. In many cultures, one cannot be 'disabled' for the simple reason that 'disability' as a recognized category does not exist. There are blind people and lame people and 'slow' people, but 'the disabled' as a general term does not translate easily into many languages. . . . The concepts of disability, handicap, and rehabilitation emerged in particular historical circumstances in Europe.

This is not surprising since, as was noted earlier in this chapter, Euro-American values differ from those in many other parts of the world. The emphasis on the importance of the individual and on individual work and achievement as a measure of accomplishment and status were important factors in the development of the goals of rehabilitation. Furthermore, social institutions in Europe gradually assumed many of the activities formerly performed by the family and this was important in the historical development and acceptance of hospitals, clinics, and other medical facilities. Sick people – and that often meant people with disabilities as well as those with short-term acute illnesses – were separated from their families and treated by professionals. Biomedicine replaced or sometimes coexisted with traditional methods of healing.

This has not happened in all or even most of the world's cultures. In many cultures, people with cognitive and physical disabilities still are expected to follow the same life cycle as everyone else, including initiation (if practiced), marriage, and parenthood. They are not isolated in care facilities (which may not exist) nor are they assumed to be incapable of participation in everyday social discourse. Disability does not define their status (social position) in the culture and therefore it cannot serve as the identifying and unifying characteristic of a distinct subculture. Katherine Dettwyler's (1994) description of a Malian family's attitude toward their daughter, who has Down syndrome, illustrates this perfectly. While conducting fieldwork in Mali, Dettwyler noticed a little girl with the unmistakable physical characteristics of a child with Down syndrome. She was particularly interested because her own son has Down syndrome. She described her conversation with the family:

'Do you know that there's something "different" about this child?' I asked, choosing my words carefully. 'Well, she doesn't talk,' said her mother, hesitantly, looking at her husband for confirmation. 'That's right,' he said. 'She's never said a word.' 'But she's been healthy?' I asked. 'Yes,' the father replied. *She's like the other kids, except she doesn't talk* [emphasis mine]. She's always happy. She never cries. We know she can hear, because she does what we tell her to. Why are you so interested in her?' . . . There was no way I could explain cells and chromosomes and nondisjunction to them . . . would that have helped them anyway? They just accepted her as she was . . . Children in the United States might have the freedom to attend special programs to help them overcome their handicaps, but children in Mali have freedom from the biggest handicap of all – other people's prejudice. (Dettwyler 1994, pp. 98–99)

In Mali, PWDs are part of the social life of their families and communities, but that certainly is not the case in all cultures. Sometimes PWDs remain isolated in their households because the disability brings shame on their families. This obviously limits their opportunities for social interaction outside of the family. Inaccessibility and lack of accommodation in the material culture – transportation, mobility aids, suitable housing – can add to their isolation. Any or all of these conditions make it unlikely that a subculture based on disability will develop. Membership in subcultures based on ethnicity or religion also may limit social interaction. PWDs who live in societies in which residential, educational, and social segregation of subcultures exists may have little opportunity to interact with other people who have similar disabilities, unless these people already belong to the same subculture. Linguistic diversity and separation also limit cross-cultural communication, even within the same society.

The development of subcultures of disability

Another important consideration is the tremendous number and variety of disabilities. People in subcultures share certain traits and life experiences but is this true of a person who is blind and a person who uses a wheelchair? Or do they define themselves differently? Perhaps one is of Asian descent and considers that far more important; perhaps the other is a lawyer and considers that to be most important. Having a disability is a necessary but not necessarily sufficient condition for membership in a subculture of disability. Such a subculture is most likely to develop when people in a culture consider disability to be an important or even defining part of a person's identity and status. Another important factor is the segregation of PWDs in schools, care facilities, and rehabilitation centers. Here they have many opportunities to meet and interact with other PWDs. In addition, they are in these programs and facilities because of their disabilities; this implies that disability therefore is a crucial, perhaps the most crucial, facet of their status. In such a situation, even if the PWDs belong to different ethnic groups or practice different religions, they may consider those differences secondary to the shared experiences stemming from their disability.

Cross-cultural evidence suggests that a subculture based on disability is most likely to be found in a culture in which the following conditions are present:

1. medical treatment makes survival with disabilities (both congenital and acquired) possible, even common
2. culture-wide concepts of normality and disability exist
3. cultural values stress individualism and achievement so that goals for children and adults with disabilities stress independence and autonomy
4. disability is a crucial determinant of status and possibly self-identity
5. the presence of a disability can override other possible determinants of status and identity such as ethnicity and religion
6. PWDs have opportunities to meet and interact with one another, as in care facilities and rehabilitation centers
7. PWDs have access to education, technology, and mobility aids that facilitate their interaction with others
8. the infrastructure of the culture, particularly the transportation and communication systems, is accessible to PWDs.

Almost all of these cultural characteristics are more likely to be found in the world's wealthier countries, and it is in these countries that subcultures based on disabilities, disability-rights movements, and patient-advocacy groups are most common. As Dettwyler (1994) noted above, however, it is also in these countries that attitudes toward disability present a greater handicap (or social barrier) than they do in some economically poorer countries such as Mali.

ANTHROPOLOGY, ETHNOGRAPHY, AND DISABILITY

The concept of culture was first defined and used by 19th-century anthropologists, although travelers and writers from many different parts of the world had long noted the great variation in the customs and beliefs of the world's people. Anthropological study of culture is different from casual observation because it strives to be objective, holistic, and comparative. The gold standard of anthropological inquiry is ethnographic research. This research requires that the anthropologist do fieldwork, spending extended periods of time living in the culture as a participant observer and not just as a passive recorder of information. The written descriptions of cultures which result are called ethnographies.

Ethnography

The hallmarks of ethnography are its reliance on qualitative participant observation research and its holistic perspective and analysis. It is ideal for obtaining an in-depth understanding of values and behavior but it also is demanding and very labor-intensive. Other considerations include the difficulty (or impossibility) of replication of ethnographic research, the maintenance (or desirability) of objectivity, and the importance of the skills, accuracy, and integrity of the researcher, since many ethnographers work alone. Adequate training, careful use of ethnographic research techniques, and awareness of the limitations of this research method can help the researcher avoid these problems.

'Ethnomedicine'

Ethnographic inquiry has proved useful in a wide and ever-growing number of fields, including disability studies, because, at its best, it results in a richly textured description and analysis that is very close to an insider's perspective of a culture or experience. Curing, concepts of health and disease, and theories of disease causation have always been of interest to social scientists because they are important aspects of culture. Early anthropologists usually addressed these topics under the broader categories of religion and the supernatural, although there was also interest in the material elements of curing, such as herbal medicines. Typically, the term 'ethnomedicine' was used in ethnographic analyses of these medical systems.

Disability research and medical anthropology

Much of the research on disability has been done by medical anthropologists and medical sociologists. There are multiple approaches within medical anthropology, including bioculturalism, applied medical anthropology, and critical anthropology. Arching over these various approaches is a broader division between cultural anthropology and biological anthropology, a reflection of the position of anthropology on the interface between the social and biological sciences. For the most part, ethnographic works on biomedicine analyze biomedicine as a distinct culture or subculture. Applied medical anthropology, like clinical medicine, attempts to use data and theories 'in the real world' outside of a purely research or academic environment. Applied anthropology is closely allied with the international public health movement. The last approach, critical medical anthropology, approaches biomedicine 'from the top down', analyzing it as one component of the culture as a whole and frequently emphasizing its importance as a means of social control.

Medical anthropology

By the 1960s, medical anthropology emerged as a distinct specialty, and in the last three decades, the field has grown and at the same time, fragmented. One result of this fragmentation has been the emergence of the field of disability studies.

There are multiple ethnographic studies which emphasize the importance of culture in the study of disability and rehabilitation (see, for example, Ingstad & Reynolds 1995, Albrecht 1992). There also are many applied studies which take an advocacy position, attempting to support and promote changes which would benefit PWDs. Finally, some social scientists take a macrolevel approach to the study of disability, focusing more on society-wide factors, such as the relationship of socioeconomic status and access to medical care. All three of these approaches emphasize that medical systems always reflect the cultures of which they are a part, and in addition they also exhibit many of the characteristics of a subculture (Konner 1987, Stein 1990).

Medical sociology

Medical sociology shares theories and research methods with medical anthropology, but there are some differences as well, many of them due to the fact that sociology has not had the same emphasis on holistic cross-cultural comparison.

The earliest theoretical approach to illness and disability in medical sociology was based on functionalism and symbolic interactionism. Parsons (1951) elaborated on what he called 'the sick role' – the set of behaviors expected of someone who occupies the status of a sick person. Although this does not work as well with chronic conditions as it does with acute illnesses, it led to the development of the deviance model, which has been widely used in medical sociology in work on disability. In this model PWDs are deviant because they fall outside the boundaries of normality within a particular culture. Related to this in sociology is the approach to disability that goes back to the work of Goffman (1963). Here disability is analyzed as a stigmatized identity, one which places the individual in a marginal or liminal status.

Two additional sociological theories are closer to critical medical anthropology in that they take a macrolevel approach to disability and emphasize issues of power and access to societal resources. Conflict theory, one of the dominant sociological theories, has tended to view PWDs as members of a minority group. From the perspective of this theoretical approach, minority groups have three defining characteristics: they differ from the majority group in a culturally important way, whether that refers to gender, racial or ethnic identity, sexual orientation, or disability; they are usually, but not always, less than one-half of the population; and, most importantly, they lack access to political and economic power. This view of disability has become a popular one among disability rights advocates in the USA. Finally, a few sociologists have focused on what is called 'the disability business' – private and governmental rehabilitation programs, particularly in the USA.

A review of these sociological theories and approaches reveals that they have limited utility in some cross-cultural settings because the discipline of sociology has focused on Western cultures since its beginnings in Europe in the 19th century. Each of the medical anthropology and medical sociology approaches has its proponents. Nevertheless, both clinical professionals and academic theorists must understand that no approach is particularly useful unless it is altered to reflect the relevant cultural environment.

SUMMARY AND CONCLUSIONS

Culture is a concept which originated in the emerging discipline of anthropology in the last decades of the 19th century. Anthropologists emphasize that culture is passed down from generation to generation through socialization or enculturation (it is learned) and that culture is adaptive and integrated. Numerous cultural and individual traits, including language, religion, and disability, can be social markers which maintain boundaries between people within a culture. The resulting groups are called subcultures. It is important to remember, however, that in many societies disability is not an important social marker and there may be no subculture based on disability.

Anthropologists and sociologists have studied and written about health, disease, and disability from many different perspectives. Because anthropology is by definition holistic and comparative, the work done by anthropologists on these topics also has been comparative and cross-cultural. Sociologists have focused more frequently on the experience of illness and disability in Western societies and it may be more difficult to apply sociological theories and conclusions cross-culturally.

All human experiences, including the experience of disability, are grounded in culture. Without an understanding of culture, both in general and specific terms, human communication and understanding face formidable obstacles. With this understanding, the rough edges of cross-cultural contact are smoothed out, and the process becomes more rewarding and more productive.

FURTHER READING

Erickson P A (ed) 1993 Teaching anthropology creatively. Reliance, New Delhi. *This book has two chapters which describe excellent activities for teaching and applying the concept of culture. They are P C Rice, 'Teaching the concept of culture using "the Ballantyne Logo"' (pp. 39–48), and J G Chadney, 'Back to the Basics' (pp. 49–58). The first emphasizes the three components of culture – knowing, feeling, and doing – while the second uses music to illustrate how important culture is in our interpretation of all types of communication.*

Randall-David E 1989 Strategies for working with culturally diverse communities and clients. Association for the Care of Children's Health, Washington, DC. *This text focuses on the importance of understanding one's own cultural identity and includes Bloch's Ethnic/Cultural Assessment Guide – a useful way of assessing one's own identity as well as one's responses to many different master statuses.*

There are many books on the market which try to introduce basic anthropological concepts (such as cultural relativism) to people who work in health care systems. References of this type which might be useful include:

Lynch E, Hanson M 1992 Developing cross-cultural competence. Paul H. Brooks, Baltimore

Galanti G-A 1991 Caring for patients from different cultures: case studies from American hospitals. University of Pennsylvania, Philadelphia

Boyland E 1991 Women and disability. Zen Books, London

Bates M S 1996 Biocultural dimensions of chronic pain: implications for treatment of multi-ethnic populations. State University of New York, Albany, NY

Cotler M 1996 Perspectives on chronic illness: treating patients and delivering care. American Behavioral Scientist 39(6)

Videos

There are many excellent films on disability available from Program Development Associates (5620 Business Ave., Suite B, Cicero, NY 13039). Insight Media (2162 Broadway, New York, NY 10024) has several films on relevant topics such as: Race: The World's Most Dangerous Myth *and* Cross-cultural communication in Diverse Settings. *Filmakers Library (124 East 40th Street, New York, NY 10016) has many recent films on disability issues, multiculturalism, and ethnicity. A wide variety of films is available from Films for the Humanities and Sciences (PO Box 2053, Princeton, NJ 08543-2053). Among them are* Understanding Our Biases and Assumptions *and* Understanding Different Cultural Values and Styles.

REFERENCES

Albrecht G 1992 The disability business: rehabilitation in America. Sage, Newbury Park, CA

Anderson R 1996 Magic, science and health: the aims and achievements of medical anthropology. Harcourt Brace, Fort Worth, TX

Dettwyler K 1994 Dancing skeletons: life and death in West Africa. Waveland, Prospect Heights IL

Disability Studies Quarterly 1995 15(4) Suffolk University, Boston, MA

Ferraro G P 1998 The cultural dimension of international business, 2nd edn. Prentice-Hall, Englewood Cliffs, NJ

Galanti G 1991 Caring for patients from different cultures: case studies from American hospitals. University of Pennsylvania Press, Philadelphia

Goffman E 1963 Stigma: notes on the management of spoiled identity. Prentice-Hall, Englewood Cliffs, NJ

Gropper R 1996 Culture and the clinical encounter: an intercultural sensitizer for the health professions. Intercultural Press, Yarmouth, ME

Harrison G, Tanner J, Pilbeam D, Baker P 1988 Human Biology, 3rd edn. Oxford University Press, Oxford

Ingstad B, Reynolds S (eds) 1995 Disability and culture. California, Berkeley, CA

Knutson L, Leavitt R, Sarton K 1995 Race, ethnicity and other factors influencing children's health and disability: implications for pediatric physical therapists. Pediatric Physical Therapy 7: 175–183

Konner M 1987 Becoming a doctor: a journey of initiation in medical school. Viking Penguin, NY

Lieberman L, Jackson F 1995 Race and three models of human origin. American Anthropologist 97: 231–242

Locke D 1992 Increasing multicultural understanding. Sage, Newbury Park, CA

Lynch E, Hanson M 1992 Developing cross-cultural competence: a guide for working with young children and their families. Brookes, Baltimore

Morrison F-M (producer and director) 1990 A choice for K'aila. Canadian Broadcasting Corporation

Parsons T 1951 The social system. Free Press, New York

Scupin R 1995 Cultural anthropology: a global perspective, 2nd edn. Prentice-Hall, Englewood Cliffs, NJ

Stein H 1990 American medicine as culture. Westview Press, Boulder, CO

Vang D, Finck J (producers) 1983 Peace has not been made. Rhode Island Department of Social and Rehabilitative Services

3

'Appearances' of disability, discrimination and the transformation of rehabilitation service practices

Aldred H. Neufeldt

THE VIEW FROM PLATO'S CAVE

An allegory made famous by Plato in Book VII of the *Republic* more than 2 millennia ago provides a fitting point of departure for the intent of this chapter:

Pictured is an underground cave with its mouth open towards a bright fire. Within the cave are people, chained so they cannot move, and facing away from the fire, able to see only the wall directly in front of them. The light casts shadows of the people themselves and various objects onto the wall. These shadows become equated with reality, with the cave dwellers naming and talking about them. Sounds from outside the cave are linked to movements on the wall, but what cannot be seen is not considered part of reality. Truth, for these residents, lies in the shadows as they have no other knowledge.

   One day a prisoner manages to escape his chains and leave the cave. Amazed by the world outside, he comes to realize that the shadows on the wall are but a simplistic, two-dimensional reflection of a much more complex reality. Having discovered that his previous understandings and perceptions have been limited and distorted, he attempts to share his new found knowledge with the remaining cave dwellers – but without success. All attempts at persuasion are met with ridicule. The familiar images on the wall are much more meaningful than any story about a world never seen. They see stories of a world outside as extremely dangerous, and as justification for tightening their grip on familiar ways of seeing the world. In contrast, the person leaving the cave no longer feels at home there, unable to act with conviction in relation to the shadowy reflections of reality given his new found knowledge.

In this allegory Plato has Socrates addressing the relationship between appearance, reality and knowledge. Plato, and Socrates before him, had concluded that people in everyday life tend to understand many facets of their world on the basis of superficial appearances rather than on well-founded knowledge. By appreciating this, and making a determined effort to see beyond the familiar illusions, one might free oneself from imperfect ways of seeing. However, as the allegory implies, there is a propensity by many actively to resist and even ridicule suggestions that one's ways of understanding the world may be limited. Conversely, once one has experienced a new way of understanding reality, a 'paradigm shift' occurs and it is difficult to return to the old ways of seeing things.

A variety of truths about human nature are illustrated by the allegory, none more so than that the social acceptance and inclusion of people with obvious physical, cognitive, or sensory impairments depends on an understanding of the relationships between appearance, reality and knowledge. In this context 'appearance' refers to the familiar ways of seeing disability, the social constructions created and accepted by people who live within psychic caves of common belief systems. 'Knowledge' refers to the cumulative content of observed and shareable information about both the nature and experience of disability. 'Reality', as both Plato and Socrates knew, is somewhat more ephemeral. With respect to the reality of disablement, it is probably fair to suggest that the lived experience of persons with disabilities provides the best approximation. Knowledge and reality can never be identical, though one might strive to make them so. When, as in the allegory, 'appearance' of the shadows is assumed to be the same as 'knowledge', then conventional wisdom dominates thinking, and distorted perceptions come to be assumed as 'reality'.

It is important that rehabilitation personnel have more than a passing familiarity with prevalent 'appearances' of disability, given their critical role in working with people who have motor, sensory, or cognitive impairments. Unfortunately for many people with disabilities, the social dimension of disability often is not well appreciated by rehabilitation personnel, despite recent advances in service philosophy

and the passage of disability rights legislation in countries such as Australia, Canada, the Philippines, the USA and Zimbabwe.

A doctoral dissertation study currently being completed (Sloan, personal communication, 1997) includes a phenomenological study which illustrates the continuing challenge. It describes early experiences with disablement of men with injuries of the spinal cord, from the moment of injury through the first few months. Each participant in the study recounted frequent examples of occasions on which their personal experiences with and views on their impairment were discounted by technically proficient and well intentioned rehabilitation professionals. Such discrepancies between intention and action reflect present day confusions of 'appearances', 'knowledge' and 'reality'. Based on reports from many countries, it seems a common experience for people with profound blindness, deafness, motor impairment, psychiatric or intellectual impairment to be perceived as different from the majority population in negatively valued ways (Driedger & Gray 1990).

This chapter begins with a brief exploration of the kinds of conventional thinking about disability that have existed (the 'appearances'), describes the general development of systematic perspectives of disability (the 'knowledge' as it has evolved), and sets out data on the extent to which the acceptance of social 'appearances' and 'knowledge' have contributed to creating discriminatory environments in which people with disabilities live (the 'reality'). The chapter concludes with a set of guidelines to assist rehabilitation personnel in linking 'knowledge' with realities of disability.

'APPEARANCES' OF DISABILITY AND SOCIETAL VALUES

To thoroughly examine the nature and depth of societal attitudes about disability and its impact is not possible in one brief chapter. It is possible, however, to provide a sampling of the kinds of attitudes that have existed over the centuries so as to illustrate the extent to which they are embedded in cultural value systems.

The pervasive role of belief systems in shaping understandings of disability has been apparent to thoughtful analysts of social environments for quite some time. The notable research of Foucault (1973), Scheerenberger (1983) and Wolfensberger (1969, 1980), among others, documents the various ways in which disablement has been perceived over the past 200 years. Scheerenberger and Wolfensberger have described the different, usually negatively valued characterizations of people with intellectual impairments common throughout history, and Foucault traced the ways in which people with psychiatric impairments have been systematically excluded by Western societies. Others examining similar issues in some depth have included Barnes (1991), Hanks & Hanks (1980), Neufeldt & Luke (1984), Oliver (1990), Scheer & Groce (1988), and Thomas (1982).

History

Though attitudes towards disability probably have not been homogeneous in any ethno-cultural context, and some periods in history seem to have been more benign than others (Neufeldt & Luke 1984, Scheerenberger 1983), there is strong evidence of a consistent bias. Sometimes such actions have been justified by the view that disability is the consequence of some evil force. At other times, people with disabilities simply have been viewed as of little worth to society. Hurst (1992) and many others have noted that many 'tribal societies talk about the disabled person as being bewitched, possessed of evil spirits'. While tribal societies continue with such notions (Nicholls 1993), traditional societies have not been unique. Even great reformers of their era, such as Martin Luther, succumbed to the view that significantly disabled people were devil possessed and, in at least one instance, suggested such a person ought to be drowned (Luther 1652). Luther reflected what clearly has been a deeply embedded attitude in many societies. Aristotle, in his *Politics*, wrote: 'As to the exposure and rearing of children, let there be a law that no deformed child shall live'. From Aristotle to the present, the killing of people with disabili-

ties has been sanctioned from time to time on a variety of rationales in most parts of the world. In the 20th century, during the German Third Reich, the most extreme of actions was justified on the more sanitized, pseudo-scientific, but no less deadly, grounds of 'eugenics', designed to promote racial purity. During the Nazi era an estimated 90 000 people with intellectual or psychiatric impairments were systematically killed (Gruneberger 1971, Remak 1969). Even today there is considerable concern amongst members of the disability community that eugenics rather than personal choice is often at the heart of the selective use of reproductive technologies, particularly prenatal diagnostic services combined with abortion, in Europe, North America, Southern Asia, China and other regions (Disability Awareness in Action 1997).

However, there have also been more humane and accepting cultural forces at work. The Judeo-Christian religious tradition, for example, has at various points in history strongly advocated against infanticide, and for the full acceptance of people with disabilities (Gold 1981, McGinley 1988, Neufeldt & McGinley 1997, Wolfensberger 1980). A similar concern for appropriate supports may be found in early writings of Islam (Ajuwon 1993, Myles 1981).

While significant and positive initiatives resulted from these and other voices, negative perspectives of disability have had a tendency to resume predominance after a period of time. Neufeldt & Luke (1984) identified three notable waves of reform over the past several millennia, including one currently underway. Each previous reform movement ended with a reversion to harsh treatment. As both Foucault (1973) and Wolfensberger (1969, 1980) document, there have been notable instances when people with disabilities were viewed by societies as heroic, or as 'blessed of God'. Again, these are sentiments that echo through the ages to the present. The research of both Foucault and Wolfensberger also demonstrates that it is but a short step from being identified as a 'holy innocent' or 'blessed of God' to being separated off from society. An open question is whether the impact of current reforms will be longer lasting.

The persistence of cultural intolerance

How does one explain such persistent cultural intolerance towards disability? One variable examined has been the relationship between changes in the economy and subsequent changes in publicly sanctioned practices (see, for example, Foucault 1973, Thomas 1982). However, Barnes (1991), Foucault (1973), Wolfensberger (1969, 1980) and others note there is sufficient historical and anthropological evidence to demonstrate that, while economic forces may play a part, they are insufficient as an explanation.

The fundamental and recurring factor pointed to by these and other authors is the deep-seated cultural values that have been passed on from generation to generation. In virtually all societies beauty is valued over ugliness (though the definition of 'beauty' may vary), dexterity and adeptness is valued over lack of dexterity, intellectual prowess is valued over lack thereof, and so on. The presence of a disability tends to challenge conventional thinking about these and other values.

'Archetypes' of disability

One might say that there are, embedded in cultural sub-consciousness, a number of, in Jung's (1971) terms, 'archetypes' of disability. An archetype literally means 'first image', a concept drawn from Plato. Five main archetypes of disability may be drawn from the evidence set out above; the disabled person as not able to contribute to the well-being of their society, hence *worthless*; as someone who has/is capable of heroic acts, the *hero*; as the product of some *evil*; as the product of some divine intervention, hence *saintly*; as of limited capacity to make decisions on their own, the *fool*. In more recent history, with the advent of modern medicine, there has been added the notion of disabled persons as *sick*.

These and similar images of disability have been evoked with great regularity across cultures and across time, from earliest recorded history to the present. While the situations and actions have changed over the centuries, and from one part of the world to another, the kinds of publicly told stories seem to have remained fairly well the same. The view that a blind person, or a person in a wheelchair, or with an intellectual impairment is different from the rest of society, in negatively valued ways, seems to persist as part of conventional wisdom. Neufeldt & Albright (1995, 1998), for example, studied approaches to income generation in 41 countries around the world (7 high-income and 34 low- and middle-income). Though social attitudes towards disability were not the direct focus of the study, it was evident in all countries that persistent biases existed against the inclusion of people with a disability in the economic well-being of their societies. Indeed, it was just such issues that prompted the United Nations to declare 1983 to 1992 as the Decade of Disabled Persons, the centerpiece of which was a 'World Program of Action concerning Disabled Persons' leading to the goals of 'full participation and equality' (United Nations 1982).

EVOLVING KNOWLEDGE

The medical model

A first step away from folk definitions of disability in contemporary history occurred in the late 19th century with the rise of new perspectives on science and medicine. The medical model, premised on the emerging scientific method, sought to classify and categorize human impairment, with the aspiration that appropriate treatments would then follow. From this perspective disability is seen as a 'deficit', 'loss', or 'sickness'. Successful intervention is one where the condition becomes 'cured'.

The medical/professional model (professional in that a variety of professions embraced similar points of view) has been roundly criticized by a variety of authors over the past 30 years. While the analytic approach of medicine and related sciences has brought many advances to our understanding of physiological impairment, it has had remarkably little to contribute when impairments are of an ongoing nature –

the impairment is dismissed as a 'chronic' condition. Nor has it contributed much to understanding personal experiences with disablement, as illustrated by Sloan's findings described earlier (Sloan, personal communication, 1997). These kinds of phenomena demand more than dissection, analysis and classification, since 'cure' is either a distant prospect or not considered relevant at all (Oliver 1990).

Perhaps the most fundamental problem was that adherents of the medical model forgot they too lived in Plato's cave. The scientific method, while a legitimate way of gathering and analyzing information, nevertheless relies on a particular perspective from which to make sense of such information. It is not as value free as many scientifically trained individuals at one time thought. It is intensely 'intra-personal' in its perspective, with relatively little room for alternative ways of viewing personal experience with disablement. For example, while the important role of either the physical environment or social attitudes in relation to disability is acknowledged, these remain seen as factors which contribute to either sustaining an impairment or its treatment, rather than as phenomena which independently influence the experience of disablement. Furthermore, professionally trained individuals have not demonstrated themselves immune from traditional assumptions about people with disabilities as being worth less than people not so impaired.

The interactionist/social model

A second step in the evolution of knowledge was taken when disability was redefined as a sociological phenomenon – a statistical deviance from the norm. Goffman (1961) and Wolfensberger (1972) were particularly instrumental in introducing this perspective. How does one address issues of 'deviance'? Their solution lay in redefining the attitudes of society and in helping disablement to be both seen as and included within the normal range of experience. The 'normalization principle', as Wolfensberger described it, sought to engage human service providers, policy makers and researchers in reshaping the social and physical contexts of daily life so that the presence of an impairment would not be negatively valued.

Recognizing the central importance of social values in shaping how people think about disability was arguably the biggest contribution of this perspective. Where the medical model places a premium on being value free in the assessment of relevant information pertaining to physiological impairment (though encouraging value based and ethical behavior by practitioners), the interactionist/social model of disability views social values as influencing all facets of the physical, social and policy environments within which people (with and without disabilities) live. While this interactionist approach recognized the important role of social and physical barriers in separating people with motor, sensory or cognitive impairments from everyday experiences, it too had limitations. Normalization based policies and practices did not necessarily guarantee access to resources, services or opportunities as a matter of right.

Civil rights

A paradigm shift occurred when people with disabilities themselves began speaking about their issues in terms of civil rights. The independent living movement in the USA and Canada (DeJong 1983, Enns 1993, Winter 1993) cast environmental and social barriers as forms of discrimination requiring a response based on social justice. Similar perspectives developed in Europe (Finkelstein 1980, Oliver 1986), Africa and Asia (Driedger 1989). No longer was it adequate to consider the problem as one which could be solved by having helpers and professionals with their technologies and knowledge. Nor was it legitimate to think of the problem as inherent in the people with an impairment. The issue was one of social oppression, where societal structures needed to change so that people with disabilities could function as full citizens with equal opportunities of choice in life in the same way as anyone else.

As noted elsewhere (Neufeldt & Mathieson 1995), this shift in perspective from 'intra-personal' to 'interactionist' to 'civil rights' occurred without the aid of much empirical data. Rather, impassioned, logical, moral arguments along with social action derived from personal experiences with environmental and societal barriers created the initial momentum. Statements such as: 'equality will be experienced when we are free of constructs and categories that limit and constrain our identities – when our disabilities are not our destinies' (Doe, 1992), and 'every nation must enact and implement a highly visible enforceable legal mandate that gives all people with disabilities protection from discrimination and equal access to full participation in society' (Dart 1992) have been characteristic. Legal precedents, such as those reviewed by Hendriks (1995), followed.

Current attitudes

Where are we, then, in our state of knowledge about disablement in all its dimensions? First, we have to say that the images in Plato's cave still persist. Recent research comparing the attitudes in different cultures towards disability demonstrate that reality (see, for example, Mallory 1993, Westbrook et al 1993). While these kinds of study shed some light on differences of degree from one society to another, and may be able to document whether progress is being made in encouraging more positive attitudes, they do not really address the fundamental question of why value-laden biases exist in the first place.

Second, the 'knowledge' as accumulated in its various forms is important but not sufficient for understanding disability. Both the 'intra-personal' and 'interactionist' perspectives have their place. They do not, however, replace the reality of experience with disablement. While it is plausible that progress is being made in various parts of the world, a continuing reality is that the presence of disablement contributes to discriminatory practices.

REALITY-BASED EXPERIENCES WITH DISABILITY

Bynoe et al (1991/2) define discrimination as occurring at three levels:

- Direct discrimination, which means treating people less favorably than others because of their disability
- Indirect discrimination, which means imposing a requirement or condition on a job, facility or service which makes it harder for disabled people to gain access to it
- Unequal burdens, which means failing to take reasonable steps to remove barriers in the social environment that prevent disabled people participating equally.

While there is some room for optimism that progress is being made to counter culturally embedded and negatively valued 'appearances' of disability, there still is ample evidence that the 'reality' for people with disabilities, in many circumstances, is one of discrimination being practiced.

Types of discrimination

Several recent studies have examined the extent and kinds of discrimination based on the above definitions. Barnes (1991) made an in-depth study of discrimination in Britain across a variety of domains, including employment, education, and health care; Hendriks (1995) examined a wide range of legal cases of discrimination around the world, though most notably in high-income countries; and Neufeldt & Mathieson (1995) examined the empirical evidence for discrimination from a number of high- and low-income countries, with particular attention to discrimination in educational opportunity, employment and assault. The consistent evidence from these studies is that systematic discrimination exists in many forms across the regions of the world. In a number of countries steps have been taken in the form of equal rights legislation, various administrative acts and through public education to reduce the amount of direct discrimination. However, indirect discrimination and discrimination as a result of unequal burden continues in all countries examined. This is evident in data that shows people with disabilities to have less opportunity to be educated, less access to employment opportunities, and often to have difficulty obtaining accessible and appropriate housing. These are all considered amongst the fundamentals of a basic quality of life.

Employment

With respect to employment Neufeldt & Mathieson (1995) found the following kinds of barriers typically created unequal burdens, and not infrequently occurred in contexts where there was reasonable evidence of at least indirect discrimination:

1. Transportation to and from places of work frequently presented a problem, particularly for people with sight, mobility or intellectual impairments.
2. Workplaces frequently were not accessible by a number of criteria. Steps up and down presented problems for people with mobility impairments. Workplaces were set up with little regard for people who had difficulty reaching or moving about. People with sight, hearing or speaking impairments found that appropriate aids were not available to assist with communication. Any number of studies have shown that inexpensive adaptations are available which would improve the situation not only for people with disabilities, but also for a large portion of the non-disabled workforce. Yet, workplaces have been slow to make the changes.
3. Opportunities to learn appropriate work skills typically are much fewer for people with disabilities than for those without disabilities (particularly in the case of people with an impairment from birth or early in life). A variety of studies give evidence that such lack of learning opportunity has relatively little to do with features of the disability (for example, it has little to do with whether one might have been physically unable to participate because of the nature of one's impairment), but is rather due to

the lack of effort at overcoming minor barriers to accessing learning opportunities. The pernicious effect has been severely to limit people's ability to pursue meaningful employment options.

Similar evidence exists of systematic exclusion from educational or other resources. One might argue that actions such as those described are the result of general societal neglect, not lack of good intent. However, it is difficult to discount the evidence cited earlier on the effects of societal attitudes and values both on public policy and day-to-day practices. Comparative data on sexual assault brings this point into bold relief.

The experience of women with disabilities

Sobsey & Doe (1991) conducted a wide-ranging study. One of their findings was that women having a variety of impairments were about one and a half times more likely to have been sexually abused as children than were women without disabilities. As with all women, in the majority of circumstances the perpetrators were people known to the victim (frequently these were caregivers abusing their positions of trust), and in less than a quarter of offenses (22.2%) was the perpetrator charged. A further disconcerting statistic is that where charges were laid, convictions were secured in only 8% of cases. The significantly higher assault rate and the extremely low rate of conviction demonstrate both the relatively powerless position of these women and the negative valuing of disability.

Lest it be concluded that physical and sexual assault is primarily an issue in high-income countries, it should be observed that widespread concerns about sexual and physical assault also exist in low-income countries. Driedger & Gray's anthology (1990) provides a variety of stories arising out of such personal experiences.

One can readily conclude that underlying the above kinds of socially negligent and discriminatory actions are the attitudes of people in the marketplace, in neighborhoods and among family members. Such attitudes, though frequently demonstrated to be wrong, continue to influence all facets of the environment in which people live.

VALUES, CONSTRUCTS AND THE LANGUAGE OF DISABILITY

There is at present a discourse on the most appropriate language to use when referring to disability. The discourse is most clearly framed by the question, does one say 'person with a disability' or 'disabled person?' Though it may seem trivial, the topic touches on a much larger social issue; namely, one's construct of disability.

Present language use practices are quite confusing, both outside of and within what might be referred to as the disability movement (i.e. organizations of people who have significant and identifiable impairments). Some argue that 'person with a disability' is the most logical because it places emphasis on (hence is sensitive to) the person first and the disability second. Government documents in North America, English language professional journals, and an increasing number of business organizations insist on this phraseology. The reason is not hard to fathom. In much of Western society there has been considerable sensitization to civil rights, and there is a wish not to offend – the epitome of 'political correctness'.

However there is a group within the disability movement which argues that the phrase 'person with a disability' is fundamentally illogical (see, for example, Barnes 1991, Oliver 1986, 1990). Their reasoning is that if one follows the World Health Organization definitions of 'impairment', 'disability' and 'handicap' to their logical conclusions, then it may be appropriate to say 'person with a sensory, cognitive or motor impairment,' but that disability results when a person with an impairment encounters an inaccessible environment. It is therefore the environment which disables the person and so the term 'person with a disability' is incorrect. This argument has been focused most visibly in international fora by Disabled People's

International, an organization with observer status at the United Nations.

The debate is not merely an academic one, or one of 'political correctness'. At the heart of it is the question of how one sees the impairment as distinct from that of disability. Confusions in the meaning of terminology also lend themselves to creating mixed messages in the communication between rehabilitation personnel and people receiving the rehabilitation. The logic of Barnes (1991), Oliver (1986, 1990) and others is hard to refute. If disablement is different from impairment, what is the difference if it does not result from the interaction with the environment? Is the term 'handicap' needed at all? (See Ch. 10).

Clarification of the terminology would allow greater precision in its use. Above all, clarification of the terminology would ensure that rehabilitation personnel do not inadvertently accept into their thinking the lingering 'appearances of disability' from Plato's cave. Indeed, there have been some discussions towards that end under the auspices of the World Health Organization, involving representatives from disabled people's organizations. Clarification cannot come too soon.

TRANSFORMING SERVICE PROVIDING APPROACHES

Within the past 30 years the disability movement has taken the lead in challenging both the discriminatory practices of, and underlying attitudes embedded in, rehabilitation services as experienced by people with disabilities. As a result, we are seeing a gradual transformation of the way in which services are being framed. The historic and often criticized stance already referred to was one in which the professional defined the problem, defined the methodology, and imposed it on the consumer. Consumers, and particularly their families, were conditioned to accept this approach as the way in which services ought to be organized and run. All the power rested with the professional, and the person with a disability was put into a 'patient' role on the presumption that the patient did not have the right, the interest, or sufficient ability to play a more proactive part. That this was not the case seemed not to matter.

If one assumes that both consumers of services and providers/professionals need to be involved in shaping a service enterprise, then the question becomes one of degree. Three broad approaches seem plausible:

1. Type 1. Consumer-directed model. In this model consumers take the lead in defining the issues, methods, and so on. The role of the service provider is to be supportive. This model has the greatest cogency when the issues addressed have to do with the experience of disablement in its various forms, and the person's quality of life. Clearly, the core holders of knowledge and those with both the most to gain and/or lose, are people with disabilities themselves. Having said this, it is noteworthy that few examples of the consumer-directed model of rehabilitation exist in its ultimate form, though we are seeing the emergence of a variety of funding mechanisms in both Canada and the USA where there is a direct payment of funds to consumers so they might purchase services from amongst a number of providers.

2. Type 2. Professional-directed model. This is akin to the traditional model, but is reshaped to ensuring that consumers are meaningfully involved in all decision making as it affects them. This model has its greatest cogency in areas of professional service that involve the identification of complex or technical diagnostic approaches or interventions. Even in highly complex problem areas, however, consumers may well be encouraged to play a key role, and are likely to increasingly do so in the future. For example, as the knowledge base expands exponentially, and as service providers find it increasingly difficult to remain abreast of the variety of kinds of knowledge related to a given problem area, it is highly probable that many consumers will themselves research the existing knowledge with respect to the particular area of their concern (for example, by using internet connections) and convey that knowledge to service providers for their professional judgment. As that happens, the role of the service provider

becomes one of making an assessment of which of the findings of the consumer has the greatest and most immediate relevance to a given situation, and which service interventions are likely to have the greatest impact in the desired direction.

3. Type 3. Conjointly-directed model. In a conjointly-directed model there is a co-identification of the issue to be addressed, and similar conjoint involvement in defining the most appropriate methodology, implementing the methodology, analyzing and interpreting results, and using the results. Within the North American service sector, this model has been adopted quite widely, at least in theory, although consumers may not always agree it has been adopted in practice.

All three types of approach have potential utility within the context of rehabilitation services as noted above. However, from a service management perspective, the model with greatest flexibility is probably the conjoint model in that it allows for subsequent decisions to be made as to whether one of the alternate approaches will be more appropriate, depending on changing circumstances. An active alliance of service providers with consumers in defining problem areas and working out appropriate interventions is least likely to lead to actions which, in retrospect, seem diverted by the shadows of Plato's cave. Conversely, it has the highest probability of ensuring that the application of knowledge is appropriate to the experienced 'reality' of disablement.

GUIDELINES FOR USER SENSITIVE REHABILITATION SERVICES

If rehabilitation services are to be sensitive to their users, and providers are to be committed to a conjoint approach in determining appropriate steps, then it is advisable for there to be developed guidelines for practice. In pursuing development of such guidelines, it is recommended that a group be set up for that purpose comprised of at least as many people with disabilities as service providers.

The following guidelines might be taken into consideration for any given service context:

1. Commitment to consumer control. Service providers should:
   a. respect the values of the consumer movement
   b. take into account the knowledge and experience of service users
   c. be open to looking at their own biases and take responsibility for any interfering or oppressing biases they have
   d. acknowledge the inherent power differentials between themselves and service users, modeling effective use of personal power.
2. Responsible conduct and informed consent. Service providers should:
   a. work only with those issues and methodologies within the realm of their competency
   b. ensure the lead person in charge of services being provided is responsible for all decisions in a given situation, including decisions of subordinates
   c. at all times respect the privacy and dignity of service users
   d. begin no services without the consent of those who may be affected, ensuring the nature of services and potential risks as well as benefits are fully explained in a way that is consistent with the communication capability of the service user
   e. in seeking informed consent, clearly identify others who may have access to information
   f. if research is to be done, obtain informed consent from each participant in research as well as from such local organizations of disabled persons as may be involved
   g. apply no undue pressure to get consent.
3. Conflict of interest:
   a. service providers should declare any real or perceived conflicts of interest prior to undertaking service provision if such is potentially the case. (Conflict of interest is defined as a situation where a person or the person's family or friends might benefit materially (financially or otherwise), either directly or indirectly, as the result of actions taken.
   b. on declaring a conflict of interest, persons so involved should remove themselves from any decision-making processes.

NEW DILEMMAS OF SERVICE IMPLEMENTATION, AND CONCLUSION

Collaboration of service providers with consumers in planning for and implementing specific services, as compared, for example, to planning for and participating in research, for the most part does not seem to have many complications. Once freed from thinking about disability in terms of historical 'appearances', the biggest challenge for both service providers and consumers is to become comfortable with their new identities. Both share values relating to achieving a 'good outcome'. The potential problem, of course, is in defining what constitutes a 'good outcome'. It is here that consumer choice and decision making, by-and-large, can easily be seen to have significant benefit to both the consumer and provider.

At the same time, an increased emphasis on consumer choice raises old dilemmas in new forms. Perhaps the most significant ones are those having to do with issues of potential harm to self or others. If a consumer chooses to ignore service provider recommendations, and persists in putting his life in danger, what does the provider do? There is a great temptation for professionals to recommend some form of intrusive procedure. Yet we know that intrusiveness itself may be counter-productive; and that if service users really wish to harm themselves, it is difficult to prevent it.

The very fact that this kind of dilemma is now surfacing illustrates something of the changed nature of relationships, where a specific kind of human service problem has been elevated to a discussion between equal human beings rather than a presumed superiority of one over the other. This very change helps break the chains binding both people with disabilities and service providers within Plato's cave. The fact that there is an exchange of views between service providers and consumers, and that people with disabilities may in fact make choices which harm them in the same way that people without disabilities do, removes some presumptions associated with historic and conventional ways of thinking about disability. Having said this, service providers also need to be alert that more is not expected of a disabled person than of others.

Does this new way of thinking about rehabilitation fit in low- as well as high-income countries, and in multiple societies? Evidence gathered from both research and personal experience suggests it does. People with disabilities and rehabilitation personnel are co-participants

in the rehabilitation endeavor wherever they live. The only question is what the nature of their relationship will be. Just as there is evidence that the various 'appearances' of disability discussed earlier have had adverse effects in many societies, so too is there evidence that a conjoint approach to service planning and provision will have long term and positive impacts on all. Development of a world-wide disability movement, based on a commonly assumed right to personal choice, illustrates that the proposed guidelines for service providers are not culture bound. It is this new balance between provider and consumer which holds great promise for the reform of rehabilitation services to new levels of excellence in all countries of the world.

REFERENCES

Ajuwon P 1993 A study on quality issues: adults with visual impairment in the Nigerian population. PhD dissertation, University of Calgary, Calgary, p. 33

Barnes C 1991 Disabled people in Britain and discrimination. Hurst University of Calgary Press, London, pp. 28–61

Bynoe I, Oliver M, Barnes C 1991/2 Equal rights for disabled people, the case for a new law. Institute for Public Policy Research, Social Policy Paper No. 7, Welfare Series. Cited in: Foley C, Prattin S Access denied: human rights and disabled people. National Council for Civil Liberties, London, p. 22

Dart J 1992 Closing Comment. In: Equalization of opportunities. Proceedings of the 3rd World Congress of Disabled Peoples' International, April 21–26, Winnipeg, MB: Disabled Peoples' International p. 84

DeJong G 1983 Defining and implementing the independent living concept. In: Crewe N M, Zola I K (eds) Independent living for physically disabled people. Jossey-Bass, San Francisco

Disability Awareness in Action 1997 Newsletters 47 and 48. March and April

Doe T 1992 Independence: a definition of equality that reaches beyond normality and liberates our humanity. In: Equalization of opportunities. Proceedings of the 3rd World Congress of Disabled Peoples' International, April 21–26, Winnipeg, MB: Disabled Peoples' International p. 48

Driedger D 1989 The last civil rights movement. Hurst, London

Driedger D, Gray S Imprinting our image: an international anthology by women with disabilities. Gynergy Books, Charlottetown, PEI

Enns H 1993 An agenda for the '90s. In: Neufeldt A H (ed) Independent living: an agenda for the '90s. Canadian Association of Independent Living Centres, Ottawa, pp. 137–140

Finkelstein V 1980 Attitudes and disabled people. Monograph No. 5. World Rehabilitation Fund, New York

Foucault M 1973 Madness and civilization. Random House, New York

Goffman E 1961 Asylums: essays on the social situation of mental patients and other inmates. Doubleday, New York

Gold R A 1981 Judaism and persons with handicaps. Documencap, 15, p. 9

Gruneberger R 1971 The 12-year Reich. Holt, Rinehart & Winston, New York, p. 451

Hanks J, Hanks L 1980 The physically handicapped in certain non-occidental societies. In: Philips W, Roseberg J (eds) Social scientists and the physically handicapped. Arno Press, London

Hendriks A 1995 Disabled persons and their right to equal treatment: allowing differentiation but putting an end to discrimination. Health and Human Rights, 1 (2): 152–173

Hurst R 1992 The media's role in equal opportunities for disabled people. In: Equalization of opportunities. Proceedings of the 3rd World Congress of Disabled Peoples' International, April 21–26, Winnipeg, MB: Disabled Peoples' International

Jung CG 1971 Memories, dreams, reflections. Routledge & Kegan Paul, London

Luther M 1652 Colloquia mensalia. Cited in: Scheerenberger R C 1983 A history of mental retardation. Paul Brookes, Baltimore, p. 32

Mallory B L 1993 Changing beliefs about disability in developing countries: historical factors and sociocultural variables. IEEIR Monograph No. 53. Traditional and changing views of disabilities in developing countries. Durham, NH University of New Hampshire Press, pp. 1–24

McGinley P 1988 Religion and rehabilitation: a particular challenge for Christianity. In: Brown R I (ed) Quality of life for handicapped people. Croom Helm, London, PP. 215–234

Myles L 1981 Some historical notes on religions, ideologies and the handicapped. Al-Mushir (The Counselor) 23(4): 125–134

Neufeldt A H, Albright A 1995 An international study of strategies leading to self-directed employment. International Journal of Practical Approaches to Disability 19: 3–8

Neufeldt AH, Albright A 1998 Disability and self-directed employment: business development models. Toronto, Captus University Publications, Ottawa, 1DRC Press.

Neufeldt A H, Luke D 1984 The history we live. In: Neufeldt A H (ed) Celebrating differences. Faith and Life Press, Newton K S, pp. 42–54

Neufeldt A H, McGinley P 1997 Human spirituality in relation to quality of life. In: Brown R I (ed) Quality of life for handicapped people. Chapman Hall, London

Neufeldt A H, Mathieson R 1995. Empirical dimensions of discriminations against disabled people. Health and Human Rights 1(2): 174–189

Nicholls R W 1993 An examination of some traditional African attitudes toward disability. IEEIR Monograph No. 53. Traditional and changing views of disabilities in developing countries. University of New Hampshire Press, pp. 25–40

Oliver M 1986 Social policy and disability: some theoretical issues. Disability, Handicap and Society 1(1): 5–17

Oliver M 1990 The politics of disablement. Macmillan, London

Remak J (ed) 1969 The Nazi years. Prentice Hall, Englewood Cliffs N, pp. 133–134

Scheer J, Groce N 1988 Impairment as a human constant: cross-cultural and historical perspectives on variation. Journal of Social Issues 4: 23–27

Scheerenberger R C 1983 A history of mental retardation. Paul Brookes, Baltimore

Sobsey D, Doe T 1991 Patterns of sexual abuse and assault. Sexuality and disability 9(3): 243–259

Thomas D 1982 The experience of handicap. Methuen, London

United Nations 1982 World programme of action concerning disabled persons. UN document A/37/351/Add. 1, 13 July

Westbrook M T, Legge V, Pennay M 1993. Attitudes towards disabilities in a multicultural society. Social Science and Medicine 36(5): 615–623

Winter M 1993 The growth and development in independent living in America. In: Neufeldt A H (ed) Independent living: an agenda for the '90s. Canadian Association of Independent Living Centres, Ottawa, pp. 121–136

Wolfensberger W 1969 The origin and nature of our institutional models. In: Kugel R B, Wolfensberger W (eds) Changing patterns in residential services for the mentally retarded. President's Committee on Mental Retardation, Washington

Wolfensberger W 1972 The principle of normalization in human services. National Institute on Mental Retardation (now the G. Allan Roeher Institute), Toronto

Wolfensberger W 1980 Elemente der Identät and Perversionen des christlichen Wohlfahrtswesens. Diakonie 6(3): 156–167

4

Health beliefs and behavior towards individuals with disability cross-culturally

Nora Ellen Groce

INTRODUCTION

If rehabilitation professionals are to make a difference in the communities in which they work, it is essential that they understand and appreciate the complexity of health belief systems. These systems differ markedly from one culture to another and they tend to dictate how individuals with disability fare within their societies. Health belief systems also often dictate how, when and what type of rehabilitative care is made available to individuals with disability.

Ideas about disability are part of a larger culturally based system of health beliefs and health behaviors. All cultures have shared ideas of what makes people sick, what makes people well and how people can maintain good health through time. These beliefs help people make sense of the world around them. Both lay people and health professionals tend to combine their society's health belief systems with knowledge gained through first hand experience. These individual models of belief are often referred to as explanatory models (Kleinman 1980). Explanatory models provide a framework within which individuals sort through and make sense of illnesses, injuries and disabilities.

Understanding the issue of health belief systems and individual explanatory models is important because there are few concepts of disability that are universally believed to be true. In fact, there are considerable differences in the way disability is regarded from one society to the next. Although disability tends to be viewed negatively in many societies, this is not always the case. Moreover, different types of disability tend to be regarded differently by members of the same society, hence an individual who has a vision impairment may be considered a full and active participant of a community, while in that same community an individual with mental health problems may be shunned.

Understanding sociocultural models of disability is of more than academic interest. Unless programs for individuals with disabilities are designed in a culturally appropriate way, the opportunity to make real and effective change is often lost. This chapter is not intended to catalogue every known variation in disability beliefs, but rather to alert the practitioners to the fact that the ways in which disability and rehabilitation are conceptualized will have an impact on the manner in which rehabilitation professionals are received, regarded and able to serve their patients.

BACKGROUND

There has yet to be a society found anywhere in the world that does not have a complex system of beliefs concerning disability. Universally, societies have explanations for why some individuals (and not others) are disabled, how individuals with disabilities are to be treated, what roles are appropriate (and inappropriate) for such individuals and what rights and responsibilities individuals with disability are either entitled to or denied (Scheer & Groce 1988).

Rehabilitation professionals are too often trained to concentrate on clinical goals – restoring function in a specific set of muscles or training an individual in daily living skills, while ignoring the larger social networks and culture matrix in which those with whom they work, must live. Being aware of the weaknesses (and strengths) of the surrounding community enables rehabilitation professionals to work far more effectively with and advocate in partnership with those whom they serve.

It is important to note that there is still much that is not known about disability in society.

The cross-cultural study of disability is less than a generation old. Although there are thousands of articles and books on rehabilitation, almost all of this research discusses disability in developed nations. Moreover, the bulk of this literature focuses on biomedical factors rather than sociocultural issues (Groce & Zola 1993). Yet it is estimated that 80% of all individuals with disability today live in the developing world, and of these 60–70% live in rural areas (Helander 1993). It is anticipated that every year will bring us new information about how individuals and societies conceptualize and treat individuals with disabilities in different, and often unexpected ways. Nevertheless, there is one clear conclusion that can be drawn, even at this early date: the lives of individuals with disability around the globe are usually far more limited as a result of prevailing social, cultural and economic constraints than as a result of their specific physical, sensory, psychological or intellectual impairments.

BELIEFS ABOUT DISABILITY: A CROSS-CULTURAL PERSPECTIVE

A history of the field of rehabilitation usually begins with 19th- or early 20th-century pioneers, and a discussion of the rise of hospitals, clinics and institutions. It leaves the reader with the distinct impression that there were no provisions made for those with disability before the rise of professionals. In fact, individuals with disability have always been part of human society. Indeed, the earliest evidence for an individual surviving with a significant disability pre-dates humans. At Shanidar Cave, in Iraq, a skeleton of an elderly Neanderthal shows that he survived for many years with a withered arm and blindness in one eye. Living into his 40s, elderly by Neanderthal standards, the man eventually died and his grave site was covered by his contemporaries with flowers, indicating that he was a valued member of that small social group (Solecki 1971).

Archaelogists rarely find any skeletal population that does not have several individuals whose remains indicate some type of disability. Ancient art and pottery, early myths and legends from Greece and Rome, India, China and the Americas all show the presence of individuals with disability (Dashen 1993, Scheer & Groce 1988).

Terminology and categorization

Not only are individuals with disability found in all known societies; even more significantly, all known societies seem to have distinct ideas about how individuals with disabilities should be treated. What then can be said about disability in society cross-culturally? It might be best to begin by examining the idea of 'disability' itself. Although in English, as in some other languages, a single term (disability) is used to refer to individuals with a wide range of physical, psychological or intellectual impairments, in many languages there is no one word to refer to such individuals. One can speak of 'the blind' or 'a deaf person' but the term 'disability' which links all these people together in a single category may be missing, or little used (Rengill & Jarrow 1993, Scheer & Groce 1988).

All societies do seem to recognize individuals with disability as having some physical, psychological or sensory attribute that distinguishes them from other non-disabled members of that society. Gallagher (1990) describes this as an 'otherness'. However it is the cultural interpretations of this 'otherness' that are of concern and these cultural interpretations vary significantly from one society to the next. Moreover, disability categories used by Western health professionals are not universal. Almost all societies have specific terms and conceptual categories for individuals who have moving difficulties; seeing difficulties; hearing and speech problems; learning difficulties; and seizure disorders.

In addition, some cultures have developed specific categories of disability that are uniquely their own. For example, there are a number of psychiatric disorders, known as cultural bound syndromes, that are unknown or rarely found in other cultures. Simons & Hughes (1985) list more than 150 of them, including 'susto', a condition believed to be caused by a sudden fright which is found widely in Latin America. A victim tends to become anxious and depressed, listless, and anorexic. Women tend to be affected far more frequently than men and in its most extreme form, it is believed to be fatal. Halatime & Berge (1990) found that in northern Mali, the most 'disabling condition' for females is to be ugly. There is widespread agreement of what physical attributes make a woman unattractive. Popular beliefs hold that a man who marries such a woman will lose a day of life for each day spent in such a marriage. Given the prevailing beliefs, marriage for such women is rare, and only married women have full social status in the community (Helander 1993). While not falling into a universal category of disability, these women's lives are, nonetheless, severely restricted by a culturally defined disability.

SOCIAL INTERPRETATIONS OF DISABILITY

Societies do more than simply recognize disabling conditions in their members. They usually attach value and meaning to various types of disability. For the purposes of this discussion, these social beliefs will be grouped together in three categories that seem regularly to appear cross-culturally and which tend to allow one to predict how well an individual will fare in a given community and society:

1. causality: the cultural explanations for why a disability occurs
2. valued and devalued attributes: specific physical or intellectual attributes are valued or devalued in a particular society
3. anticipated role: the role an individual with a disability is expected to play as an adult in a community.

These three categories are ones that should be familiar to rehabilitation professionals, for they will be used as a basis upon which people's expectations and demands for (or avoidance of and passivity about) rehabilitation systems will be built. The beliefs associated with these categories will affect individuals' willingness to receive care, and family and community willingness to support and encourage the individual who is receiving care. Additionally, the categories influence priorities, policy and a community's willingness to pay for care and services. Although there are many variations, the following is an overview of the more salient issues involved in each of the above categorizations.

Causality

Societies treat individuals with disability well or poorly based in part on culturally based beliefs about why a disability occurs. Divine displeasure, witchcraft or evil spirits, reincarnation and biology are all given in the ethnographic record as the reasons why disability occurs (Scheer & Groce 1988).

The birth of a child with a congenital anomaly is often considered a sign of divine displeasure with the child's parents or with the community. Disability which occurs later in life may also be considered a sign of divine displeasure with the individual who becomes disabled or is chronically ill. For example, disobedience to God's law was so strongly linked to disability in the Old Testament that individuals with disability were not allowed to approach the altar. In the New Testament, Christ, upon restoring sight to the blind man, is reported to have said 'go and sin no more,' firmly tying the man's inability to see to the tradition of divine punishment (Gallagher 1990).

Interestingly, the belief that God selects who will be disabled is not always negative. One study of Mexican-American parents found the belief that God wills a certain number of disabled children to be born. Being merciful, however, God chooses parents who will be particularly kind and protective for these 'special' children (Madiros 1989). A similar finding is reported in Botswana, where the birth of a disabled child is viewed as evidence of God's trust in specific parents' ability (Ingstad 1988).

The supernatural figure need not be a divine one. For example, marital infidelity on the part

of the father (Ingstad 1990), or intercourse with too close a family member, a demon or an animal by the mother (Scheer & Groce 1988) are often cited as reasons why a disabled child born. The belief that an offended witch or spirit has caused a child to be born disabled, or an adult to have a disabling accident, is widely reported from regions where witchcraft is a traditional explanation for ill health or misfortune. A victim of witchcraft is not always seen as an innocent victim. He or she may have done something to antagonize a spirit and the individual who is disabled is often avoided for fear that close association with such a person will put others at risk.

Reincarnation, the belief that one's current physical and social state is a reflection of one's conduct in a previous life, often leaves individuals who are disabled in a particularly difficult situation. Their current status is seen as earned – and there may be less sympathy and less willingness to expend resources on their behalf.

Not all societies believe the cause of disability is divine or supernatural. The idea that a disability can be 'caught', either by touch or by sight, is found widely. New brides and pregnant woman, in particular, are discouraged from seeing, hearing or touching someone with a disability, for fear that they may give birth to a similarly disabled child. Examples can be found from Sri Lanka (Helander 1993) to rural USA (Groce 1985, Newman 1969). This idea of contagion is so strong that some Native American parents continue to discourage their children from even touching assistive technology devices, such as wheelchairs (Thomason 1994). Similarly, in Kenya, huts for adults who are disabled are still built at some distance from the rest of the settlement, and utensils and other objects belonging to these individuals are not mixed with those of the rest of the family (Nicholls 1992).

Modern medicine has redefined disability causation and looked for explanations in the natural world: genetic disorders, viruses and accidents are now commonly accepted as explanations for why a person is born with or becomes disabled. But if modern medicine has replaced older causation concepts, it has often not done so completely. The idea of blame, inherent in most cultures for centuries, often reappears in more 'scientific' forms. For example, if a child is born with a disabling condition, both professionals and lay people are quick to ask whether the mother smoked, drank or took drugs. If a young man is disabled in a car accident, many are anxious to know if he was driving too fast, or whether drugs or alcohol were involved. Some of these factors certainly can cause a disability to occur, but such inquiries often go beyond simple scientific curiosity. What seems to occur is a resurfacing of the older need to determine whether the individuals thus affected are in some way responsible for their current condition or the condition of their children.

It has been hypothesized that part of this interest may be a psychological distancing – individuals try to establish a logical reason why a disability has occurred to reassure themselves that something similar will not happen to them. But another issue here is the continuation of the almost universal practice of determining causality in order to determine what demands the individual with a disability and that individual's family may justifiably make on existing social support networks and community resources. Sympathy and support is much more readily given to an individual whose disability is believed to be caused by a genetic anomaly, chronic illness, or random accident that, it is believed, could potentially affect anyone.

Causality continues to be important even in the most modern of medical systems. For example, in the USA, someone in military combat who receives a severe spinal cord injury has access to far greater social, medical and economic supports than an individual with an identical injury who acquired it in a drunk driving accident. The deciding factor here is not the disability itself, but the specific circumstances surrounding the occurrence of the injury.

Cultural explanations about causality are intriguing, but they must be used with some caution. Nkinyangi & Mbindyo (1982), doing work in Kenya, found that although witchcraft was regularly offered as an explanation, only 2% of their informants with disabilities believed that witchcraft was the reason why they themselves were disabled. In the Bahamas, although supernatural causes were traditionally associated with disability, nowadays that explanation is usually cited only to confirm the bad opinions about persons or families that were held prior to the onset of the disability (Goerdt 1989). Conversely, in the USA or Canada, parents may inform friends and relatives that their child has been born with a particular randomly occurring genetic syndrome, only to have these people speculate behind the parents' backs about the possibility of maternal drinking or incest being present.

Few societies have only one explanation of why a disability occurs. Rather, different types of disabling conditions are accounted for by different explanations. Profound deafness may be attributed to marital infidelity, whereas a disabled limb may be considered the result of personal 'bad luck' and 'fate'.

Valued and devalued attributes

The underlying factors that determine how well an individual with a disability will fare in any given society will depend not only on how that society believes a disability is caused, but also on what personal attributes a society finds important. Those individuals who are unable to demonstrate these attributes will be considered more severely disabled (Wolfensberger 1983). This will in turn be reflected both in the manner in which these individuals are treated and in the society's willingness or unwillingness to allocate resources to meet their needs.

For example, in societies where physical strength and stamina are valued, those with significant physical disabilities are at a particular disadvantage. When one's status in the community depends in large measure on how well one can hunt or fish or farm, difficulty in walking or in lifting will diminish one's social status. Conversely, in a society where intellectual endeavors – the ability to work in an office or deliver a speech – are considered important, the fact that one uses a wheelchair or crutches to get around will be far less significant. Factors will vary from one society to the next. In many Native American groups, calling attention to oneself is considered improper. A valued attribute is to blend into the larger community rather than to stand out. Having a disability that automatically makes one stand out from one's peers, in such a community, is considered to be particularly stressful.

In societies' willingness to allocate resources based on anticipated adult roles, disability issues often intersect with other social concerns, such as that of gender. The willingness of families to expend scarce resources on a girl with a disability might be substantially less than for a comparably disabled boy. In Nepal, for example, although polio affects males and females in equal numbers, there are almost twice as many boys reported as disabled by polio as girls. At issue is not who gets polio, but who survives in the years following the illness (Helander 1993).

Anticipated roles in communities as adults

Finally, the willingness of any society to allocate resources for individuals with disability, including resources for rehabilitation efforts, will also depend in large measure on the anticipated role individuals with disability are to play in the community as an adult.

At one extreme end of the continuum, a society might refuse to allocate any resources for those with disability and not allow them to live. However, infanticide, even of severely disabled newborns, is exceptionally rare in the ethnographic literature (Scheer & Groce 1988). Only a small handful of groups seem to have regularly practiced it. Historically, in such cases, death is usually brought about by abandoning the infant on a remote hillside or cave shortly after birth. Smothering infants or otherwise causing death at the time of delivery has been reported in Western midwifery, where families were usually informed that the child had been stillborn or died immediately following delivery (Helander

1993). In more recent years, the use of amniocentesis, genetic counseling, and the withholding of medical care in the delivery room, while touted as medical advances by some, are viewed by many disability activists as a more technologically sophisticated form of infanticide (Asch 1990, Hahn 1989).

Even if infanticide were practiced on a regular basis, it would eliminate only a small percentage of all those having a disabling condition. Most types of congenital disability, such as deafness or mild mental retardation, are not discernible in infancy, and accidents and chronic illness can occur at any point in the life cycle. The intentional killing of individuals with disability beyond the first 2 weeks of life is all but unheard of in the ethnographic record. The killing of infirm or disabled elderly is reported from several societies, although it should be noted that such practices are quite rare and usually take place during periods of extreme hardship for the group as a whole, such as a time of food shortages, or exceptionally severe winters. Although there are isolated accounts of elderly infirm individuals being put to death for humanitarian reasons, the only known systematic elimination of disabled children and adults occurred in Germany during the Nazi era when, in an attempt to purify genetic stock, 300 000 German citizens with physical or psychiatric disorders (85% of Germany's institutionalized population) were systematically put to death (Gallagher 1990). Renewed discussion of the 'right to die' and prolongation of life due to modern medical technology has stirred new debate on these issues around the subject of disability.

While infanticide is rare, medical and physical neglect which results in death is extremely common. It is not unusual in many countries for infants and children with disabilities to be 'allowed' to die for want of food, medicines or other types of care in a way that would be considered neglect if they were withheld from comparable non-disabled peers (Groce 1990). Predictions that such children and adults will not live long, nor be healthy can become self-fulfilling prophecy.

Medical neglect can take many forms. Parents with limited resources may be slower to take their disabled child to a physician or healer should the child appear ill, hoping that the illness will clear on its own. They may be less willing to carry a disabled child several miles to ensure participation in the local immunization drive. Families that already have few resources may want to invest little in a child with a significant disability.

The issue of social inclusion, over and above inclusion in medical care, is a complex one. Survival is not the only measure of social attitudes. In some societies, individuals with disability are kept alive but hardly welcomed. In the Micronesian island of Paulau, someone with mental retardation is called 'ultechei' which means 'substitute' or 'replacement', a less-than-fully-human being. While such individuals are maintained within the kinship system, they are considered a burden on the family and community and their presence is not welcome (Rengill & Jarrow 1993).

It is not uncommon for individuals with significant disabilities to be considered a disgrace to the family, hidden from public view in the backroom or inner courtyard of a family house. This is particularly true in societies where disability is said to be caused by parental sin or God's displeasure. In some cases, while individuals with disability are valued within their own homes, they can anticipate no outside role in the community. They will be provided basic medical services, they will be fed, housed and cared for by relatives, but there is no provision made for their participation in society. Indeed, it is assumed that they will not want to or be able to participate in society. In such instances, educating these individuals, training them to earn a living, arranging for a marriage or even expending time and energy to locate medical and rehabilitative services for them may be considered an unreasonable drain on a family's resources, particularly if such resources are very limited.

Some have argued that in such societies an individual's inability to contribute to the family's economic needs is the deciding factor in what status he or she maintains in the household and in the community. However, calculating a person's contribution in terms of formal employment, even marginal employment, outside the home, may be misleading. Many individuals with a disability who do not work outside their own homes or family units do make significant contributions to their family's economic well-being. All but the most significantly disabled of individuals can contribute some work – they watch children, cook, clean and do housework and farm work, they help assemble parts for piecework or crafts brought to the marketplace in someone else's name.

Indeed, they may be regularly assigned tasks that others do not want. Greene (1977) reported that rural families in Ecuador were concerned that newly introduced iodized salt would eliminate the birth of children with iodine deficiency syndrome. These children, born with hearing loss and mild mental retardation, were regularly given the task of herding animals, collecting firewood and drawing water. Who would do these onerous tasks, they asked, if such individuals were no longer born in their villages?

Individuals with disability are often allowed partial inclusion in society. They are given limited roles and responsibilities. Specific roles for disabled individuals are often found. For example, blind people become potters, broom makers, market vendors and musicians in many cultures. By far the most common role assigned to individuals with disability, however, is that of the beggar. Worldwide, the only way many individuals with disability may have to support themselves and their families is that of begging outside churches, temples and mosques, in marketplaces and railway stations. As Helander (1993) insightfully points out, for those who live in dire poverty, there is often little choice but to exploit their condition. The more obvious the disability, the greater the chance of receiving alms. In such instances, rehabilitation may be avoided by some concerned that their improved physical abilities might lower their chances of feeding themselves and their families. More research is needed on this and many other issues that affect disability among the very poor.

A full adult role in any community implies not simply employment, but also the ability to marry and have a family of one's own, to decide where one will live, with whom one will associate; and it implies having a voice in decisions made in the community. Although societies differ as to where, when and how individuals carry out these roles, a good rule of thumb for professionals evaluating the status of those with disability in any community is whether such individuals are participating in such activities at a rate comparable to that of their non-disabled peers (i.e. individuals from comparable socioeconomic and ethnic/minority backgrounds).

In some societies, individuals with disability are given a special role. Used as symbols, they are sometimes believed to be particularly close to God, or to bring or hold good luck, or it is believed that their existence satisfies evil spirits (Nicholls 1992). In some societies, individuals with disability are thought to be inspirational, and although ill treated on a day-to-day basis, at certain times of the year or on certain ceremonial occasions they become the center of attention (Christmas is such an example in the West). A special or reserved status is not, needless to say, necessarily an equal status.

Full acceptance, that is, status and treatment comparable to one's non-disabled peers, is relatively rare, but it does exist and is important. For example, a number of tribal groups around the world, such as the Azandi in East Africa and the Ponape of the Eastern Carolines in the southern Pacific, warrant comment because of their general kindness and acceptance of children born with obvious impairments (Gallagher 1990).

Indeed, communities may interpret even significantly disabling conditions in a positive light. On the island of Martha's Vineyard, off the northeast coast of the USA, a gene for profound hereditary deafness led to the birth of a number of deaf individuals. Because deafness was so common, it was in the best interests of the hearing islanders to learn and use sign language and most did. With the substantial communication barrier – the very thing that most regularly blocks deaf individuals from full participation in society – breached, it is perhaps not surprising that deaf individuals on Martha's Vineyard participated vigorously in the life of the small villages in which they lived. They were not considered to be (nor did they consider themselves to be) 'handicapped' (Groce 1985). The fact that individuals with a disability assume roles comparable to all other members of a society is a good indication that real integration has been achieved.

Obviously, the more that the local health beliefs support the idea that individuals with disability are fully participating members of a community, the more demands may be placed upon rehabilitation professionals to assist such individuals. There may also be an opposite reaction. If a disabling condition is fully accepted and thought to be caused for a specific reason (especially if it is thought to occur because of divine will), individuals and families may be less anxious to seek rehabilitation to eliminate traits which they do not perceive as a problem.

Finally, the social role that an individual holds in society may well change over time, as societies modernize. For example, in societies where most members live by manual labor, where people live by tilling the land or watching the flocks, many chores and jobs can be found for many who are mildly retarded. (Indeed, many who are severely retarded can also make significant contributions to their families and communities in such places). In technologically sophisticated societies, where all children are required to attend school for a number of years, it has become important to identify at an early stage those children who fall below certain standardized test levels. Once identified, these children are likely to be singled out from their peers. Their ability to compete in the work force as adults is considered to be so compromised that in many countries they are placed on a formal pension system at the age of 18 – a system that will maintain them for the remainder of their life. The difference here is not in the mental retardation of the individual, but in the socioeconomic structure of the society into which that person has been born.

WHY REHABILITATION PROFESSIONALS NEED TO UNDERSTAND BELIEF SYSTEMS

The discussion about variation in the ways disability is conceptualized and dealt with cross-culturally is of more than passing importance for the rehabilitation professional. It has significance for virtually every part of the process of rehabilitation, from basic diagnosis, to treatment, to developing policy. Traditional diagnostic categories of disabling conditions, folk interpretations of the causes and consequences of living with a disability and willingness to follow prescribed medical and rehabilitative courses of action will all reflect local health belief systems.

Even an action as simple as early childhood screening for disability and census taking to locate individuals with disability, so that planning can begin for rehabilitation programs, may be complicated by such belief systems. In many cultures where shame is attached to being disabled or having a disabled family member, reporting the presence of such an individual to the local health care provider or census taker may expose families to censure. When disability is connected with a sin or breaking a taboo, parents may avoid seeking early diagnosis and treatment in order to prevent drawing attention to that child or stigmatizing the family.

HEALTH CARE PRACTICES AND TREATMENT

Rehabilitation professionals must be cognizant of traditional medical systems and health seeking behaviors, recognizing that they often have much to offer. Not only is disability itself universal, but all societies have health care practices that in some way address various types of disabilities.

There is often an inherent tension between traditional and modern medical practices, with practitioners from both groups advocating competition rather than cooperation. This is unfortunate. Traditional medical practices may be effective, ineffective, or ineffective in clinical terms, but of great benefit in psychological terms. A number of traditional folk practices, including massages and relaxation techniques, may be of help to individuals with disabilities (in fact, the National Institutes of Health in the USA have recently established a program to look specifically at what they call 'Alternative Medicine' and to study the potential benefits of non-Western forms of medical care).

In many cases, rehabilitation professionals might be well advised to try to combine the best of both traditional and Western techniques and practices. Patients are often already combining these practices, with or without the permission of their physicians and therapists. A survey of one of the largest and most modern rehabilitation hospitals in Indonesia revealed that over 85% of all those with physical disability were also making use of traditional healers or remedies. In many Native American communities, chronic illness and disability are seen as the outward manifestation of disharmony between the individual, the family or the community and the surrounding universe (Thomason 1994). In such instances, the issue to be first addressed is not the specific clinical or rehabilitative needs of the individual, but the restoration of some sort of harmony or balance between the individual and the surrounding universe, a process that can only be done by a traditional healer. Only after that are rehabilitation questions able to be dealt with.

Decisions on whether to go to traditional healers or to seek help from Western practitioners or clinics, or to combine the two forms of healing, will be based on a variety of factors. The type of disease or disability for which care is sought may be important; some types of illness may be believed to be treatable by Western medicine, other types may not. The availability and accessibility of care is equally important. If rehabilitation programs require travel over considerable distances or if they are considered too costly, a local traditional practitioner may be sought, even if Western trained practitioners are believed to be more effective. Social networks also play an important role. If the local health practitioner is a cousin on whom you rely for financial aid in time of need, or who is responsible for helping you arrange the marriage of your son or daughter, or whose wife serves as the village midwife, going outside the community to seek help from a rehabilitation professional may seem unwise. In such a case, it is not that the rehabilitation professional has nothing to offer, but rather that in seeking care for one individual in your family, you have effectively severed important social support systems that reverberate throughout the rest of your family's social network.

Furthermore, the need for clinical and rehabilitative services for those with disability will rarely exist in isolation from social needs, such as in cases of extreme poverty or lack of education. Rehabilitation professionals must therefore do more than simply deliver services in a clinical setting. Rehabilitationists must also take it upon themselves to learn what life is like in the community for the individuals they serve. Much can be learned by just talking (and listening) to individuals with disabilities and their families.

CONCLUSION

Individuals with disability and their rehabilitation can no longer be put at the end of a long list of competing social needs, such as basic education, clean water, sufficient food supplies or safe housing. Individuals with disabilities stand in as much need of the other social necessities as all other members of the community. Rehabilitation professionals, with an understanding of the sociocultural ramifications of living with a disability, can contribute a great deal to this dialogue. For if prevailing social attitudes are not changed, much that rehabilitation professionals attempt to do will be fruitless. Extensive rehabilitation may allow a young woman with cerebral palsy to walk to the end of her street and back, but if she cannot do so without adults muttering insults and children throwing stones, not much has been accomplished.

A cautionary note should be added here. There is often a tendency for policy makers, families and communities to turn to professionals for the definitive word on systems of care and service for those with disability. It is vitally important to remember that those in rehabilitation should assist individuals with disability to represent their own claims in the community. They can help empower individuals with disability and their families to address and change traditional health beliefs and social attitudes, but they should not become their voices.

In urging rehabilitation professionals to bring people's attention to the potential of individuals with disability, it is imperative that they first become familiar with traditional belief systems and health seeking behaviors. Culturally based beliefs about disability are often both strongly held and locally interpreted in a way one needs to understand in some detail before setting out to make changes.

There have also been a number of successful adaptations to disability and there are without doubt many more as yet undocumented, that represent real strengths and provide decided advantages for disabled members of the community. In some communities, strong and supportive family structures, special roles and adaptations and a general acceptance of a specific type or types of disabilities may provide a solid foundation upon which individuals with disabilities should build. Many of these adaptations might be quite local – perhaps specific to a small community or remote region. Even professionals in the nearby city or regional hospital may be unaware that they exist. Hence, rehabilitation workers need to ask what is traditionally done locally before they set out to make changes. Modernization and Westernization can affect traditional health and disability beliefs and behaviors, but not necessarily dictate what old beliefs are retained, what new beliefs are added, or how the old and new belief systems will recombine. A new approach to disability may, in fact, be no better than the more traditional belief systems. As traditional community supports dissolve with growing urbanization, individualization and a shift to a monetary economy, where the value of what a person is is reflected by how much he or she can produce, the future is not necessarily clear or bright.

Attempts to introduce new ideas by rehabilitation professionals must therefore be carefully monitored.

In conclusion, it must be argued that although many types of physical or intellectual impairments are universal, a person's experience of *being* disabled is largely shaped by the health and social beliefs of the culture in which the individual lives. Issues of class, gender, family structure, economics, education and regional/national development all will have implications as to who is considered to be disabled, what is expected of that individual and how that individual with a disability fares in his or her own society

REFERENCES

Asch A 1990 Reproductive technology and disability. In: Cohen S, Nadine J (eds) Reproductive laws for the 1990s. Humana Press, Clifton, N J

Dashen V 1993 Dwarfs in Ancient Egypt and Greece. Oxford, NY

Gallagher H 1990 My trust betrayed: patients, physicians, and the license to kill in the Third Reich. Henry Holt, NY

Goerdt A 1989 Social integration of the physically disabled in Barbados. Social Science and Medicine 22(4): 459–466

Greene L Hyperendemic goiter, cretinism and social organization in Highland Ecuador. In: Green L (ed) Malnutrition, behavior and social organization. Academic Press, NY

Groce N 1985 Everyone here spoke sign language: hereditary deafness on Martha's Vineyard. Harvard University Press, Cambridge, MA

Groce N 1990 Traditional folk belief systems and disabilities: an important factor in policy planning. Rehabilitation International/UNICEF, NY. One in Ten 9(2): 2–7

Groce N, Zola I K 1993 Multiculturalism, chronic illness and disability. Pediatrics 91(5) 1048–1055

Hahn H 1989 Theories and values: ethics and contrasting perspectives on disability in ethical issues. In: Ethical Issues in Disability and Rehabilitation, (report) Oakland CA World Institute on Disability

Halatime F, Berge G 1990 Perceptions of disabilities among Kel Tamnsheq of Northern Mali. In: Brunn FJ, Ingstad B (eds) Disability in a cross-cultural perspective. Working paper no. 4. Department of Social Anthropology, Oslo

Helander E 1993 Prejudice and dignity: an introduction to community-based rehabilitation. United Nations Development Programme, NY

Ingstad B 1988 Coping behavior of disabled persons and their families: cross-cultural perspectives from Norway and Botswana. International Journal of Rehabilitation Research 11: 352–359

Ingstad B 1990 The disabled person in the community: social and cultural aspects. International Journal of Rehabilitation Research 13: 187–194

Kleinman A 1980 Patients and healers in a cultural context. University of California Press, Berkeley

Madiros M 1989 Conception of childhood disability among Mexican-American parents. Medical Anthropology 12: 55–68

Newman L 1969 Folklore of pregnancy: wives' tales in Contra Costa County, California. Western Folklore 28(2) 112–135

Nicholls R 1992 An examination of some traditional African attitudes towards disability. Traditional and changing views of disability in developing societies. Monograph No. 53. National Institute of Disability and Rehabilitation Research, Durham, NH

Nkinyangi J, Mbindyo J 1982 The condition of disabled persons in Kenya: results of a national survey. University of Nairobi, Kenya, Institute for Developmental Studies, Nairobi

Rengill Y, Jarrow J 1993 Culture and disability in Palau. International Exchange of Experts and Information in Rehabilitation. Newsletter January 1993. University of New Hampshire

Scheer J, Groce N 1988 Impairment as a human constant: cross-cultural and historical perspectives on variation. Journal of Social Issues 44(1): 23–37

Simons R, Hughes C 1985 The culture-bound syndromes: folk illnesses of psychiatric and anthropological interest. Reidel, Boston

Solecki R 1971 Shanidar: the first flower people. Knopf, NY

Thomason T 1994 Native Americans and assistive technology. In: Murphy J H (ed) Technology and persons with disabilities. Proceedings of the 9th Annual Conference. California State University, Northridge

Wolfensberger W 1983 Social role valorization: a proposed new term for the principle of normalization. Mental Retardation 21: 234–239

5

Some influences of religions on attitudes towards disabilities and people with disabilities

M. Miles

NO COOKBOOK

To get anything from this chapter requires readers to do some thinking of their own – which may have incalculable results. At any rate, there are no cookbook answers here. In discussion, people normally use terms like 'disability', 'disabled', quite loosely. In what follows, 'disability' and 'people with disabilities' (PWDs) will be more in line with the Impairment-Disability-Handicap triad, developed in the 1950s by Riviere (1970) and colleagues, than with the politically-charged 'Social Model' dyad of Impairment-Disability. (The dyadic term supports the view that difficulties arising from impairments are largely due to the oppressive way in which society operates and environments are designed. It is a powerful campaign slogan, but rather oversimplifies the experiences of PWDs.) The term 'attitudes' is highly problematical, and will not be used very much. Attitudes can mean the sort of changeable muddle of hopes, feelings, dispositions and beliefs that we all experience in our dealings with other people. If afterwards we examine coolly how we actually behaved in a given situation, and compare our behavior with what we thought was our 'attitude' to that sort of person or situation, we may often be surprised. . . .

This brief chapter cannot encompass all the insights of the world's major religions on issues of disability, suffering, compassion, rights. Disability and world religions is a recent field of studies. There are a few students, but no experts. Further, I doubt if one can write about disability or religious belief with a truly neutral stance, and I do not pretend to. I write as a Western student of Asian disability history, whose thinking has been shaped, but not perhaps fixed, within the cultural traditions of Judaism, Christianity and Islam. I also doubt if very much can be understood about religions without some active, personal engagement with one of them, or with a political ideology or other belief system having some of the characteristics of a religion.

All the religions I have come in contact with have some points or incidents concerning disability that look rather positive to a Western eye. All have some negative sides or stories or historical practices. A selection will appear below. Yet most people in whichever religious group spend very little time thinking about the meaning of disability, or the teaching of their religion about disability. So it is unwise to generalize, e.g. that 'Sikhs think this about disability', or 'Christians think that'. In the long run, the world religions have shown some capacity to take in new ideas, or rediscover old ones, integrate them with their teaching, and make them available to new generations. The results are not all predictable, and are sometimes quite surprising.

REFLECTIONS

Rachel, a community-based therapist in a Western country, parks her car near the house of a child with a disability, referred to her for a professional visit. The family name sounds Asian. In the optional space for 'Religion' in the referral notes, someone has marked 'Hindu'. Rachel knows that she usually succeeds in making a friendly start with families having all sorts of backgrounds. For a moment she pauses, and questions flood in:

Hindus. What do they believe about disability? Will there be a problem about physical contact with the child? Are there not many different sorts of Hinduism? But they all believe in reincarnation, including animals, don't they? It's a very old religion . . . and this is a modern family, living in a Western city. How much of the traditional beliefs will they hold, and how much will they think 'modern'?

Rachel reflects for a moment that her own beliefs also belong within an ancient religious tradition. Some of her beliefs do not fit comfortably with parts of her professional knowledge and training – so she keeps them in separate compartments in her mind . . .

Is that perhaps what modern Hindus do? Maybe it would be good to ask them. But you have to be careful, with questions of religion. And people are sensitive around disability. It doesn't really make any difference to what you hope to do with the child. But should it make a difference maybe? After all, community-based work aims for a partnership between professional and family, within the context of the local community, so it's important to learn how the family thinks . . . supposing that they all think alike. Maybe the child is growing up in two worlds. On the other hand, the family may have been here 100 years already . . .

Another country. Two counselors in friendly argument. Mohammed Nasir has cerebral palsy. Wellington Smith has a visual impairment. These guys have known each other for years. They aren't usually so polite – but not to offend readers, this is a cleaned-up version . . .

MN: Bugs me that people in West write books and make big noise about rights and do best thing by disabled people like it was something new. In Islam we had right idea from way back. By Will of Allah maybe I got some problem, muscles on me do things different like, I don't complain, it is test for me, like challenge, I grow strong in my mind. But in Islam it is also duty and test for the community to fix things like so I get my food and gear, I get chance of training, I get to do some job of work. Not charity like. No-no. It is for community own good that everyone get chance to do something, nobody fall in gutter, nobody count as worth nothing. Community itself is disabled if fails to take right action to advance forward one who is falling behind.

WS: Right brother, okay, so do we see it? You know, this country, access law is there, politician speech is there, Christian Father say and say, Muslim Maulvi say and say. So the result? Disabled person come for counseling, you see I see any day, no school, no training, not allow this, rule against that, can't go there, sorry boy, very sorry missy, not allow, for your own good, we have to protect, you might fall down, safety thing, regular customer don't like. You ask boss can we fix collecting box by door, charity appeal for disabled, religious duty, most often boss say okay. Ask boss any chance a job this blind girl, not charity, smart girl, she type fast, take note fast, answer phone real good, after three day you don't know she got any problem at all. Most often boss say no chance. Christian boss, Muslim boss, Hindu boss, nothing different. Sure, you got historical stuff in Islam, pretty good. We got stuff in Christian Church, pretty good. Do we see it on street?

Mohammed Nasir and Wellington Smith are right. Relevant historical material exists in the three allied monotheisms, Judaism, Christianity and Islam. Some of it would seem quite 'modern' if people knew of it and decided to act on it.

THE MONOTHEISMS

Wertlieb (1988) discusses a range of evidence about disabilities and attitudes towards them in the Talmud. Her work aims to refute the charge that Judaism historically reflected a negative view of PWDs; but the study covers a lot of other useful ground. Background material on disabilities and Judaism is given in detail by Preuss (1978), who showed the extensive legal restrictions imposed on PWDs, practices which were inherited and continued within Christianity and Islam.

Down the centuries, all three religions have slowly discovered ways of modifying these burdens, sometimes by returning to the original purpose of the restriction. For example, the Jewish priest had the task of examining sacrificial animals, so that what was offered should be without blemish. This required good eyesight, and was a justification for excluding visually impaired people from the priestly office. It was not a justification for dismissing other abilities which a visually impaired person might have. Thus, for example, to memorize sacred texts and declaim portions of them on public and private occasions has been an honored occupation for blind men, especially within Islam.

Christian texts record healings of people with various disabilities, often showing some reticence. These stories sometimes involve touchy points of religious doctrine or protocol, or had

the result of impeding the mission of Jesus (see for example Mark 1:40–45; 7:31–37; 8:22–26; and Luke 5:12–26). In John's gospel (9:1–41), Jesus rejects his companions' question, whether a certain man was born blind through his own, or his parents', sin. The answer was neither. This blind man was to serve as a demonstration of the works of God.

Instantaneous healing, as a response to disabilities, has remained elusive down the ages; but records of the Christian church offering practical, caring services for PWDs began AD *c.*360, when Eustathios, bishop of Sebasteia in Lesser Armenia, set up a hostel 'specifically to serve persons afflicted with disfiguring or disabling diseases' (Miller 1985, p. 79). This was soon followed by services organized by Basil of Caesarea (Miller 1985, pp. 85–88), and similar efforts slowly spread westwards over several centuries, reaching even the cold, foggy islands off the coast of Northern Europe (Orme & Webster 1995, pp. 15–31).

Christian theologians have long pondered the meanings of disability, without reaching definite answers. Augustine, for example, used the occurrence of 'feeble-mindedness' to support his view that 'fallen' human nature was transmitted down the generations. Elsewhere, the example of a person with mental retardation who revered Christ was given by Augustine to refute believers in reincarnation who thought mentally retarded people must have been very sinful in previous lives. Such issues seldom engage modern Christians, but they are still relevant to theologians of other major religions.

Linguistic review may bring a different understanding of some ancient scriptures. The revelation of God as one 'visiting the sins of the parents upon the children' (Exodus 20:5; 34:7) is hard for Jews and Christians to comprehend, but may remain in the minds of some parents with disabled children. The Hebrew *poqed*, translated as 'visiting', could equally be remembering', or 'bearing in mind'. It may then be understood as a more merciful judgment on the children, taking into account the morally vitiated environment in which they were raised. Some children, for example, are born with impairments as a result of their parents' substance abuse. They may have a difficult life; but need not bear the additional burden of thinking that a vindictive deity has punished them for their parents' failings. On the contrary, their struggle through life may be attended by divine mercy, bearing in mind their flawed inheritance.

The reformer Martin Luther is sometimes criticized for being negative about disability, on the basis of a casual suggestion about drowning a grossly disabled and 'unmanageable' child. The problem was that he did not think such children could actually be human (Luther 1964–68, vol. 54, pp. 44–45; pp. 396–397). Elsewhere, Luther recorded vigorous arguments for better care of pregnant women (Luther 1964–68 vol. 5, pp. 381–382) and consolation of women after miscarriage (Luther 1964–68, vol. 43, pp. 245–250), and displayed solicitude for premature babies (Luther 1964–68, vol. 54, p. 58), contradicting the claim that he lacked compassion.

By the 7th century, the vigorous new religion of Islam was spreading across the Middle East. Muslim jurists were soon to develop an intricate debate about the civil rights of people with mental retardation. Some Muslim law schools maintained that such people were not legally empowered to handle their own property, because, like children, they lacked the ability to do so sensibly. Others argued that to deprive adults of this right of action was to do them more harm than anything they could suffer by losing property (Hamilton 1963, pp. 526–527; Miles 1992). Even now, a thousand years later, such questions have not finally been resolved.

SUFFERING AND DISPASSION

A foundational story within Buddhism tells of a prince who has been brought up unaware of pain, disease and death. He desires to go out for a drive, beyond the royal palace. The king's servants clear the highway of all 'blind, lame or crippled beggars, sick and decrepit old people', so that the illusion of pain-free perfection can continue. However, the gods intervene and cause the prince to see suffering. When he

demands an explanation, his driver reveals the truth. Perceiving human suffering, Prince Gautama is driven to embrace it, to leave his protected lifestyle and to search for the right way to live in the world (Cowell 1894, pp. 27–35).

The resulting 2500 years of Buddhist teaching and literature, in their enormous variegation, can hardly be summarized in three paragraphs. They constitute a rewarding field of study, especially for the monotheisms underpinning Middle Eastern and European civilization. The cherished Western notion of the autonomous individual self is challenged by those parts of Buddhist thinking that stress the interdependence and interexistence of all. To take up the religious life, a dedicated Buddhist may welcome some disfigurement and enter the self-humiliation of dependence on others, thus becoming more aware of the illusoriness of self, the folly of pride, the transience of earthly desire (Tachibana 1992, p. 178). Such exercises have also been known in the Christian monastic tradition. They contrast sharply with those forms of Christian teaching in which spiritual 'feel-good'ness, body healing, wholeness of mind, financial success, career advancement and a good public image can be part of the package.

Buddhism's rather cool, intellectual image in Western countries would not immediately connect with the world of disability service provision or the rights movement. Yet a Buddhist civilization was providing asylums for PWDs in Sri Lanka, centuries before the time of Jesus (Smith 1920, pp. 66, 162, 317–318, 324) in an age when northern European societies were primitive. Buddhist missionaries to China found that by offering medical treatment they could win a hearing for their teaching (Unschuld 1979), some 1400 years before Catholic and later Protestant Christian missionaries to China used a similar strategy. Christian influences in Buddhist nations in the past two centuries have motivated Buddhists to rediscover their own heritage and to develop distinctively Buddhist formulations in response to the disability movement in the West. Those formulations, still awaited, are unlikely to be a simple endorsement of Western slogans.

THE HINDU HERITAGE

The classical literature of Hinduism has many references to disabilities. Some are exhortations to charity. Others suggest the exclusion of PWDs, who seem on the whole to be fixed in the role of people who are undesirable, but who serve the function of receiving charity and thereby enabling donors to gain merit. For example, the great Indian epic *Mahabharata* refers several times to rulers' duties to cherish 'like a father, the blind, the dumb, the lame, the deformed, the friendless' (Ganguli 1993, Sabha Parva 5). This is given more substance when, during diplomatic shuttling before the great battle scene, Yudhishthira, oldest of Pandu's sons, sends elaborate greetings to the court of his uncle Dhritarashtra, who is himself blind and whose queen, upon her marriage, adopted a blindfold out of respect to her husband (Ganguli 1993, Adi Parva 110). Yudhishthira includes greetings to 'the many hump-back and lame ones' among the servants. He asks after the welfare of those who are 'defective in limb, those that are imbecile, the dwarfs to whom Dhritarashtra gives food and raiment from motives of humanity, those that are blind, and all those that are aged, as also to the many that have the use only of their hands being destitute of legs' (Ganguli 1993, Udyoga Parva 30).

This kindly display of concern seems in contrast with the counsel later given to Yudhishthira, that there must be 'no dwarfs, no hump-backed persons, no one of an emaciated constitution, no one who is lame or blind, no one who is an idiot, no woman, and no eunuch, at the spot where the king holds his consultations' (Ganguli 1993, Santi Parva 83). A similar exclusion appears in the *Laws of Manu* (Doniger & Smith 1991, p. 143). One reason might be the custom of employing spies either with disabilities or disguised as PWDs (Ganguli 1993, Udyoga Parva 195), as recommended in the *Arthashastra*, classic manual of Indian statecraft (Rangarajan 1992, pp. 506–509). Such spies, trading on the custom of royal charity, could gain access to court. The King had to protect himself against those who might be spying for a rival ruler. Keeping these tricks in mind, a more complex picture emerges of the status of PWDs, and of the attitudes deemed correct towards them.

The three works cited above have been key parts of the heritage of Hindu literature through two millennia. They convey a broad message that charitable provision is a duty of the state, and kindly concern is the duty of kings and their subjects. Yet there is also an undertone that the state, the king, and his subjects should keep a wary eye on PWDs. The ambivalence continues in later literature. Bowker (1987, pp. 203, 206), writing on suffering in the world's religions, notes that the goddess Nirriti is 'the personification of misery and suffering'; yet she also protects those who 'by being born into evil families, are handicapped, and yet who, despite that remain virtuous.' The Buddhist manual *Puggala-Pannatti* portrays such people, living in extreme poverty and also 'swarthy, ill-featured, hunchbacked, a prey to many diseases, purblind, or with a crooked hand, lame or paralysed,' yet who are well-doers in thought, word and deed. Their reward will be 'a happy destiny in the bright worlds' (Law, n.d., p. 71).

DISABILITY AS SOMETHING 'GIVEN'? (see Ch. 4)

Religious beliefs have been associated at many times and places with the idea that a person's disability is 'given' by an agent, with purpose. There are a number of essentially 'negative' views, which may see a disabling impairment being given as:

1. Punishment
2. Inescapable consequence
3. Statistically probable consequence
4. Casual (not necessarily *causal*) outcome, of:
   a. disabled people's own
   b. their parents'
   c. their society's
   d. humankind's:

  i.   sinful actions
  ii. ignorance and foolish actions
  iii. accidental actions
  iv. mistaken beliefs:
       w. in the present life
       x. in a previous existence
       y. in earlier centuries
       z. since the human race began.

Clearly there are many possible combinations available in the above sets. Person A might hold view 1.b.i.w., common to much 'traditional' religious belief, that the child's disabling impairment is a punishment to its parents for their sins. The view 3.b.ii.w., that the child's disabling impairment is a predictable consequence of its parents' foolish actions (e.g. in alcohol abuse, or failure to immunize the child), might in certain cases represent a modern scientific analysis by Person B, who scorns religious beliefs. Yet it would also be possible for Person C to combine both these thoughts in her head. Further, it would be extremely hard to predict, who of Persons A, B and C, might best be able to keep their views to themselves and be a friendly and supportive counselor to the parents, or teacher to the child.

The 'giver' in the above cases is usually understood to be the deity, fate, karma; or sometimes a lesser force such as the offended spirits of ancestors, or microbial agents such as polio viruses, to which insufficient respect has been offered. However, some other views of 'given' disabilities offer a different picture. They may see disability as:

1. an open-ended challenge for the strengthening of a person's soul
2. a specific lesson to be learnt, to enable the soul to make progress
3. a challenge to the disabled person's family or other carers
4. an opportunity for the deity's power or love to be demonstrated
5. an opportunity for individual or neighborhood charitable action.

These last five pictures would be counted by many people as more 'positive' than the views listed above; yet they have also come under strong attack in recent decades from Western groups of PWDs, and they may be rejected very bitterly by some individuals in almost any country.

There are some systems of thought or belief in which disability is not actively 'given'; it 'arises' randomly or from the complex interplay of many factors. Having 'arisen', the disability can be perceived as an individual challenge; or interpreted as a form of oppression by a 'disabling' society, which must be resisted.

In another quite widespread belief system, identification of certain disabling conditions is done in a curious ceremony performed by people in white gowns. Drops of blood, taken from the suspected person's arm, are smeared on slabs of glass and are viewed through a tube. The person looking at the blood claims to be able to count different spots and shapes, though these are not visible to ordinary people. Elaborate stories are built up around these spots and shapes, and predictions are made about the future of the person whose blood has been used. Sometimes blood from their ancestors is also studied for comparison, if it can be obtained. Predictions by the white-gowned people have often come true, and the belief system has a strong hold on its adherents, however odd it may seem to the rest of the world. As in most strongly-held systems, adherents are inclined to see their beliefs as 'The Truth', even though disability obviously has many aspects which cannot be examined with a microscope in a science laboratory, and which do not have spots or shapes.

RELIGION OR PERSONALITY?

Historically, the dominant religion in a particular region used to constitute a large part of the 'social environment'. You might believe its tenets more or less fervently; you might practice its morality more or less closely; but what you could not easily do was to pick and choose the bits that took your fancy, while leaving other parts aside. Religion, culture, socialization, the communal life of your neighborhood, were all closely interwoven. While some people probably had questions and private opinions in the back of their minds, it was seldom wise to express them openly. In such times and places, a religious teacher, especially in a small community, could say that 'Our religion teaches X and Y about disability' – and that was it. That was the teaching. To reject it, even on one point alone, would be taken as a rejection of the teacher's authority, sometimes equivalent to a rejection of the religion. It was hardly a rational option.

Between 1 and 2 billion people live in such a religious environment in the 1990s. At the other extreme, in much of the Western world and among some urban dwellers in all countries, the dominance of any one religion as a 'social environment' has practically disappeared. Modern believers choose the teachings that attract them or make sense to them, leaving aside the bits they do not like or cannot believe. Many people have no formal religious beliefs at all. In between, there are 2 or 3 billion people who are in critical periods of transition, where traditional authority and beliefs are under serious threat, and alternative patterns and choices are becoming attractive to some. Families are, of course, often divided between an older generation with traditional beliefs, their grandchildren with 'modern' views, and the middle generation caught uneasily in between. We should remember also that the world religions have all gone through considerable evolution in past centuries, with changes of understanding that may look small now with hindsight, but seemed immense and threatening at the time.

Some studies in the past suggested that people with certain sorts of personality may have a lot of attitudes in common, regardless of the particular doctrines of their religion or philosophy. For example, people who seek strong, clear, authoritative religious or ideological statements and doctrines may find themselves happiest among other Christians, or Muslims, or Hindus, or socialists, holding 'fundamentalist' or 'traditionalist' beliefs. Such people are often found engaging whole-heartedly in socially useful and compassionate work, regardless of the particular religion or ideology in which they believe. On the other hand, the term 'fundamentalist' has in many groups become associated with extremes of behavior, including sharp intolerance towards other beliefs. People who see their lives and beliefs in very clear-cut terms, with individuals and their actions sharply categorized as good or bad, may share in common certain clear-cut attitudes towards disability and PWDs, and may resist experiences or evidence that suggests complexity or ambivalence. However, such studies have been criticized by Söder (1990). He finds that most studies of attitudes towards disabilities, or towards PWDs, are constructed in such a way as to constrict the range of possible answers. They thus eliminate the actual ambiguity of feeling, thought and action reflected in the way most people behave. Söder's insight suggests also the need for caution in thinking about the influence of religions on attitudes.

THERAPISTS AND BELIEFS: IN PRACTICE . . . .

It is hardly the therapist's job to try to change a client's fundamental beliefs – to do so might be seen as unprofessional conduct. Yet for most therapists, their work is more than a bag of techniques and gadgets. The therapist cannot avoid some engagement with clients' efforts to make sense of their disabilities, or those of their relatives. To listen attentively and with understanding requires the competent therapist to have some broad awareness of the range of human beliefs in the disability area, and at least an outward tolerance of some that may seem personally repugnant. One benefit of studying a little further is that it may be possible to hint at paths that would take clients toward a more positive position within their own belief system.

Clients may believe, for example, that disabilities are given by Allah as a trial to be endured, and that it would be an act of rebellion to try to avoid the test. For a non-Muslim to contradict this would be unwise. Yet one might, with all due respect to clients and their beliefs, enquire about the well-known saying, 'For each illness,

Allah has provided a remedy.' Since Allah does mercifully provide remedies, and bestows knowledge and skill on doctors and therapists, would it be an act of rebellion, or perhaps instead an act of thankfulness, to avail oneself of this mercy?

When parents lament the fact that their child has a disability, and attribute it to some wrong-doing of their own, it may be unwise to contradict such a position directly – yet one might at another time mention that families in some parts of the world consider it an honour to be 'given' a disabled child. They believe that the deity, when sending babies to families, chooses a special family who will take loving care of the extra needs of the disabled child. A thought such as this, offered gently, not insisted upon, would be likely to be acceptable to people of almost any religion, whether or not they actually believed it. For some, it might begin a re-evaluation of their own child and their attitudes toward it.

Another benefit of studying further is that the therapist might reach the point of understanding something important from a client with different beliefs. What the major religions have to offer is not all patent. What appears on the surface often seems rather disappointing, until the meaning of the religious language or symbols has become familiar.

IN CONCLUSION

We left our community-based therapist, Rachel, a few pages back, reflecting on religion, change, Hinduism and uncertainty. By now, maybe she is asking her client's family some polite questions. Maybe she buys this book and reads it. Maybe she tries her local library. Maybe she finds a quiet place to meditate or pray. Maybe she rejects it all as 'superstitious nonsense'. Maybe she gets scared, and retreats inside her professional *persona*.

Whatever her own beliefs and feelings and practices, the one thing Rachel cannot do is to find a world where all her clients and their families have the same religion, and have simple beliefs within that religion, and see a straightforward connection between the religious beliefs and their approaches to disability. If Rachel is going to continue to mature as a therapist and as a human being, she must swim in the multi-cultural, multi-religious, multi-ideological ocean of modern and post-modern society.

Biographical note: Mr Miles has studied Mediterranean languages and religions, and spent 12 years in Pakistan developing disability resources. Since 1992 he has been studying Asian disability history.

FURTHER READING

Bowker J 1987 Problems of suffering in religions of the world. Cambridge University Press, Cambridge
Groce N E, Zola I K 1993 Multiculturalism, chronic illness, and disability. Pediatrics 91(5: 2, Supplement): 1048–1055
Lynch EW, Hanson M J (eds) 1992 Developing cross-cultural competence: a guide for working with young children and their families. Brookes, Baltimore (see pp. 79–80, 105–106, 142, 168–169, 285–287, 309–312, 340–343)
Miles M 1995 Disability in an Eastern religious context: historical perspectives. Disability and Society 10: 49–69

Morgan P, Lawton C 1996 Ethical issues in six religious traditions. Edinburgh University Press, Edinburgh
Ninomiya A H 1986 Japanese attitudes towards disabled people – religious aspect. Japanese Christian Quarterly 52: 202–206
Preuss J 1978 Biblical and Talmudic medicine, translated by Rosner F (German original published 1911). Sanhedrin Press, New York (see especially pp. 206–209, 230–239, 270–293, 299–320)
Wertlieb E C 1988 Attitudes towards disabilities as found in the Talmud. Journal of Psychology and Judaism 12: 192–214

REFERENCES

Bowker J 1987 Problems of suffering in religions of the world. Cambridge University Press, Cambridge

Cowell E B (trans) 1894 The Buddha-Karita of Asvaghosha. In: Müller F M (ed) Sacred books of the East, vol. 49. Clarendon Press, Oxford

Doniger W, Smith B K (trans) 1991 The laws of Manu. Penguin, London

Ganguli K M (trans) 1993 The Mahabharata. Munshiram Manoharlal, New Delhi

Hamilton C (trans) 1963 The Hedaya or guide. Premier Book House, Lahore

Law B C (trans) (n.d.) Designation of human types (Puggala-Pannatti). Pali Text Society, London

Luther M (1964–68) Works, ed. Pelikan J, Lehmann H L. Concordia, Philadelphia

Miles M 1992 Concepts of mental handicap in Pakistan: toward cross-cultural and historical perspectives. Disability, Handicap and Society 7: 235–255

Miller T S 1985 The birth of the hospital in the Byzantine Empire. Johns Hopkins University Press, Baltimore

Orme N, Webster M 1995 The English hospital, 1070–1570. Yale University Press, New Haven

Preuss J 1978 Biblical and Talmudic medicine, trans. Rosner F. Sanhedrin Press, New York

Rangarajan L N ed. and trans. 1992 Kautilya. The Arthashastra. Penguin, New Delhi

Riviere M 1970 Rehabilitation codes, Classification of impairment of visual function, Final Report 1968. US National Institute of Neurological Diseases and Blindness

Smith V A 1920 Asoka, the Buddhist emperor of India, 3rd edn. Clarendon Press, Oxford

Söder M 1990 Prejudice or ambivalence? Attitudes toward persons with disabilities. Disability, Handicap and Society 5: 227–241

Tachibana S 1992 The ethics of Buddhism. Curzon, London

Unschuld P U 1979 The Chinese reception of Indian medicine in the first millennium AD. Bulletin of the History of Medicine 53: 329–345

Wertlieb EC 1988 Attitudes towards disabilities as found in the Talmud. Journal of Psychology and Judaism 12: 192–214

6

Poverty and health: an international overview

Rebecca Reviere
Kevin Hylton

One of the burdens of poverty is poor health. People who are poor have more disabilities, higher rates of both physical and mental illness, and lower life expectancies than those who are not poor. People with money have access to quality health care and rehabilitation services, live in cleaner, safer environments, and have healthier diets and more control over their lifestyles. These relationships know no boundaries; they hold across and within national borders. Individuals living in richer industrial countries are healthier than those living in poorer developing countries. Within countries, those with more financial resources are healthier than those with fewer financial resources. This is most grimly illustrated by mortality statistics; it is estimated that two-thirds of the variability in death rates across the globe relates to the distribution of income. Life expectancies range from 43 in Guinea to 76 in the USA, and infant mortality rates vary from 168 per 1000 live births in Mali to 5 in Japan (Baker & van der Gaag 1993).

The 20th century has been a time of vastly increasing wealth for much of the world; lifestyles and access to goods and services have improved dramatically. In addition, as sanitation, housing, and diet have improved, death rates from infectious diseases have dropped rapidly. However, this progress has not been equitable. Much of the fruit of global economic growth has gone to the already fortunate; in the past 30 years the rich have become richer and the poor more desperate (Durning 1990). Further, while health conditions have improved in developing countries, these improvements have slowed compared to pre-1960s (McEvers 1980). In a rich nation such as the USA, differences in life expectancy between those in higher and those in lower socioeconomic groups have also increased in recent years (Pappas et al 1993).

Ideally, a clearer understanding of these connections leads to concrete changes in government policy that can help raise living and health standards for those truly in need. More simply, it can sensitize therapists and health care providers to the complexities and consequences of economic inequality on health. This chapter first discusses the definition and distribution of poverty and issues of comparability to outline the general parameters of the issue. Next, it presents reviews of three major areas that reveal basic links between poverty and ill health, including disability: the health care system, the environment, and individual lifestyle.

DEFINING POVERTY

Poverty is the inability to achieve a minimum standard of living or purchase a minimum basket of the goods and services needed to satisfy basic needs (Meso-Lago 1992). It can be defined in either absolute or relative terms. Absolute poverty, a minimum standard required for physical survival (Blackburn 1991), is associated with inadequate shelter, under- or malnutrition, unemployment, illiteracy, and importantly here, high rates of morbidity, disability, and mortality. In 1988, the World Bank estimated that 900 million people lived in a state of absolute poverty, with the majority of these in Africa, Asia, and Latin America.

Absolute poverty is a more appropriate term for places where famine or war is an issue; it fits less well in countries where basic survival is not of such immediate concern. Relative poverty exists when people may be able to afford some basic necessities but are unable to maintain an average standard of living. It is relative to a middle- or upper-class standard and includes access to meeting both physical needs, such as food and shelter, and social needs, such as buying a child's birthday present (Blackburn 1991).

DISTRIBUTION OF POVERTY

During the 1980s, the proportion of the world's population living in poverty decreased, but the number of poor people increased due to rapid population growth. Rural dwellers (except in Latin America) and those living in urban slums are particularly likely to be impoverished (World Health Organization 1993). Importantly, families of people with disabilities suffer a disproportionate risk of poverty (Blackburn 1991). Specialized and expensive supplies, equipment, and treatment are often needed. At the same time, if the person who is disabled is an adult, earning capacity may be reduced.

Poverty is not randomly distributed through the population; it is strongly related to gender, age and race or ethnicity. Despite dramatic social changes in many parts of the world, women (regardless of race or ethnicity, urban or rural residency, age or labor force participation) are more likely than men to be poor (Parales & Young 1987) (Figs 6.1 and 6.2). The 'feminization of poverty' (Pearce 1978) is a result of inequalities in pay, responsibilities for children, and hiring discrimination. In India, for example, women work fewer hours for lower wages than men, and they have fewer employment opportunities (Rajuladevi 1992). In Russia, women earn about 71% of what men earn (World Bank 1995). In addition, in parts of the developing world, women have suffered economically from agricultural modernization. Women's access to

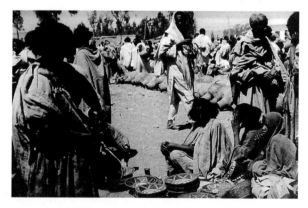

Fig. 6.1 Ethiopian women trying to sell their home-made baskets to earn some money. Photo courtesy: Ronnie Leavitt.

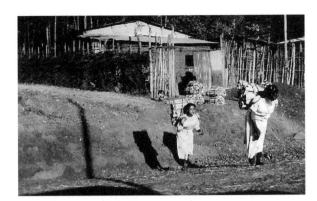

Fig. 6.2 Ethiopian women carrying firewood. Photo courtesy: Ronnie Leavitt.

land, technology, and employment has been replaced by private ownership and industry in which women have little part (Vlassoff 1994).

This culture of inequality has direct effects on women. In some countries, for example, women and female children are nutritionally deprived because cultural beliefs legitimize giving adult males the best and the most food (Giorgis 1981). Young adult women, those most likely to be pregnant or nursing, or caring for a child with a disability, often get the smallest and worst share in times of food shortage (Santow 1995). Further, girls (including those with a disability) are less likely to be treated by medical professionals than boys (Santow 1995, Zaidi 1988).

More than any other group, children are at risk of living in poverty. It is estimated that in the USA 20% of all children are growing up in relative poverty (Williams 1993) and that perhaps two-thirds of the world's absolute poor are under the age of 15 (Durning 1990). Because poverty is a family rather than an individual characteristic, children live in poverty because of the economic conditions of their parents. In India, 90% of street children have families but are on the streets due to poverty. The others have few family ties or have been abandoned and neglected (Nigam 1994). Children of female-headed households are generally the poorest of the poor. Many poor children who survive the deprivation of childhood are physically and/or mentally disabled as a result of chronic malnutrition, early disease, and poor health care.

In many countries, the likelihood of being poor is strongly related to race. In the USA, roughly 67% of African-American families and 46% of Hispanic families live in poverty, compared with only 31% of white families (Current Population Reports, 1992). Because other countries are more racially homogeneous, however, the issue is largely unexplored from a global perspective.

Because poverty is not equally distributed, the poor health outcomes associated with poverty are not equally distributed. Throughout the developing world, women, particularly pregnant women, and infants and children are at high risk for poor health (McEvers 1980). In countries where data are available, race has also consistently been related to health. For example, African-Americans have shorter life expectancies, higher rates of chronic disease and disability, and poorer perceived health than their white counterparts.

ISSUES OF COMPARABILITY

It is difficult to compare directly either the extent of poverty or the health status of different societies. Ideally, governments carry out surveys to determine the range of income within their countries and then set numerical standards defining poverty. This is expensive and time consuming and therefore rare in developing countries. Describing the health status of populations is equally problematic. Even among developed countries there is no single method for recording vital statistics, defining infant mortality, or maintaining disease registers, although there are attempts at standardization (see Percy & Muir 1989). Comparing rates of disability is particularly difficult due to:

1. disagreement on what disability means and on what states of health should be measured
2. differences in how disability surveys are conducted
3. the need to interpret disability statistics in a cultural and social context (Office of Technology Assessment 1993).

This lack of consensus can seriously undermine international comparisons of health (Office of Technology Assessment 1993). (See Ch. 10 for further discussion of the classification of impairments, disabilities, and handicaps, and Ch. 12 on the epidemiological considerations in the assessment of disability.) The difficulty of obtaining valid and reliable information on health indicators from developing countries further complicates the picture.

Comparability of terms and statistics is important to researchers, academics, and practitioners. Without agreed definitions, it is almost impossible to generalize treatment procedures, communicate among professionals and between therapist and client, and further the knowledge base. Problems of comparability mean that assumptions and practices that fit in one society may or may not fit into another. The following discussion of the links between poverty and health is therefore necessarily general.

HEALTH CARE DELIVERY SYSTEM

Patterns and timing of health care utilization are very different for the poor and nonpoor. For many poor people, health care is simply unavailable. It is estimated, for example, that in Africa nearly 250 million people (Clay 1994) and in Mexico 7 million are without health care (Sherraden & Wallace 1992).

Differences in availability result in part from funding priorities; in most countries, the government finances and manages health care services. Although urbanization is rapidly increasing among poorer countries, less than 35% of the population now lives in urban areas (United Nations 1989). At the same time, 70% of government health spending in these countries goes to urban hospitals, and these facilities are still often overcrowded and short of supplies and personnel (Baker & van der Gaag 1993). As a result, community health centers and rural clinics, where preventive care might be available to the poorest, are underfunded (Durning 1990). It is estimated that in Kenya, for example, 10% of physicians serve rural areas while over 70% have urban private practices; in Afghanistan

only about 18% of the rural population has a health facility within easy reach (Phillips 1990). In these and other countries, some private and public health care services are available from missionary hospitals, religious and charitable groups, as well as from nongovernmental organizations and international aid agencies (Wang'ombe 1995). But in times of political insecurity, the only health care available to a population may be through the military (Phillips 1990). In countries where physicians and clinics are rare, rehabilitation services may be non-existent (Leavitt 1992).

If health care facilities do exist, problems of utilization still may remain based on:

1. accessibility – can they be reached?
2. affordability – can medical care be paid for?
3. willingness – is there a desire to reach the facility?

Accessibility

In some countries, as little as 10% of the population has access to modern health services (World Bank 1995). Individuals living in slum settlements within or around cities have little access to urban hospitals, and the problem is critical for rural dwellers as well. Most studies have found that as distance to medical facilities increases, utilization decreases (Phillips 1990). This distance decay, as it is known, is complicated by other factors. Long distances, poor roads, unreliable public transportation, regional conflicts, and expense can all make travel to a medical facility a major undertaking (Fig. 6.3). Even in the USA, transportation can be a barrier to use of services for both rural and urban dwellers (Miller et al 1989).

These difficulties are exemplified with pregnant women. While good obstetrical care relates directly to maternal and infant health outcomes, the first time many women with no easy access to modern health care see a physician is when it is time to give birth (Spector 1984). This lack of access to prenatal care leads to more complicated deliveries and higher rates of prematurity (Puentes-Markides 1992), eventually leading to greater risk of disability.

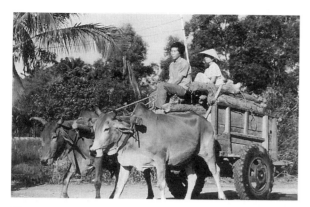

Fig. 6.3 Typical mode of travel in rural Vietnam. Photo courtesy: Ronnie Leavitt.

Affordability

Economic factors directly exclude many people from receiving quality health care. In some cases the poor can only secure services that are free and nearby (Green 1991). Many people see health care services, and especially something like rehabilitation where a positive cost–benefit ratio may be less obvious, as a luxury they simply cannot afford when faced with the more immediate needs for food, clothing, and shelter (Spector 1984).

Health insurance can lighten the economic load of illness and disability when it is an option. It affects the ability to pay for health services and, consequently, the types, quality, and intensity of care delivered (Office of Technology Assessment 1993). In Norway, Australia, Canada, the United Kingdom and other countries, public health insurance covers most of the population; on the other hand, 13% of the people in the USA have no health insurance (Office of Technology Assessment 1993). It has been hypothesized that financial considerations play a role in the rising mortality rates for African-Americans. For example, inability to pay for hypertension medication is associated with worsened blood pressure control (Shulman et al 1986). Even insurance, however, often does not pay for assistive devices and services important to individuals who are disabled. Countries with universal health insurance have reduced but not eliminated all inequalities of access, even as

they have lowered the chances of becoming impoverished as a result of disability-related needs (Starr 1993).

Willingness

Poor individuals may feel little motivation to use health care services. Having little success in other endeavors, they often feel hopeless in the face of negotiating an unfamiliar medical bureaucracy, and for good reason. The facilities available to the poor are often crowded public clinics where service is fragmented, providers discourteous and impersonal, and waits interminable. Studies from Uganda, Nigeria, and the Ivory Coast report that patients may spend between 2 and 8 hours waiting for a few minutes of attention (Baker & van der Gaag 1993). When attention is forthcoming, the interaction is often controlled by staff who directly and indirectly indicate status and knowledge differences. These encounters can leave the individual feeling out of place and unserved. The inhospitality of these settings, coupled with travel and financial problems, can discourage the poor from visiting medical offices early or often. As a result, treatment is often delayed until the problem is much more serious.

Economists use equity and efficiency as the yardsticks to measure the performance of health care systems (Starfield 1991). Clearly, modern health care facilities for the poor fall short by both standards. It is not surprising then that people turn first to family care and then alternative forms of health care. In some countries, individuals can buy 'controlled' Western pharmaceuticals in informal drug markets. These markets are appealing to the poor because, although unregulated, they are handy and cheap (Geest 1987). Other options are spiritual healers, herbalists, technical specialists such as bone setters, and traditional birth attendants who serve large numbers of the rural poor in the developing world. In Swaziland, for example, 85% of the population utilizes the services of traditional healers; in some rural settings traditional birth attendants may attend 90% of all births (Phillips 1990). The decision to seek care from a traditional healer is often prompted by financial considerations. Folk healers do not always ask for money; many will treat patients for other forms of payment or on credit (see Ch. 4).

THE ENVIRONMENTAL LINK BETWEEN POVERTY AND HEALTH

One benefit of adequate wealth is the ability to secure relatively safe, clean, and uncrowded surroundings. The poor are left crowded into areas considered uninhabitable by others. Their living conditions are often dangerous, dirty, and, for the city dwellers, densely populated. Rapid urbanization in many parts of the world has left neighborhoods heaped with garbage and solid waste. In addition, the poor must contend with improperly maintained buildings; for example, children fall from upper floor windows because there are no screens. People who live in neighborhoods in deteriorating central cities must deal with high levels of violence. Four aspects of the environment increase risks of disability for the poor: poor housing, unsafe water, inadequate waste disposal, and pollution.

Housing

Living conditions may influence health status, especially for the elderly and children who spend more time in the home (Office of

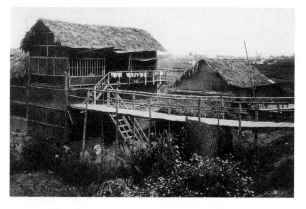

Fig. 6.4 A type of housing in Vietnam. Photo courtesy: Ronnie Leavitt.

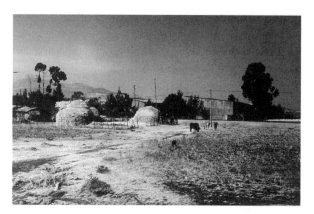

Fig. 6.5 Typical housing in Ethiopia. Photo courtesy: Ronnie Leavitt.

Technology Assessment 1993). It is estimated that around 1 billion people across the world live in grossly inadequate housing (Goldstein et al 1990). With household crowding, healthy individuals increase their risk of infection when they share space with the sick. Airborne diseases such as pneumonia, influenza, and tuberculosis account for roughly 20% of total mortality in some areas (McEvers 1980). In many countries women cook on open fires or old-fashioned stoves, increasing risks from fire and smoke-related respiratory problems. (Figs 6.4 and 6.5)

The poor in industrialized countries also have health problems associated with housing conditions. Inner-city residents are exposed to twice as many health hazards as people living in the suburbs; these include smog, polluted water, asbestos, lead paint, and the problems associated with crime and drugs. The effects of these assaults are enormous: inner-city residents suffer from hypertension, heart disease, chronic bronchitis, emphysema, sight and hearing impairments, and cancer at a rate of 50% higher than their wealthier neighbors (Watson 1993). The most extreme example is homelessness, with its multitude of associated health problems.

Water

For maximum well-being, a population must have access to a safe, clean and ample water supply for drinking, cooking, and bathing (Fig. 6.6).

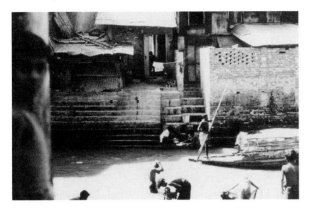

Fig. 6.6 Bangladesh – people using contaminated water for washing their bodies, clothes and dishes. Photo courtesy: Ronnie Leavitt.

Unsafe water can carry disease; clean water can prevent it (Phillips 1990). In industrialized countries, access to relatively pure water is generally a matter of turning on a tap. Developing countries, however, differ substantially in the availability of clean water, despite the fact that the 1980s was the International Drinking Water and Supply Decade. It is estimated, for example, that well over 200 million people in Africa are suffering from severe water shortages (Dasgupta et al 1994). An unsafe or inadequate water supply can result from drought, problems with pipes, pumps, and other equipment, pollution from human waste or toxic chemicals, unclean home storage, or regional conflicts that disrupt accessibility. In some rural areas, over half of the households lack ready access to safe water, and women spend hours carrying water. This system limits the amount available and can introduce impurities during handling. Whatever the reason, the health risks are clear: households without piped water have substantially higher rates of infant mortality and diarrheal disease (Zaidi 1988).

Waste disposal

The disposal of human waste is often a major problem in developing countries, especially in rural areas and urban slums, and is closely tied to the domestic water supply. When tap water is available, mothers are much more likely to dispose safely of their family's waste (Curtis et al 1995). Poor sanitation practices and the resulting soil and water contamination are responsible for diseases such as typhoid, cholera, enteritis, and dysentery that are among the major causes of infant and child mortality. In many countries the subject of human defecation is taboo, and misconceptions abound. For example many women believe that children's feces are 'harmless' (Elmendorf 1981) and act accordingly. Education, particularly for women, is crucial in eliminating dangerous beliefs. But even with knowledge, if working pipes and pumps are not available, inadequate sanitation and its related health problems will remain.

Pollution

The poor of the world are also at great risk from illness or disability related to pollution. For example, exposure to toxic chemicals can increase the risk of cancer or produce genetic damage (Vaughan 1993). While industrial pollution is evident across the globe, pollution disasters such as the chemical spill in Bhopal seem to be more frequent in poorer countries where regulations are less strict (Phillips 1990). On a daily basis, migrant workers absorb pesticides, and subsistence farmers eat food from tainted soil. Environmental justice movements in industrialized countries have highlighted the frequency with which toxic waste is dumped in poor neighborhoods. Recent studies in the USA have revealed that the poorer the neighborhood and the darker the skin of the residents, the more likely it is to be near a toxic waste dump. More than half of all African-Americans and Hispanic-Americans live in communities with at least one toxic waste dump (Durning 1990).

LIFESTYLE LINKS BETWEEN POVERTY AND HEALTH

Lifestyle is closely linked to income, education, and occupation. As a result, lifestyles of the poor are sometimes dramatically different from lifestyles of the rest of society, and researchers have increasingly looked to these differences to explain persistent differences in health.

Lifestyle factors have gained this attention for three main reasons. First, causes of mortality in much of the world have shifted from infectious diseases of childhood to chronic degenerative diseases of aging that are strongly influenced by behaviors over a person's lifetime. Second, some contemporary, infectious diseases, such as AIDS, clearly relate to individual behavior. Third, differences in rates of morbidity, mortality, and disability remain in countries with national health insurance for all residents.

One longitudinal study identified factors related to life expectancy and health; people reporting more of a number of practices were healthier and lived longer (Berkman & Breslow 1983). Lifestyle factors related to physical well-being include: not smoking cigarettes, not drinking excessive amounts of alcohol, eating a healthy diet, wearing seat belts, practicing safe sex, exercising regularly, engaging in preventive medical care, coping well with stress, and avoiding firearms. Interest in these factors is well-founded. As the Office of Technology Assessment (1993) reports:

- Cigarette smokers die at twice the rates of non-smokers through middle age, and nearly 20% of deaths in industrialized countries are attributable to the effects of smoking.
- Throughout the industrialized world, alcohol contributes to chronic diseases and to injuries that lead to disability and death. As many as one-half of all automobile crash fatalities are alcohol-related.
- In the USA automobile accidents are a major cause of death, yet it is estimated that up to one-half of these fatalities could be prevented with proper use of lap-shoulder belts.

Although evidence suggests that positive health behaviors are becoming more common across all economic groups, the poor of the industrialized world generally practice fewer of these good health habits than do the more affluent. For example, young men in the USA with the least education and income have relatively high risks of suffering injuries and death from violence (Singh & Yu 1996), and smoking is more common among poorer individuals, at least in the USA and UK (Feinstein 1993). The poor are also more likely to work in hazardous occupations.

Research on lifestyle is absent in societies where much of the population lives in absolute poverty. However, two of the more widely studied and relevant health practices are diet and preventive medical care.

Diet

The World Bank Food Council estimated that there were about 1 billion chronically hungry people in the mid-1980s. Poor nutrition increases vulnerability to viral, bacterial and parasitic infections (Zaidi 1988), and malnutrition and starvation are major causes of death for young children. Dietary deficiencies in young children can lead to a permanent reduction in brain cells and permanent stunting of the central nervous system (Bengtsson & Gunnarsson 1994), both of which are major causes of disability. Food supplies have improved for much of the world, as cereal grain production has hit record highs (World Health Organization 1993), but food does not reach all regions equally. Distribution problems brought on by military conflict have resulted in famine or near-famine for some parts of Africa. In addition, erosion and nutrient depletion of soil, flooding from deforestation, crop damage from pollution, and changing climates make providing food for a rapidly growing population more problematic (Brown & Young 1990). Malnutrition is clearly a problem of poverty, not of food.

Preventive medical care

Preventive health care can have a wide-ranging influence on the levels of disability and health of a population, but its role in developing countries (and some industrialized countries) is small (Baker & van der Gaag 1993). Moreover, individuals with inadequate food, water, and housing are unlikely to place a priority on even fairly simple preventive interventions. Nonetheless, measures such as childhood immunization and prenatal care are both inexpensive and effective. It is estimated, for example, that the lives of roughly 4 million children were saved in the 1980s by large-scale immunization projects (Phillips 1990). Increasing vaccination rates for children has become an important goal for international health agencies, which often view it as a proxy for well-child care in general (Miller 1993, Office of Technology Assessment 1993). Regional variations in immunization rates, especially urban and rural differences, are large. Differences in immunization rates exist even among industrialized nations: the USA, for example, lags behind other industrialized countries by almost 35% (Miller 1993).

IMPLICATIONS

Words and numbers have little use for the poor unless the meanings behind them can be understood and palliative action taken. There are efforts to improve the health of the citizens of the world. For example, in 1978, the World Health Organization and United Nations Children's Fund (UNICEF) announced a plan, Health for All by the Year 2000, to reduce inequities in health and health care throughout the world (World Health Organization 1993). The importance of this platform may lie more in its idealism than its reality. Poverty causes disease, disability, and death because the poor lack basic resources – knowledge, power, money, and social connections – to avoid risks and to reduce the impact of disorders when they occur. Because these resources connect so broadly to all aspects of life, social inequalities translate into health inequality (Link & Phelan 1996). If they want health for all their citizens, governments must act to reduce rates of poverty.

Even governments unwilling to redistribute wealth can make significant progress in improving health. Differences in availability, accessibility, and affordability result in a dual-system of health care for much of the world. Private well-stocked clinics and well-trained staff and doctors exist for middle- and upper-income groups, while public hospitals, clinics, and emergency rooms exist for the poor (Dutton 1978). But inequality does not have to be the case. When national governments give priority to health, good care is widely available. Costa Rica, for example, has low per-capita income but reliable health care systems for most of its citizens.

In addition, program changes can make a difference. For example, education is strongly linked with good health and healthy lifestyles. Women are the primary health care providers for a family, and their knowledge often translates directly into more healthy behaviors for others, particularly their children. Research in Tanzania has shown that children of mothers with no education have half the chance of survival of children of mothers with 5 or more years of school (Giorgis 1981). A healthy population is also dependent on its natural resources. Programs that promote clean environments, sustainable development, and family planning are important, though more indirect, routes to healthier populations.

Further, targeting the most vulnerable groups and most impoverished areas could funnel services and supplies to those most in need (Meso-Lago 1992). Targeting requires good research and foresight. The aging of the population, for example, will require that new approaches to alleviate disease and disability be available. In addition, actively soliciting community involvement in all aspects of health care and development could insure that new ideas and practices are widely circulated and accepted (Levin 1992). Under-utilization of facilities can be linked to decreased knowledge, comfort, and accessibility, but often providing these is not enough to entice individuals to take advantage of services. The lessons from community based rehabilitation efforts suggest that full and democratic grassroots involvement and thorough integration of indigenous health workers can facilitate community participation in both planning and implementation of health projects (Lysack 1995). Only when projects and personnel are sensitive to local norms and values will they truly be accepted.

The effects of poverty are far reaching, and one main purpose of this chapter is to illustrate how thoroughly poverty impacts the health of the poor. Much of the world's population is poor, as are many persons with disabilities. One critical issue for rehabilitation professionals involves recognizing that practices and attitudes that work well with middle- and upper-class clients may not work well for poor clients who lack basic resources. In addition, therapists must see beyond the individual client to the larger social and cultural context from which that person comes. Full integration into society includes getting a job, going to school, and receiving medical and rehabilitation interventions when needed. These activities are simply more difficult for poor persons. Finally, poverty is not an individual problem, it is a global problem, and while it exists everyone is impoverished.

REFERENCES

Baker J L, van der Gaag J 1993 Equity in health care and health care financing: evidence from five developing countries. In: Doorslaer E D, Wagstaff A, Rutten F (ed) Equity in the finance and delivery of health care. Oxford University Press, Oxford, pp. 356–394

Bengtsson T, Gunnarsson C 1994 Population, development, and institutional change: summary and analysis. In: Lindahl-Kiessling K, Landberg H (eds) Population, economic development, and the environment. Oxford University Press, Oxford, pp 1–23

Berkman L, Breslow L 1983 Health and ways of living: the Alameda County study. Oxford University Press, Fairlawn, N J

Blackburn C 1991 Poverty and health: working with families. Open University Press, Philadelphia

Brown L R, Young J E 1990 Feeding the world in the nineties. In: Brown L, Durning A, Flavin C et al (eds) State of the World 1990. W W Norton, New York, pp. 59–78

Clay R 1994 A continent in chaos: Africa's environmental issues. Environmental Health Perspectives 102(12): 1018–1023

Current Population Reports 1992 Poverty in the United States: 1992. Consumer Income Series P-60, No. 185. Bureau of the Census, Washington, DC

Curtis V, Kanki B, Mertens T, Traore' E, Diallo I, Tall F, Cousens S 1995 Potties, pots and pipes: explaining hygiene behavior in Burkina Faso. Social Science and Medicine 41(3): 383–393

Dasgupta P, Folke C, Mäler K G 1994 The environmental resource base and human welfare. In: Lindahl-Kiessling K, Landberg H (eds) Population, economic development, and the environment. Oxford University Press, New York, pp. 25–50

Durning A B 1990 Ending poverty. In: Brown L, Durning A, Flavin C et al (eds) State of the World 1990. W W Norton, New York, pp. 135–153

Dutton D B 1978 Explaining the low use of health services by the poor: costs, attitudes, or delivery systems. American Sociological Review 43: 348–368

Elmendorf M L 1981 Women, water, and waste: beyond access. In: Blair P W (ed) Health needs of the world's poor women. Equity Policy Center, Washington, DC, pp. 93–95

Feinstein J S 1993 The relationship between socioeconomic status and health: a review of the literature. Milbank Quarterly 71(2): 279–322

Geest S 1987 Self-care and the informal sale of drugs in south Cameroon. Social Science and Medicine 25(3): 293–305

Giorgis B W 1981 Africa: health requires advancement for women. In: Blair P W (ed) Health needs of the world's poor women. Equity Policy Center, Washington, DC, p. 15

Goldstein G, Novick R, Schaefer M 1990 Housing, health, and well-being: an international perspective. Journal of Sociology and Social Welfare 17(1): 161–181

Green R H 1991 Politics and poverty: health for all in 2000 in the Third World? Social Science and Medicine 32(7): 745–755

Leavitt R L 1992 Disability and rehabilitation in rural Jamaica: an ethnographic study. Associated University Press, Cranbury, NJ

Levin L S 1992 Listen to the community. World Health May–June: 10–11

Link B G, Phelan J C 1996 Editorial. Understanding sociodemographic differences in health – the role of fundamental social causes. American Journal of Public Health 86(4): 471–473

Lysack C L 1995 Community participation and community-based rehabilitation: an Indonesian case study. Occupational Therapy International 2: 149–165

McEvers N C 1980 Health and the assault on poverty in low income countries. Social Science and Medicine 14C: 41–57

Meso-Lago C 1992 Health care for the poor in Latin America and the Caribbean. Scientific Publication No. 539. Pan American Health Organization and Inter-American Foundation, Washington, DC

Miller C A 1993 Making a difference in the health of children. In: Rogers D E, Ginzberg E (eds) Medical care and the health of the poor. Westview Press, Boulder, pp. 91–106

Miller C L, Margolis L H, Schwethelm B, Smith S 1989 Barriers to implementation of a prenatal care program for low income women. American Journal of Public Health 79(1): 62–64

Nigam S 1994 Street children of India. Journal of Health Management 7(1): 63–67

Office of Technology Assessment 1993 International health statistics: what the numbers mean for the United States. OTA-BP-H-116. US Government Printing Office, Washington, DC

Pappas G, Queen S, Hadden W, Fisher G 1993 The increasing disparity in mortality between socioeconomic groups in the United States, 1960 and 1986. New England Journal of Medicine 319(2): 103–109

Parales C A, Young L S 1987 Women, health, and poverty. Women and Health 12(3–4): 259

Pearce D 1978 The feminization of poverty: women, work, and welfare. Urban and Social Change Review 11(1/2): 28–36

Percy C, Muir C 1989 The international comparability of cancer mortality data. American Journal of Epidemiology 129(5): 934–946

Phillips D R 1990 Health and health care in the Third World. John Wiley, New York

Puentes-Markides C 1992 Women and access to health care. Social Science and Medicine 35(12): 619–626

Rajuladevi A K 1992 How poor are women in rural India? Asia-Pacific Journal of Rural Development 2(1): 1–34

Santow G 1995 Social roles and physical health: the case of female disadvantage in poor countries. Social Science and Medicine 40(2): 147–161

Sherraden M S, Wallace S P 1992 Innovation in primary care: community health services in Mexico and the United States. Social Science and Medicine 35(12): 1433–1443

Shulman N B, Martinez B, Brogan D, Carr A A, Miles C G 1986 Financial cost as an obstacle to hypertension therapy. American Journal of Public Health 76(9): 1105–1107

Singh G K, Yu S M 1996 Trends and differentials in adolescent and young adult mortality in the United States, 1950–1993. American Journal of Public Health 86(4): 560–564

Spector R 1984 Ethnicity and health: a study of health care beliefs and practices. Urban and Social Change Review 12(2): 34–37

Starfield B 1991 Primary care and health: a cross-national comparison. Journal of the American Medical Association 266(16): 2268–2271

Starr P 1993 The politics of health care inequalities. In: Rogers D E, Ginzberg E (eds) Medical care and the health of the poor: Westview Press, Boulder, pp. 21–32

United Nations 1989 World population reports 1988, United Nations, New York

Vaughan E 1993 Individual and cultural differences in adaptation to environmental risks. American Psychologist 48: 673–680

Vlassoff C 1994 From rags to riches: the impact of rural development on women's status in an Indian village. World Development 22(5): 707–719

Wang'ombe J 1995 Public health of cities in developing countries. Social Science and Medicine 41(6): 857–862

Watson S D 1993 Health care in the inner city: asking the right question. Paper presented at the symposium, The Urban Crisis: The Kerner Commission Report Revisited.

Williams D 1993 Barriers to achieving health. Child and Adolescent Social Work Journal 10(5): 355–363

World Bank 1995 Toward gender equality: the role of public policy. World Bank, Washington, DC

World Health Organization 1993 Implementation of the global strategy for Health for All by the Year 2000. Eighth report on the world health situation. World Health Organization, Geneva

Zaidi S A 1988 Poverty and disease: need for structural change. Social Science and Medicine 27(2): 119–127

7

Understanding racial prejudice, discrimination and racism and their influence on health care delivery

Joseph W. Smey

Alice had never seen such a strange croquet-ground. It was covered with ridges and furrows, the balls were live hedgehogs, the mallets were live flamingoes, and soldiers bent over to make the wickets.

In this well known story from Lewis Carroll's *Alice in Wonderland*, Alice's flamingo mallet would twist its head around and look up at her whenever she wanted to strike her hedgehog ball with it. Her hedgehog ball ran away, everyone played at once without waiting their turn, and the soldiers serving as arches walked off to other parts of the ground. The only thing that seemed clear to Alice was that the game was hardly worth finishing; the Queen of Hearts would always win.

Alice's frustrations help us to understand what people of color, individuals of African/Black, Asian, Hispanic/Latino or Native American ancestry, experience as they struggle to achieve equity within societies with long histories of racial prejudice and discrimination. The USA is a primary example, but this same analogy holds true for the UK, Brazil, South Africa, Germany, and other nations that have struggled with race relations. While the USA was built upon the premise that all individuals are created equal, a great many people argue that those in control of the nation's institutions (i.e. government, industry, education, religious and civic groups) are treated more equally than others. As with Alice and her croquet match, people of color often report feeling helpless as they play by someone else's rules. They frequently feel confused and often betrayed as they witness inconsistencies and contradictions between what people from the white majority say and do. While some claim that the USA is now largely a color-blind society, many people of color see the rules continuously changing to benefit those in power, leaving people of color the losers in the game of life (Whitaker 1993).

INTRODUCTION

This chapter explores issues pertaining to race, race relations, health care equity, and the nature of attitudes and beliefs and their relationships with human behavior. It describes prejudice and discusses its expressions and consequences. It delineates the need for rehabilitation professionals to learn more about their own prejudices and possible manifestations of these prejudices; and it suggests strategies that can lead to better health and rehabilitation care for all members of society.

The effectiveness of patient care depends a great deal upon the ability of health care practitioners to serve as a primary source of motivation and to build positive helping relationships with their patients. Furthermore, the health care delivery system is changing to rely more on horizontal rather than vertical divisions of labor, and it is adopting the interdisciplinary team as a common model of care. With these changes, skills such as communication, team interaction, and an ability to build trust and rapport with coworkers also become increasingly critical to the delivery of effective health care. Understanding one's own self and the perceptions others have of you is an essential step toward developing effective interpersonal relations with patients and an ability to work successfully with coworkers. Critical to this self-understanding is taking time to examine one's own true attitudes and beliefs, particularly as they relate to individuals from different racial and ethnic groups.

DEMOGRAPHIC CHANGES AROUND THE GLOBE

Almost a third of the population of the USA traces its ancestry directly to Europe and to white men, women, and children who came through Ellis Island between 1892 and 1954. However, today the complexion of the USA is changing, making improved race relations more important. More than 80% of the immigrants in the 1980s and 1990s trace their ancestry from Central and South America and from Asia. Today, one out of every four people in the USA is a person of color. By the year 2010, given current birth rates and immigration projections, the Asian population will increase 22%, the Latino population 21%, and the African-American population almost 12%. Over this same period, the white population is expected to increase just over 2%. It is estimated that the population of people of color in the USA will double by 2020 while the white population will not increase at all. Whites will be in the minority by the year 2050 (Henry 1990, Kinney 1990, Oxford 1990).

The trend is the same around the globe. White people in 1900 represented approximately 30% of the total population worldwide. This steadily shrinking number is projected to be 9% by the year 2010. These changes, which are quite significant, are well within the lifetime of most people alive today (Henry 1990, Hodgkinson 1985, Oxford 1990). They are also occurring at a time when national boundaries are decreasing in significance and the notion of the world as a global village is becoming a reality.

One does not need to be a fortune teller to recognize the implications for the rehabilitation professions. However, while these great demographic changes are occurring worldwide, diversity in the health professions remains largely unchanged. As a result, the individuals who compose the rehabilitation professions less and less reflect the diversity of the communities they serve. In the USA, a largely white population of professionals still takes responsibility for the health and well-being of all segments of society. With limited data available through licensure and professional association membership, it appears that across the USA about 7.7% of occupational therapists, 6.2% of physical therapists and 7% of speech-language pathologists are people of color (Walker & Brand 1993, American Speech-

Language-Hearing Association 1996). People of color are under-represented across all the health professions. Increasing diversity within the health care professions is one part of the solution to improving health care services to the under-served (Schroeder 1996).

RACIAL INEQUITY IN THE USA

Soon the total number of individuals in the USA who identify themselves as African American, Latino, Asian American, or Native American will equal those who are white, but other vital statistics relating to race are changing less rapidly. Recent Bureau of Census reports dealing with health, education, and employment reveal a dramatic level of inequity for people of color in the USA. Life expectancy is shorter, and infant mortality for blacks is more than twice that of whites. Mortality rates due to heart disease for blacks are nearly twice that of whites, those due to cancer are 34% higher, for chronic liver disease and cirrhosis 70% higher, and for homicide they are more than four times greater than for whites (USDHHS 1986, Council on Interracial Books for Children 1982, Coughlin 1988, Kington & Smith 1997). Black women are 13 times more likely to have AIDS than are white women and black men 4 times more likely than white men. AIDS contracted through intravenous drug use in 1996 was 17 times more common among black women than white women and 14 times more common among black men than white men (CDCP 1996; Leland 1996).

In the past, the 'all American' child came from an intact middle-class family unit; today's reality for people of color is dramatically different. While only 15.2% of white households are run by single parents, 48.8% of African-American and 47.9% of Latino households have only one parent present. In 1988, 55% of all births to black women were to teenagers. The percentage of Latino (23%) and Native-American children (25%) living below the poverty line is more than twice as great as that for white children (9%). The percentage of African-American children living below the poverty line (31%) is more than three times that for white children (Hodgkinson 1985, NOW 1984, Morganthau et al 1992, USDHHS 1986).

Although 76% of whites graduate from high school, only 71% of African Americans and 63% of Latinos graduate (Green 1989). While 20.5% of all white adults 25 years and over complete 4 or more years of college, only 10.7% of African-Americans and 8.6% of Latinos of comparable age complete 4 or more years (Record 1988, Rothman 1988).

African Americans are twice as likely to be victims of robbery, car theft, and aggravated assault. Homicide is the leading cause of death among African-American males between the ages of 15 and 34 years. Nearly half of all prison inmates in America are black, and there are currently more black men in prison than in college (Council on Interracial Books for Children 1982, Coughlin 1988, Morganthau et al 1992).

An increasing number of upwardly mobile people of color have been able to move into the middle class. However, the fact remains that equity does not exist for all Americans. The data above clearly illustrate that, for millions, the land of opportunity has been elusive. For people of color, social reality has been in stark contrast to America's social ideology. The cost to society will be astronomical should the gap in health care, education and income in the USA persist as the demographics continue to change.

DOES COLOR MAKE A DIFFERENCE?

The American Medical Association's board of trustees authorized a search of the literature on racial and ethnic disparity in health care in the decade from 1984 to 1994, restricting the study to articles, commentaries, and letters in the *New England Journal of Medicine* and *Journal of the American Medical Association* (AMA 1995). The review consistently found that the poor and African Americans received care that differed from that of whites. African Americans were less likely to receive hip and knee joint replacements, have cardiac surgery for heart disease, or obtain organ transplants and sophisticated testing procedure but were more likely to undergo hysterectomies and amputations. Gornick et al (1996) studied 26 million Medicare beneficiaries in 1993 and determined that both race and income have effects but that race was the overriding determinant of disparities in the level of health care received. Broad and systematic evidence indicated that racial disparity existed for people of color in health care (Geiger 1996, Schroeder 1996).

It has been argued that no relationship exists between the kind of health care people receive and the race of their care givers, but two recent studies would disagree. Komaromy et al (1996) found that California communities with high proportions of African-American and Latino residents were far more likely to have a shortage of physicians, independent of the population of the community, and that African-American physicians were more likely to treat African-American patients and Latino physicians Latino patients. A similar nationwide study by Cantor et al (1996), conducted in 1987 and 1991, found that physicians who were people of color were much more likely than others to serve other people of color and the poor.

Although race, independent of economic status and health insurance, may be the single overriding variable accounting for the differences in the health care people receive, no evidence indicates the precise cause of this inequity. The problem is likely to be the interactions of numerous confounding variables, including patient preferences, lack of communication, unspecified cultural differences, and racial prejudices. As Escarce et al (1993) note, 'Race . . . may influence physicians' clinical decisions in ways that physicians do not even recognize but that are not justified by medical need.' That is, racial prejudice may be a factor, although thoughts and resultant actions are more likely to be subconscious and not overt.

Behavior in the clinical setting

This author studied relationships between the racial attitudes and behavior of white physical therapy students during a simulated clinical intervention similar to those commonly used to prepare students in the rehabilitation professions to interact with actual patients (Smey 1983). A series of tests to measure racial prejudice was administered to participants prior to the simulations, which all utilized the same African-American client. Videotape records of the simulations were analyzed to judge the use of both verbal and nonverbal interpersonal skills. Observations from this research suggested that relationships did exist between the attitudes of students and their behavior during a health care intervention with an African-American patient. Surprisingly, this study demonstrated that the more prejudiced subjects used a greater percentage of verbal communications skills that are known to facilitate trust and rapport than did their less prejudiced counterparts. However, the results were the opposite when it came to nonverbal communication. The more prejudiced subjects maintained greater distance between themselves and the client than did their less prejudiced counterparts, moving toward the client less often and away more often. Movement closer to the client conveys a feeling of interest, trust, and love; movement away conveys lack of interest and concern (D'Augelli et al 1981).

Katz & Benjamin (1960) also found that in biracial situations prejudiced whites tended to demonstrate stronger communication skills, as judged by their accepting more suggestions from African Americans, and showed trends toward greater compliance on tasks requiring group decisions. They concluded that this suggests 'the presence of internal controls so powerful as to produce behavior opposite their hostile impulses.' A similar conclusion can be drawn from the verbal communication exhibited by the more prejudiced subjects participating in the simulated clinical interventions described above. The exact effect of the inconsistencies between the positive verbal and negative nonverbal communication cues on the African-American client who participated in the stimulations was never determined. Perhaps the conflicting messages, if telegraphed to the client, would be perceived as discriminatory and logically would have serious implications in the therapist–client relationship. In the context of the review conducted by the American Medical Association, which reveals that race by itself is an important variable in the health care one receives, it is clear that more work needs to be done to understand better the relationships between the racial attitudes of providers and the health care they deliver.

Exploring the role of racial prejudice in the clinical teaching environment, Haskins et al (1997) looked at physical therapy practitioners. The physical therapists (73 white, three African-American, and seven Latino) serving as subjects all read an identical case study about a patient; they were then asked to rate one of four video-taped presentations by physical therapy students on two factors: clarity of presentation and overall rating. The students selected for videotaping (one white, one Latino, one Asian, and one African-American) all read the exact same case study about a patient. The white, Latino, and Asian students received higher ratings by their physical therapy evaluators than did the African-American student on clarity of presentation and overall rating. Written comments by the evaluators were organized into two groups: those pertaining to the students' personal style and those pertaining to the content of the students' presentation. The African-American student received the highest number of negative comments about her personal style and the lowest number of negative comments about the content of her presentation. The white student received the highest number of negative comments about the content of her presentation and the lowest number of negative comments about her personal style. Haskins et al (1997) concluded that racial or ethnic bias may influence the opinions of physical therapy practitioners.

These findings were consistent with those found by Powell & Collier (1990), which discovered bias in the oral performance scoring of Latino, Asian, and African-American college students as compared to white students. Powell & Collier concluded that the white students' mainstream speaking style caused them to be perceived as more competent and that the non-white students were negatively criticized because of their accents or communication styles. Similarly, Haskins et al (1997) thought that the African-American student's lower ratings might be due to her accent and the negative stereotypes associated with that style of speech.

RACIAL PREJUDICE AND RACISM DEFINED

Prejudice stems from the Latin *praejudicium*, which means pre-judge or form an opinion without sufficient knowledge or experience. As defined by Allport (1954), racial prejudice is a negative attitude toward people solely on the basis of skin color. It is thought to be learned from family and cultural influences. By the age of 4, according to Allport (1954), children establish a sense of white superiority as they select, accentuate, and interpret sensory data from their experiences with parents, schools, and religious and social organizations (Allport 1954). Whites with racial prejudice have unfavorable attitudes and negative beliefs toward people of color that are not founded upon actual experience but rather upon notions that are shared and transmitted within a particular society. These negative feelings and thoughts are generalized by one's racial identity, as determined principally by skin color, the shape of one's nose, and the features of one's hair (Allport 1979, Allport & Kramer 1946, McDonald 1970).

The practice of making sweeping generalizations about members of outside groups without regard to individual differences is known as stereotyping. Stereotyping goes hand-in-hand with poor race relations and is symptomatic of the closed and rigid thinking associated with racial prejudice. According to Allport & Katz (1931), with stereotyping we respond to individuals as a personification of the symbols we have attached to them as a result of fixed values, attitudes, and beliefs. These stereotypes are sustained, according to Allport (1954), by selective perception and selective forgetting. Common stereotypes in the USA ascribed to Asians are that they are smart and work hard, to African-Americans that they are very good at sports and dancing, and to Latinos that they are good lovers.

Kramer (1949) and Katz & Stotland (1959), Rokeach (1968) and Secord & Blackman (1964) defined different levels of racial prejudice. These authors, using what Kramer (1949) called an 'age-old trichotomy,' described prejudice in terms of three distinct levels: cognitive, emotional, and conative. Allport's definition cited above contains the elements that are essential to racial prejudice and give this particular attitude its three-dimensional character:

1. Reference is made to an unfounded judgement. This is the 'cognitive' dimension and deals with thought processes that incorporate unsubstantiated information to develop perceptions, beliefs, and expectations with regard to particular individuals and groups. The styles of thinking associated with racial prejudice are 'close mindedness' and inflexibility. Opinion is unlikely to change in the face of data to the contrary.

2. The often strong feelings associated with racial prejudice give this attitude its 'emotional' dimension. These feelings stem from a variety of early life experiences involving family and friends and the way people of color are portrayed through such communication vehicles as the news media, television, movies, and advertising. This emotional element includes a general unfriendliness and various associated feelings that give this attitude a strong affective coloring.

3. The 'conative' dimension includes a desire or an impulse on the part of an individual for action involving the stimulus object, regardless of whether the impulse is carried out. This component is not an action or behavior but instead an attitude suggesting how one might act in certain situations involving a racial group or 'typical' individuals belonging to that group (Harding et al 1969).

The complex nature of racial prejudice

The most commonly noted characteristic of racial prejudice is its extreme complexity (Adorno et al 1950, Kramer 1949). Historians insist that racial prejudice in the USA has resulted from, among other factors, the failure of society to understand the beginnings of slavery, resistance of whites to racial integration, and class differences that formed along racial lines. Sociologists claim that the social structure itself and cultural patterns cause racial prejudice, while psychologists look toward personality characteristics and the inability of people to recognize individuals for what they are. Regardless of the approach, research into racial prejudice has been troubled by the serious failure to thoroughly consider the interrelations of the dimensions of racial prejudice and the relationships of this attitude to racial discrimination and other associated behaviors (Ashmore and DelBoca 1976, Brighman et al 1976, Ehrlich 1973, Rokeach 1968).

Adorno et al (1950), nearly a half century ago, portrayed the structure of an individual's ideology as a series of levels: 'What the individual consistently says in public, what he says when he feels safe from criticism, what he thinks but will not admit to himself, what he is disposed to think or to do when he feels safe from criticism, what he is disposed to think or to do when various kinds of appeals are made to him' (Adorno et al 1950, p. 4). These complex levels constitute one personality structure which may not be totally integrated but may contain many contradictions and inconsistencies. These contradictions and inconsistencies in large part result from the interactions of this powerful attitude with other critical intrinsic and extrinsic factors associated with an individual, such as culture, language, social class, education, and the economic and political environment. Although nearly 50 years have passed since Adorno et al (1950), a full and complete understanding of this very complex attitude still eludes historians, sociologists, and psychologists.

Understanding racial prejudice, discrimination and racism

Like all attitudes, racial prejudice cannot be observed directly; it can only be inferred from what people say and do regarding certain individuals or groups in society. Action that is prejudicial and directed categorically rather than individually is defined as discrimination (Webster's Ninth New Collegiate Dictionary 1988, p. 362). Discrimination stemming from racial prejudice is called racial discrimination, and one particularly oppressive type of racial discrimination is called racism. Racism involves the use of power or influence (economic, political, emotional) differentially to the advantage of one racial group and the disadvantage of another. Racism is defined by James Jones (1972, 1981, 1986, 1988) as 'the exercise of power against a racial group defined as inferior . . . with the intentional or unintentional support of the entire culture' (Jones 1981, p. 28).

The term racism is used to describe behavior that can result from the interaction of racial prejudice with key personal variables such as authority, status, and control. It has existed for centuries and is thought to have had a profound sociological and psychological effect on life around the globe. Conscious or unconscious, racism is behavior that is the consequence of the interaction of racial prejudice with power and is characterized by systematic discrimination by members of one group in an effort to maintain their power and influence over others in society.

The PDI model

Because of the complex nature of racial prejudice, many theoretical problems remain unresolved. More than a half century of research on race relations and prejudice has not produced a theory capable of unifying the literature in this area. However, one particular model of 'personal identity' advanced by scholars in the counseling profession has considerable utility for those struggling to understand racial prejudice. The Personal Dimensions Inventory (PDI), developed by Arredondo et al (1996), sheds light on how a single attitude – racial prejudice – can appear so complex. It does so by placing race in the context of other variables that contribute to individual differences and shared identity. Arredondo et al (1996) have used the PDI to define competencies required of those in the counseling professions relating to cultural, ethnic, and racial differences. By explaining the interaction of multi-cultural group identity and other dimensions of human diversity, the PDI provides direction for all those seeking to improve their interpersonal effectiveness in today's multi-cultural society.

The PDI model suggests that race, along with the other important variables that contribute to personal identity, can be categorized in three dimensions:

- The A dimension includes race along with age, culture, ethnicity, gender, language, physical disability, sexual orientation, social class and other variables. Like race, each of these factors is largely a characteristic that one is born with or grows into. These characteristics are fixed and quite visible differences that engender stereotyping and labeling as a result of the lack of cultural awareness.
- The C dimension, on the other hand, encompasses historical moments or eras that profoundly influence society. These are events over which one has little control: economic depressions, armed conflict, or political swings for example. The C dimension places individuals in context, grounded in historical, political, sociocultural, and economic events. According to Arredondo et al (1996), the C dimension suggests that there are many factors that surround us and over which we have no control, but which nevertheless affect us.
- A number of qualities over which one may have some influence (for example educational background, geographic location, income, marital status, religion, work experience, citizenship status, military experience, and recreational interests) are part of the B dimension. This B dimension is included last because it theoretically represents the 'consequences' of the interaction of the A and C dimensions. Historical,

political, sociocultural, and economic events in the C dimension, together with race, age, culture, ethnicity, gender, language, and physical disability from the A dimension, intersect and enhance or limit what happens to the individual along the B dimension. Despite the myth of self-control and self-reliance, considering the interaction effect of the A and C dimensions gives a better appreciation that what people become is not totally within their control.

The three dimensions of the PDI model illustrate the complexities of humanity. The model helps place race in a broader and more complete framework and makes it easier to appreciate why the stereotypical labels of identity are limiting and counterproductive. For the rehabilitation professions, the PDI model provides direction for those who wish a fuller understanding of themselves, their coworkers, and patients and who desire to become more culturally competent health care providers.

STRATEGIES FOR CHANGE

Over the last decade there has been considerable interest and much controversy over initiatives to establish a more culturally diverse yet integrated society. While conservative and liberal thinkers differ on the need to promote diversity, leaders in business, industry, and government, as well as civic and volunteer organizations, have taken action. They have implemented programs to increase understanding and promote positive relations among employees and customers with different backgrounds. Cross-cultural training has now taken its place as an essential component of human resource management as organizations compete in an ever more diverse society. To remain competitive in the health care marketplace and to foster improved patient care, health care administrators have increasingly begun to recognize the critical value of maintaining an appropriate mix of employees with the prerequisite knowledge, skill, and cultural adaptability to function in today's changing society.

In the USA, Western Europe, and Australia, where whites control the wealth and political power, there is a disproportionally large number of whites in health care. Given the evolution and the status the rehabilitation professions enjoy, it is not surprising that these practitioners are educated principally through traditional educational models that espouse white middle class values and beliefs. Considering the communities in which they were raised, the educational, public, and professional institutions in which they have participated, and their current neighborhoods and circles of friends, it is safe to assume that most white rehabilitation professionals have very little exposure to the needs and difficulties of people of color. It is also safe to conclude that, no matter how well intentioned these individuals are, most have been inculturated in a racist society, and none are exempt from racial prejudice. This attitude may not be conscious, yet research has shown that it differentially affects the way whites interact in a multi-cultural environment.

Individuals and organizations have taken many approaches to increase cultural awareness and sensitivity. Judging from these prejudice-prevention, racism awareness, and work-team development interventions, successful initiatives are multi-faceted and ongoing. Bruhn (1996), Nemetz & Christensen (1996), and Pedersen & Pedersen (1989) have all proposed strategies directed at preventing prejudice and improving attitudes and behaviors of whites toward people of color.

Common themes

A review of the various interventions that claim success include several commonalities transcending the various models. While there are unique aspects to each approach, the following six themes appear critical:

1. *Believing in the need for change.* No element is more important than this first one – establishing a felt need for change. Change is very difficult, especially when it involves longstanding attitudes and behaviors. While many may believe that conditions have

dramatically improved for people of color, the statistics do not concur. A thorough exploration of objective facts and figures pertaining to the health, education, housing, economics, and social status of people of color serves to create the necessary internal disequilibrium required for change.

2. *Understanding the dynamics of racial prejudice and racism.* Interventions linked directly to the dynamics of racial prejudice are effective in reducing this attitude (Crawford 1974, Goldberg 1956, Carlson 1956). Not until the origin and nature of racial prejudice are understood can meaningful change occur. Manifestation of the cognitive and emotional aspects of this attitude must be explored as should relationships of racial prejudice and racism.

3. *Embracing diversity and cultural differences.* Progress depends to a large extent upon one's ability to recognize ethnocentrism as a force that narrows viewpoints and limits perspective. Emphasis should be placed on learning as much as possible about cultural differences. The goal is to begin to accept and embrace differences rather than expect that people of color should assimilate into the dominant white society.

4. *Experiencing self-assessment and self-insight.* Individuals should be stimulated to undergo introspective examination of personal value systems relating to people of color. A high level of self-involvement is necessary for this to be effective. Individuals must also seek to recognize personal values and behaviors that may clash with the values of various cultural groups and to understand the potential cultural biases that could affect behavior.

5. *Remaining open and striving for feedback.* There are a multitude of views on racial prejudice, racism, and preferential politics and practices targeting the disparity that exists for people of color. It is critical to anticipate that as individuals take on a new set of values and beliefs concerning a multi-cultural society, they will face feelings of discomfort and anger. The importance of remaining open and continuing to learn from individuals with differing viewpoints must be emphasized. As people attempt to integrate aspects of their new found sensitivity and awareness with the harsh realities of the real world they must be ready to receive feedback from friends and foes alike. Progress will rarely be easy.

6. *Pursuing ongoing change.* Change is a long and arduous process. Racial awareness is a life-developmental process, and success will require many years of hard work, considerable frustration, and constant introspection and reassessment. Feeling comfortable and secure with one's own identity while simultaneously appreciating other racial groups takes time. Societies evolved from centuries of racial prejudice and racism cannot change overnight.

CONCLUSION

One would think that individuals whose livelihoods depend upon their ability to interact with others would do everything in their power to improve their interpersonal skills and effectiveness in working with their patients and health care colleagues. However, most health care practitioners who appreciate the need for life-long learning typically concentrate most on keeping their clinical skills current. Too often, they fail to make self-awareness, communication skills, and knowledge of the social and community context of health care a continuing education priority. This is especially true as it relates to dealing with attitudes that may not be completely conscious. Workshops, seminars, and conferences dealing with communication, cultural awareness, sensitivity, race relations, and racism are seldom sponsored: when they are, they draw far less participation than do programs concentrating on clinical skill development.

Introspection and self-insight training in race relations is particularly vital for rehabilitation professionals because they frequently spend considerable time with patients who depend upon them for their welfare. Few other professions offer the resources or the opportunity to make such a profound difference in the lives of so many. Pragmatically, individuals in the rehabilitation professions would profit immensely by becoming more cognizant of how their own attitudes, beliefs, and behaviors toward people from other racial or ethnic groups might differentially affect the care they render. While, consciously, health care providers commit themselves to a code of ethics that calls for non-discrimination and the protection of the rights and dignity of all people, unconsciously they may be letting their prejudices influence treatment outcomes.

REFERENCES

Adorno T W, Frenkel-Grunswick Levinson D J, Sanford R N 1950 The authoritarian personality. Harper, New York

Allport G W 1954 The nature of prejudice. Addison-Wesley, Reading, MA

Allport G W 1979 The nature of prejudice. Addison-Wesley, Reading, MA

Allport G W, Katz D 1931 Students' attitudes. Craftsman Press, Syracuse

Allport G W, Kramer B M 1946 Some roots of prejudice. Journal of Psychology 22: 9–39

American Medical Association 1995 Board of Trustees report 50-1-95, November 1995, Chicago

American Speech-Language-Hearing Association 1996 ASAH membership highlights and trends. American Speech-Language-Hearing Association, Rockville, MD

Arredondo P, Toporek R, Brown SP et al 1996 Operationalization of the multicultural counseling competencies. Journal of Multicultural Counseling and Development 24: 42–78

Ashmore R D, DelBoca F K 1976 Psychological approaches to understanding intergroup conflict. In: Katz P A (ed) Toward the elimination of racism. Pergam Press, New York

Brighman J C, Woodmansee J J, Cook S W 1976 Dimensions of verbal racial attitudes: interracial marriage and approaches to racial equality. Journal of Science Issues 32: 9–21

Bruhn J G 1996 Creating an organizational climate for multiculturalism. Health Care Supervisor 14(4): 11–18

Cantor J C, Miles E L, Baker L C 1996 Physician service to the underserved: Implications for affirmative action in medical education. Inquiry 33: 167–180

Carlson E R 1956 Attitude change through modification of attitude structure. Journal of Abnormal and Social Psychology 52: 256–261

Centers for Disease Control and Prevention 1996 HIV/AIDS surveillance report, 8 (No. 2): pp. 11–12

Coughlin E D 1988 Conditions of black men in American society presents challenges for behavioral sciences, psychologists at meeting agree. Chronicle of Higher Education, September 1

Council on Interracial Books for Children 1982 Fact sheets on institutional racism. Council on Interracial Books for Children Inc., New York, NY

Crawford T J 1974 Sermons on racial tolerance and the parish neighborhood context. Journal of Applied Social Psychology 4: 1–23

D'Augelli A R, D'Agelli J F, Danish S S 1981 Helping others. Brooks/Cole, Monterey

Ehrlich H J 1973 The social psychology of prejudice: a systematic theoretical review and propositional inventory of the American social psychological study of prejudice. Wiley and Sons, New York

Escarce J J, Epstein K R, Colby D C, Schwartz J S 1993 Health care reform and minorities: why universal insurance won't equalize access. Leonard Davis Inst. Health Policy Res Q 3: 1–2

Geiger J H 1996 Race and health care – An American dilemma? New England Journal of Medicine 335: 815–816

Goldberg A L 1956 The effects of two types of sound pictures on the attitudes of adults toward minorities. Journal of Educational Sociology 29: 386–391

Gornick M E, Eggers P W, Reilly T W et al 1996 Effects of race and income on mortality and use of services among Medicare beneficiaries. New England Journal of Medicine 335: 791–799

Green M F 1989 Minorities on Campus: A handbook for enhancing diversity. American Council on Education, Washington, DC

Harding J B, Proshansky H, Kutner B & Chein I 1969 Prejudice and ethnic relations. In: Lindzey, Aronson G, Aronson Ed (eds) The handbook of social psychology, 2nd ed. Vol. 5. Addison-Wesley, Reading, MA

Haskins A R, Rose-St Prix C, Elbaum L 1997 Covert bias in evaluation of physical therapist students' clinical performance. Physical Therapy 7: 155–162

Henry W H 1990, April 9 Beyond the melting pot. Time, pp. 28–31

Hodgkinson H C 1985 All one system: demographics of education, kindergarten through graduate school. National Institute of Independent Colleges and Universities. NAICU Press, Washington, DC

Jones J M 1972, Prejudice and racism. Addison-Wesley, Reading

Jones J M 1981 The concept of racism and its changing reality. In: Bowser B J, Hunt R G (eds) Impact of racism on white Americans. Beverly Hills, CA, Sage, pp. 27–49

Jones J M 1986 Racism: a cultural analysis of the problem. In: Dovidio J F, Gaertner S L (eds) Prejudice, discrimination, and racism. Academic Press, Orlando, FL, pp. 279–314

Jones J M 1988 Racism in black and white: a bicultural model of reaction and evolution. In: Katz P A, Taylor D A (eds) Eliminating racism: profiles in controversy. Plenum, New York, pp. 117–135

Katz I, Benjamin L 1960 Effects of white authoritarianism in biracial work groups. Journal of Abnormal and Social Psychology 61: 448–456

Katz D, Stotland E D 1959 A preliminary statement to a theory of attitude structure and change. In: Koch S (ed) Psychology: a study of a science, Vol. 3: Formulation of the person and the social context. McGraw Hill, New York, pp. 423–475

Kington R S, Smith J P 1997 Socioeconomic status and racial and ethnic differences in functional status associated with chronic disease. American Journal of Public Health 87: 805–728

Kinney D G 1990 Reopening the gateway to America. Life (September): pp. 26–38

Komaromy M G, Grumback K, Drake M 1996 The role of black and Hispanic physicians in providing health care for underserved populations. New England Journal of Medicine 334: 1305–1310

Kramer B 1949 Dimensions of prejudice. Journal of Psychology 27: 389–451

Leland J 1996 The end of AIDS? Newsweek (December 2): pp. 64–73

McDonald M 1970 Not by the color of their skin. International Universities Press, Inc., New York

Morganthau T, Mabry M, Washington F et al 1992 Losing ground. Newsweek (April 6): 20–23

National Organization for Women 1984 Combating racism: facts at a glance (June). National Organization for Women, Washington, DC

Nemetz P, Christensen S 1996 Challenge of cultural diversity: harnessing a diversity of views to understand multiculturalism. Academy of Management Review 21: 434–462

Oxford E 1990 Ellis Island: monument to memories. US Air Magazine (September)

Pedersen P, Pedersen A 1989 The cultural grid: a framework for multicultural counseling. International Journal for the Advancement of Counseling 12(4): 299–307

Powell R P, Collier M J 1990 Public speaking instruction and cultural bias: the future of the basic course. American Behavioral Scientist 34: 240–250

Record 19.9 1988 Percentage of adults holding college degrees. Chronicle of Higher Education (September 28)

Rokeach M 1968 The nature of attitudes. In: Rokeach M (ed) Beliefs, attitudes and values. Jossey-Bass, San Francisco

Rothman R 1988 Carter-Ford panel says race issues moving backward. Education Week (June)

Schroeder S A 1996 Doctors and diversity: improving the health of poor and minority people. Chronicle of Higher Education, B5 (November 1)

Secord P F, Blackman C W 1964 Social Psychology. McGraw-Hill, New York

Smey J W 1983 A model to improve racial attitudes and relationships of racial prejudice with behavior during a health care intervention. Unpublished doctoral dissertation. Clark University, Worcester, MA

US Department of Health and Human Services, Public Health Service Health Resources and Services Administration, Bureau of Health Professions, Division of Disadvantaged Assistance 1986 Health status of disadvantaged: chartbook. DHHS Pub. No. (HRSA) HRS-P-DV86-2

Walker P W, Brand M K 1993 The status of data on minority practitioners in selected allied health professions. Journal of Allied Health 22: 1–7

Webster's Ninth New Collegiate Dictionary 1988 Dictionary of the English language. Merriam-Webster, Springfield, MA

Whitaker M 1993 White & Black Lies. Newsweek (November 15): pp. 52–54

8

Cross-cultural communication

Alejandro Brice
Lynda Campbell

Communication and language are at the core of service delivery. They are vital to the interactions of the clients of health care professionals and to the services that are delivered. Communication, the process by which others come to know what another person thinks and feels, involves language and is culturally bound and influenced. Thus, it is important to understand the role and significance of both language and communication in understanding and delivering clinical services. This need is magnified by the growth of the culturally and linguistically diverse population to be served.

Traditionally, the assimilationist or 'melting-pot' view of communication and interaction has been widely accepted as the norm (Brice 1995, Campbell 1994a, 1994b). This view centers on the notion of diverse cultures blending together to form a single homogeneous one. Typically, persons from the prevailing dominant culture expect others, such as individuals from 'minority' and diverse cultural and linguistic backgrounds, to adapt their beliefs and become 'one' with them.

In contrast, a culturally pluralistic philosophy of communication welcomes the notion of maintaining one's native culture, communication patterns, and world view while acquiring and becoming proficient in the dominant culture. That is, the group maintains some of its own cultural values and does not completely acculturate to the dominant culture. This view is often referred to as a 'tossed salad' or 'painting mosaic'.

Clearly, communication and culture are ambiguous concepts, yet they are both vital to the effective delivery of rehabilitative services. Communication is not an isolated activity. As communication is both a social and a language phenomenon, carefully studying the sociolinguistic environment of the patient's language and culture is necessary for providing therapy services (Anderson 1997). As health care providers deliver services to persons from different cultures, they must overcome potential communication barriers to service provision. Hence, a review of cultural communication variables is necessary. It is the purpose of this chapter to examine communication and culture and how these two interrelate and their potential impact on the delivery of health care services. It will also suggest strategies to minimize communication conflicts.

LANGUAGE, COMMUNICATION AND CULTURE

Language, communication, and culture are intertwined and inseparable. As stated by Levine (1984), culture is an 'inherited system of ideas that structures the *subjective* [added emphasis] experience of individuals' (Levine 1984, p. 20). Haslett (1989) maintains that 'culture and communication are acquired simultaneously: Neither exists without the other' (Haslett 1989, p. 20). Haslett has also said that 'culture constrains what is acquired and how it is acquired' (Haslett 1989, p. 20). Hence, culture as viewed through communication can be ethnocentric and act as a barrier to providing health care.

Communication is 'a basic social process and that as such, it is influenced by the philosophical foundations and value systems of the society in which it is found' (Yum 1994, p. 75). Cultural actions are reflected in how language is used and what language is used (Brice 1994, Mulvaney 1994). A person's native language affects a person's view of the world. It is the means by which one's experiences are encoded into words (Fantini 1991). It reflects views such

as harmony or human-centeredness and other value orientations.

Language, or one's means of communication, can liberate or constrain one's view as it is learned in the context of the environment. That is, the environment influences how language is acquired; however, language also influences and affects one's concept of culture (Vygostksy 1962). Language is a collective organization of life. According to Edward Sapir: 'The fact of the matter is that the "real world" is to a large extent unconsciously built onto the language habits of the group. No two languages are nearly ever sufficiently similar to be considered as representing the same reality' (Mandelbaum 1949, p. 162).

Pennington (1985) states that, 'Language is the medium through which a culture expresses its world view. Like culture in general, language is learned and it serves to convey thoughts; in addition it transmits values, beliefs, perceptions, norms and so on' (Pennington 1985, p. 33). Fantini (1991) maintains that 'language is a medium (or paradigm) which directly influences our entire lives. This notion is known as "language determinism and relativity". In other words the mother tongue acquired in infancy influences the way we construct our vision of the world' (Fantini 1991, pp. 110–111).

Much of communication involves unconscious scripts. These scripts are habitual and typically we are oblivious to them unless we examine them (Gudykunst 1991a). These unconscious scripts may become barriers to communication in the health care community. We are often unsuspecting of how we use these scripts and to what degree culture influences their use. Gudykunst emphasizes this point: 'When we engage in habitual or scripted behavior we are not highly aware of what we are doing or saying' (Gudykunst 1991a, p. 26). He also maintains that when we are communicating with others of differing cultures, we base our interpretations on our own cultural symbolic systems, which involve speaking–listening and verbal–nonverbal behavior scripts. Thus, ineffective communication may result. As Gudykunst states (1991a): 'Our culture and ethnicity influence the attributions we make about others' behavior' (Gudykunst 1991a, p. 30).

Language serves as a means of solidifying a group. Gallois et al (1988) state that 'members of subordinate class, ethnic and cultural groups signal solidarity with their group by selective use of ingroup language, dialect, accent, or vocabulary' (Gallois et al 1988, p. 164). If the members of a linguistic group believe that its linguistic identity is in jeopardy, then 'they may use their ingroup's speech style more frequently and show stronger loyalty to it (Gallois et al 1988, p. 165). They are, in essence, using their native language as a 'we code' (Gumperz 1982).

THE ELEMENTS OF CULTURAL VARIABILITY

Individualistic (I) versus collectivistic (we) cultures

As communication is both a cultural and a language phenomenon, it is necessary to study carefully the patient's culture, in order to provide culturally appropriate therapy services and to retain patients in therapy (Anderson 1997). For example, the difference between East Asian and North American communication patterns is the difference between the focus on social relationships (Asian) versus the focus on individualism (North American) (Yum 1994).

Ting-Toomey (1994) refers to individualism as:

the broad value of tendencies of a culture to emphasize the importance of individual over group identity, individual over group rights, and individual needs over group needs. In contrast, collectivism refers to the broad value of tendencies of a culture to emphasize the importance of the 'we' identity over the 'I' identity, group obligations over individual rights, and ingroup-oriented needs over individual wants and desires. (Ting-Toomey 1994, pp. 360–361)

In individualistic cultures (Triandis 1995), the self is defined independent of the group; one should do what is enjoyable and required by contacts with others. The focus is on the person and individual. Individualists rely on internal

attributes to explain behaviors (Triandis 1995). There is stress on the 'autonomous self' (Ting-Toomey 1994), while 'face', the outer portrayal of oneself, is self-oriented (Gudykunst 1991c).

Direct communication is more predominant in individualistic cultures than in collectivistic cultures. Strangers or outsiders establish communication relationships more easily (Gudykunst et al 1988). Highly individualistic values have been found in the USA, Australia, the UK, Canada, the Netherlands, New Zealand, and Italy (Gudykunst et al 1988, Ting-Toomey 1994). 'Loose' cultures are associated with individualistic cultures. Looseness in culture 'occurs in heterogeneous societies where people get rewarded for independent action' (Triandis 1995, p. 53). Looseness is associated with creativity. Language and speech reflect this as the speaker tries to be clever with words and puns (this is very characteristic of Cubans and their speech (Brice 1993)).

By contrast, collectivism stresses the importance of the 'connected self' or connectedness to the group (Ting-Toomey 1994). High collectivistic values have been found in Indonesia, Columbia, Venezuela, Panama, Ecuador, and Guatemala. In addition, China, Korea, Japan, Hong Kong, Indonesia, and Mexico have also been identified as collectivistic group-oriented cultures (Gudykunst et al 1988, Ting-Toomey 1994). First generation immigrants from all of these countries, such as Asian immigrants in the USA, may keep their group-oriented values (Ting-Toomey 1994).

Ting-Toomey identifies several aspects of collectivistic cultures. First and foremost is the concept of 'face' being other-oriented. The concept of giving 'face' to others with higher status is important in collectivist cultures. (Gudykunst 1991c). Collectivists see ambiguous groups as outgroups (Triandis 1995). However, some collectivistic cultures, such as the Chinese, Japanese, and Columbian, are more equitable with members outside their group than are people in the USA, which is highly individualistic (Gudykunst et al 1988).

Membership in a collectivistic group includes the right to get involved in the affairs of others

(Triandis 1995). Collectivists use norms to explain behaviors. For example, they may use the norm of arriving late for appointments as the expected behavior. A sense of fate is common and prevails. Collectivistic cultures show tendencies to be closely (as opposed to loosely) connected (Triandis 1995).

Asian collectivists use apologies as social lubricants. The apologies are usually reciprocated so that 'face' is saved, with both parties taking the blame (Triandis 1995). An apology is a social function and should not be taken literally – outrageously incorrect statements do not matter as long as they protect the other individual (Triandis 1995). In summary, the focus of collectivistic cultures is on relationships.

Low context versus high context communication

In understanding cultural variability, health care professionals need to consider the concept of low-context and high-context communication, which was initially introduced by Hall (1983). Low-context communication relies little on the surrounding context for interpretation; rather, most of what is communicated is found in the verbal message. Low-context communication reflects linear logic, direct verbal interactions and styles of speech, overt intention, and sender-oriented values. It is typically found in individualistic cultures (Ting-Toomey 1994).

Individualistic, low-context cultures tend to be more sensitive to a person's values, attitudes or dispositional characteristics and to attribute behavior to their individuality and personality. By contrast, high-context communication and cultures are highly sensitive to situational and context features of communication. High-context cultures tend to attribute behavior according to the situation or factors that are external to the person (Gudykunst 1991c). High-context communication refers to a spiral logic or interaction approach that uses indirect styles of speech. It consists of indirect verbal negotiation, use of subtle nonverbal nuances, and a receiver-listener focus. Figure 8.1 presents an illustration of a linear-low-context communication versus a high-context spiral communication pattern.

High context spiral communication pattern

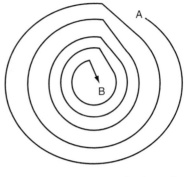

Low context linear communication pattern

A ————————▶ B

Fig. 8.1 Low context versus high context communication patterns.

Collectivistic cultures tend to use more high-context communication patterns. Brice (1993) notes that Cubans and Cuban Americans reflect the spiral method of communication in particular: 'Social greetings are exceedingly important within the Cuban society. A more indirect approach of getting to the topic is exhibited with the Cuban society, i.e., more spiral vs. linear. Discussions of family, friends, and employment always precede any formal discussion' (Brice 1993, p. 4). This approach has also been noted in other Latino-Hispanic cultures (Langdon 1992).

Indirect communication is also used in collectivistic cultures. For example, Cuban-American medical doctors will typically not inform a patient that they have a life-threatening disease if they do not see that such knowledge is in the patient's best interests. They may, however, inform a family member.

To reduce uncertainty, individuals from collectivistic cultures wish to know about the other's status and background. 'This,' for example, 'leads Japanese to introduce themselves saying things like "I belong to Mitsubishi Bank" and immediately asking, "What is your job?", "How old are you?", and "What is the name of your company?" ' (Gudykunst 1991c, p. 97). In health care settings, this may translate to such questions as, 'I am Columbian, are you Cuban?', 'What is your position in this rehabilitation company?', or 'You look young to be a doctor, how long have you been working?' (It should be noted that in Latino-Hispanic cultures many health care providers are referred to as doctor regardless of their actual credentials.)

Horizontal versus vertical cultures

A third element in cultural difference, the horizontal versus vertical distinction, relates to both individualistic and collectivistic cultures. Thus, a collectivistic culture may be either horizontal or vertical. Horizontalism places an emphasis on people being similar or parallel on most attributes, especially those involving status (Triandis 1995). Verticalism accepts inequality and rank. In vertical societies rank has its privileges (Triandis 1995).

Horizontal individualism (same/independent) is evidenced when a culture emphasizes sameness and uniqueness (individuality or independence). Sweden has this orientation. The elderly in Scandinavian countries do not live with their offspring; and living apart (an individualistic characteristic) is highly valued (Triandis 1995).

Vertical individualism (different/independent) is achievement-oriented. Triandis (1995) notes that, 'They [vertical individualists] want to be distinguished and to "stick out," and they behave in ways that tend to make them distinct' (Triandis 1995, p. 46). They also frequently ask questions. Many middle- and upper-class people from the USA tend to be orientated this way.

Horizontal collectivism (same/interdependent) occurs when the culture is cooperative and there is a sense of social cohesion and of oneness with members of the group. Members of Israeli kibbutzim are horizontal collectivists: 'They neither want to stand out nor to dominate others in a group, and they value community needs more than individual needs' (Triandis 1995, p. 46).

An example of vertical collectivism (different/interdependent) exists in a culture noted by its dutifulness. Japanese society is one example

of vertical collectivism. The word *giri* signifies the concept of duty, honor, obligation, and burden all in one. A strong sense of hierarchy, noted by specific language forms for each type of status relationship with others and for specific social engagements, is used. For example, a Japanese person may be less critical of an 'insulter' from an outgroup if that person is of higher status. Vertical collectivists rarely ask questions.

By placing the collectivistic (high-context) versus individualistic (low-context) continuum on one level and an intersecting continuum of horizontal versus vertical cultures on another level, one can construct a model of four quadrants. Thus, four cultural attributes emerge: horizontal collectivist, vertical collectivist, horizontal individualistic, and vertical individualist.

Figure 8.2 illustrates collectivistic and individualistic vertical and horizontal cultural attributes of the four quadrants.

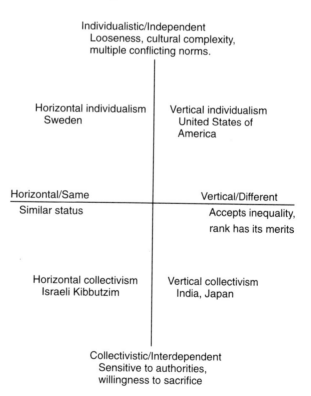

Fig. 8.2 Collectivistic and individualistic, vertical and horizontal cultural attributes.

Monochronic vs. polychronic time views

Yet another set of cultural differences affecting communication concerns time. Monochronism is the orientation that events happen in chronological order and that adherence to schedules is important. Monochronic views predominate in individualistic, low-context cultures. Monochronic cultures, as exemplified by the USA or Germany, subdivide time schedules, and individual needs from group needs (Hall 1983). Task orientations (e.g. work) are separated from social orientations (e.g. socializing). Monochronic cultures are more future conscious than present or past conscious.

Polychronism is the orientation that events can happen concurrently and that a fixed timeliness to schedules is not important. Polychronic views predominate in high-context, collectivistic cultures. The focus is on people and on completing transactions rather than adherence to specific time schedules. For example, it is often expected that a Cuban therapist will periodically pause to converse with the client about non-therapy related topics, or a client's daughter may bring coffee for an anticipated break during the therapy session. Polychronic cultures are more conscious of past and present than the future. Polychronic cultures include Latin-American cultures, Middle-Eastern cultures, and Asian, French, and Greek cultures (Hall 1983).

BARRIERS TO EFFECTIVE COMMUNICATION: STEREOTYPING, BIAS, AND ETHNOCENTRISM

If the therapist and client approach the rehabilitation process from different cultural perspectives, then ethnocentrism and bias are likely to increase barriers to communication. To reduce stereotyping and ethnocentrism, health care providers must remember that variations exist within and across cultural groups (Campbell 1996).

Language

Use of the native language by families may be a barrier for many health care professionals. Many health care professionals make no attempt to communicate with families in their native language, for example, by saying a few words or greetings. It is not uncommon to find families speaking their native language when confronted with an adverse situation such as when a family member is hospitalized. Ideally, the therapist should converse with the patient and family in the language with which the client feels most comfortable. Many healthcare settings require clinicians to be bilingual, especially when the community is highly bilingual (for example, Miami, Florida, in the USA). The therapist or clinician should not view the use of the native language as a threat to his own professional identity.

Reducing bias

Rehabilitation professionals can overcome the biased attributions or stereotyping that are made about other cultures and languages. Therapists and clinicians must adopt the view that culture is highly variable and recognize and appropriately manage the diversity through effective language and communication.

Gudykunst et al (1988) state that cultural stereotypes are less likely to be retained if there is a willingness to move in and out of friendship exchanges. Therefore, establishing a friendship with clients may reduce one's own bias. Cook (1978, cited in Gudykunst et al 1988) maintains that bias is reduced among groups when five conditions exist:

1. The individuals have near equal status
2. Negative stereotypes are not reinforced and hence confirmed
3. Cooperation exists among individuals – a joint goal or common goal may assist this effort
4. Encounters have high degrees of shared alliance
5. There is a supportive clinical environment.

Gudykunst (1991c) states that, 'When members of different groups are working together and fail their task, members of the ingroup usually blame the outgroup for the failure' (Gudykunst 1991c, p. 87). Prejudice is reduced not by the total amount of contact but rather by the disposition or type of contact, such as in friendships. Prejudice occurs when others attribute negative aspects to personal characteristics, especially when negative outcomes are experienced. However, if positive outcomes occur, then 'our tendency is to treat the person as an "exception to the rule"' (Gudykunst 1991a, p. 87).

UNDERSTANDING FAMILIES

Working with families involves working with spouses, children and caretakers, parents of children with disabilities, other relatives, and even close family friends. All these relationships will be considered under the category of 'family'. Family style of interaction and communication may differ from the rehabilitation professional's own communication style. Styles must match to a reasonable degree in order to foster a successful intervention. A rehabilitation therapist must adopt the cultural variables of the family, for example, taking a collectivistic viewpoint in communicating important information if the family is from a collectivistic culture.

The members of a family interact with each other in a variety of ways (Turnbull & Turnbull 1986). Aspects of family relationships involve cohesion (enmeshed vs. disengaged), adaptability, chaos, and rigidness.

Cohesion (enmeshment vs. disengagement)

Family cohesion consists of 'the close emotional bonding that members have toward each other and the interdependence of an individual within the family system' (Turnbull & Turnbull 1986, p. 61). Enmeshment is one end of the continuum of cohesion. Within highly enmeshed families the personal and role boundaries are blurred or weak. Characteristics of highly enmeshed families include abundant involvement with protection. Family members have difficulty developing their own individuality, with

reduced risk taking for all family members including the patient. These families organize all interactions around the disability and handicap. What appears to be overprotection and over-involvement within one family (e.g. in an individualistic family) may be the norm for another (e.g. in a collectivistic family). Thus, abundant protection and involvement must be evaluated within the family's culture.

Similarly, adult children with a mother receiving therapeutic services from a highly enmeshed family may frequently accompany her to therapy and insist on being a part of each session. The adult children may not allow the mother to speak for herself and may answer all questions directed to her. The adult children may exaggerate progress at home as a result of protection and possible denial. Protection may also come in the form of demanding the 'best'; hence, adult children may 'shop' for the best clinician or therapist.

Disengagement is the other end of the family cohesion continuum. It is characterized by very rigid role and personal boundaries. Specific characteristics include limited family involvement and input into decision making. A disengaged family may be rarely seen with the client. A spouse may bring his wife to therapy and yet never inquire as to her progress or well-being. Many personal or family decisions may be left up to the clinician or therapist. Limited involvement in the disengaged family will be a major obstacle to overcome if carryover of objectives into other settings and the involvement of family members are required.

Adaptability (chaos vs. rigidity)

Adaptability is another component of family relationships. It is the ability to change in response to new demands placed upon the family, such as those that may be necessary during a period of rehabilitation. For instance, families may react to stress along the continuum of chaos versus rigidity. Chaotic families display low degrees of control and structure. Interactions are characterized by few rules, which in turn are seldom enforced. Other characteristics include unkept promises and commitments (for example, being unable to keep appointments for therapy), and the absence of a family leader.

In a chaotic family, the perception of what has been recommended may be quite different from that of the clinician. Such issues complicate matters when carryover of therapy techniques and strategies into the home is required. To illustrate, the mother and grandmother of a child with a disability may demand specific services but may refuse recommendations made for the specific therapy, for example, total communication (sign language and oral language) for a child with hearing impairments. This may occur even after initial cooperation and agreement. Hence, a word of counsel is to write down all recommendations. Chaotic families may often break promises and agreements. Drop out and discontinuation of therapy are common occurrences.

Rigid families display a high degree of control and structure. Rigid families also tend to develop rules and be rule-oriented. The family's interactions are characterized by many strictly enforced rules. The power structure within the family is highly delineated, with little room for change. Although rigid families may also drop out and discontinue therapy, a helpful strategy is to explicitly state rules at the onset of service delivery, such as hospital or rehabilitation center rules, absences, or payment.

COMMUNICATION CONFLICTS

In attempting to establish and maintain effective intergroup communication, health care professionals should be aware that cross-cultural communication will result in occasional conflicts. Ting-Toomey (1994) stated that, 'conflict is inevitable in all social and personal relationships. Intercultural conflict usually starts off with miscommunication' (Ting-Toomey 1994, p. 360). When conflict occurs, determining its nature is important. Professionals should attempt to resolve conflict and build community by the simple act of communicating. Table 8.1,

Table 8.1 Conflict as interpreted by individualistic and collectivistic cultures

Individualistic cultures	Collectivistic cultures
An opportunity to clear and 'air out' differences. Conflict such as scheduling with the family is dealt with directly	Conflict is damaging to social 'face'. Conflict with the patient and family should be dealt with between the parties
Conflict is dysfunctional and functional	Conflict is dysfunctional
Conflict is dysfunctional when it is repressed. Emotions, wants, and patient desires must be communicated directly	Conflict demonstrates a lack of self-discipline. Patient or therapist outbursts are signs of immaturity and put the therapy relationship into jeopardy
Conflict is functional when opportunities for problem solving discussion with the patient occur	Conflict provides for skillful 'face' negotiation procedures
Task issues and patient emotional issues are handled separately	Task issues and patient emotional issues are handled together
Conflict resolution can be a win situation for the therapist and the patient/family	Conflict resolution can be a win situation for the therapist and the patient/family

for health care professionals, lists several examples of conflict as interpreted by individualistic and collectivistic cultures.

To illustrate, for individualistic cultures, bargaining and talks may revolve around individual self-esteem, self-centered based emotions, and autonomy (Ting-Toomey 1994). In particular, individuals with disabilities may need to be accommodated in terms of their emotions, pride, and what they would like to obtain from therapy.

In order to minimize conflict, rehabilitation professionals should be aware of differing communication styles and nuances and how these differences might have a discriminating influence on the interaction and unintentionally cause misperceptions and hence conflict. Box 8.1 summarizes some general differences in communication styles for Latino-Hispanic, African-American, and Native-American cultures (Brice 1995, Campbell 1994b).

Box 8.1   Differences in communication styles (Brice 1995, Campbell 1994b)

Latino-Hispanic
Communication:
- Hissing may be used to gain another's attention.
- Official or business conversations are preceded by social greetings. Conversations may switch between official and social language.
- Interruption during conversations is usually tolerated.
- Raising one's voice is used to gain the conversational floor.

Touching:
- Touching between two people in conversation is common.

Eye contact:
- Avoidance of eye contact is a sign of attentiveness, respect; sustained eye contact may be perceived as a sign of threat or challenge to authority.

Distance:
- Distance between two speakers is relatively close.

African-American
Communication:
- Distinction between 'arguing' and 'fighting'. Arguing can involve verbal abuse, while fighting can be physical.
- Asking personal questions of someone one has just met is perceived as inappropriate.
- Indirect questions are sometimes seen as harassing.
- Interruption during conversations is usually tolerated.
- Conversations are considered to be private between participants.

Touching:
- Touching another's hair may be perceived as offensive.

Eye contact:
- Preference for indirect eye contact during listening; direct eye contact during speaking.

Asian-American
Communication:
- It is considered impolite for children to interrupt in conversation.
- Addressing others is regulated by hierarchies as seen in language and behaviors.
- Social status is established by one's age, sex, job status, and marital status. Therefore, it is common to ask questions related to these factors.
- Kinship terms are very important in establishing the relationship between two family members. These terms may extend beyond the family to include community members.
- Facial expressions are composed.
- Giggling when embarrassed may occur.
- Finger beckoning is used for small children and not adults.

Touching:
- Touching and hand holding between members of the same sex is acceptable.
- Hand holding and kissing between members of the opposite sex in public is unacceptable.

Eye contact:
- Avoidance of eye contact is a sign of attentiveness, respect; sustained eye contact may be perceived as a sign of threat or challenge to authority.

Native-American
Communication:
- Personal questions may be considered snooping or prying.
- It may be acceptable to ask the same question several times.

Eye contact:
- Avoidance of eye contact is a sign of attentiveness, respect; sustained eye contact may be perceived as a sign of threat or challenge to authority. Prolonged and continued direct eye-contact is undesirable.

Box 8.2   General recommendations for effective cross-cultural conflict resolution (adapted from Gudykunst 1991a, Mulvaney 1994, Wood 1994)

1. Do not assume similarities.
2. Suspend making judgments. Avoid the tendency to stereotype.
3. Recognize the vitality of diverse communication strategies. Language use will be different. What type of language is used will reflect cultural orientations.
4. Respect others.
5. Provide translation clues, make your thoughts explicit. Describe behaviors without attributing meaning. Use descriptive statements of the behavior.
6. Seek translation clues from others, have them explain their actions. Pay attention to the patient and family's feedback.
7. Metacommunicate. Tell the other person how you interpreted the message or what she/he just said.
8. Expand your communication style repertoire.

Recognize that in many cases, differences are shades of similarities. Attempt to identify common ground. Do not assume that similar words and concepts have the same meaning.

Nevertheless, conflict is bound to surface on occasion. Box 8.2 summarizes general recommendations for effective cross-cultural conflict resolution (adapted from Gudykunst 1991a, Mulvaney 1994, Wood 1994).

Table 8.2 identifies specific conflict resolution strategies for persons from individualistic and collectivistic cultures.

Table 8.2 Conflict resolution strategies for working with persons from other cultures

Individualistic cultures (A*)	Collectivistic cultures (B*)
Become aware of face maintenance and face saving strategies	Become aware of strong problem solving orientations
Address problems before they escalate to major conflicts	Focus on the issues of conflict
Give 'face' and give the other party options for resolution (i.e., give them room for 'face saving' or negotiation)	Engage in more assertive, direct style of conflict management. Collectivists need to avoid hierarchical management styles and deal with others on the same horizontal level
Be aware of and incorporate quiet observation of the events surrounding the conflict	Own the resolution process
Practice active listening skills	Provide active, verbal feedback
Use less direct language, such as using qualifiers, disclaimers, tag questions, tentative statements. In refusing a request, do not attempt to use the blunt and direct 'no', which carries a high 'face' threat to the other person/party	Use more direct and integrative language
Let go of the conflict if the other person/party does not want to deal with it directly	Commit time and effort to resolving the conflict

*Category A refers to people from an individualistic background working with collectivistic cultures and category B refers to those from a collectivist background working with individualistic cultures.

MAXIMIZING THE INVOLVEMENT OF FAMILIES AND SIGNIFICANT OTHERS

A principal element of open communication and an optimal therapeutic relationship with clients is the development of trust. Developing trust is a first step toward reducing conflict and involving families in rehabilitation therapy. In a cross-cultural encounter, development of trust may be more difficult to establish than when two parties are from a similar background. A presumed history of bias and ethnocentrism may be difficult to overcome. Also, the cultural variability, in and of itself (for example individualistic or collectivistic culture) makes trust less natural.

Luterman (1991) lists three elements in building trust: caring, consistency, and credibility. He also states that, 'Caring is conveyed to the client in any number of ways, not the least of which is active and sensitive listening' (Luterman 1991, p. 37). Health care professionals must become non-judgmental listeners and be able to take a 'receiver attitude' such as that displayed by many collectivistic cultures.

From practical experience, it becomes evident that many clients display respect only after the health professional shows caring. In fact, caring may be a high priority, on the same level as the actual therapy. The rehabilitation professional should take time to talk about events that the client may deem to be important.

Consistency and credibility are both important in developing trust. Consistency can be displayed by working on the same therapy objectives with clients and by demonstrating the techniques used in therapy to the family. Although credibility may initially be garnered through use of a professional title, it can also be earned by demonstrating experience and expertise to family members and others in the community.

Suggestions for building trust and maintaining credibility with culturally and linguistically diverse families include the following:

1. Speak the client's native language when possible (even if it is only some words of greeting).

2. When possible, provide written messages and materials in the family's native language.

3. Use members of the community as representatives for initial contacts in developing relationships.

4. Encourage families to share with you their view of the situation. This may reinforce the notion that you are sincerely interested.

In addition, family involvement, especially prevalent in collectivistic cultures, requires respect and open communication. General suggestions for health care professionals who want to maximise family involvement include:

1. Accept families as they are – most families are composed of competent individuals and competent caregivers.

2. Recognize and respect the rights and beliefs of families (this includes religious and spiritual beliefs that accompany health care).

3. Do not ask families to compromise their beliefs or to take on the attitudes of the dominant culture.

4. Listen carefully and empathetically for the family's message and focus on hopes.

5. Help families feel comfortable by sharing information and available resources. Prepare for all meetings so that your knowledge will be apparent at the right moments.

6. Keep your word and follow through with agreements.

7. Allow the family's vitality to come through.

Changes in service delivery

Traditionally, the Eurocentric medical model, also referred to as the expert model, has been used in therapy situations with all clients from all backgrounds, regardless of appropriateness. In this model, the health care specialist assumes full responsibility for the entire process, for example, the speech-language pathologist determines the goals, selects the procedures, informs the client of those procedures, implements them, determines what changes should/need to be made, assesses progress toward goals, and counsels other health-related professionals

regarding a client's communications (Creaghead 1994). This model can often fail to be 'family-friendly' due to limited opportunities for interactions and family participation.

A more holistic and collaborative model, however, would allow for more family participation, whether families are from individualistic or collectivistic cultures. This approach is characterized by shared problem solving; that is, all participants – the family and professionals – are part of a team involved in determining if a problem exists, its nature, intervention, goals, and roles for implementing the solutions (Creaghead 1994). Characteristics of successful collaboration include:

- team members share common goals
- all members contribute equally
- leadership is distributed equally
- responsibility for implementing team decisions is shared.

Luterman (1991) states, 'The basic notion underlying all family therapy is that the family is a system in which all components are interdependent . . . any time a change occurs in one member of the family, everybody in the family is impacted' (Luterman 1991, p. 137). Involving all family members in the therapy process is part of the holistic and collaborative therapy systems model that can result in the following (Luterman 1991):

- a greater understanding of impairments and people in general for the client and family
- increased compassion for the client
- the family gaining an increased appreciation of their own health and well-being
- increased sensitivity to prejudice (as a result of experiencing or seeing prejudice toward impaired individuals) for the family
- the family coming closer together.

CONCLUSIONS

Language tends to constrain health care professionals to a specific cultural view. Yet, using language to expand the view in providing services to clients is essential. As the culturally and linguistically diverse client population continues to increase dramatically, health care professionals repeatedly face the challenge of how best to provide services. The health care professional's role of diagnostician-clinician can be more difficult when different languages and cultures are involved. Thus, health care professionals need to understand the interrelationship of language and culture used by the clients and their families.

REFERENCES

Anderson R 1997 Examining language loss in bilingual children. Communication disorders and sciences in culturally and linguistically diverse populations newsletter. 3(1): 2–5

Brice A 1993 Understanding the Cuban refugees. Los Amigos Research Associates, San Diego, CA

Brice A 1994 Spanish or English for language impaired Hispanic children? In: Creaghead N, Ripich D (eds) School discourse problems, 2nd edn. Singular Publishing, San Diego, CA, pp. 133–153

Brice A 1995 Differences in learning styles. Institute on multicultural literacy in communication sciences and disorders. Speaker for the American Speech-Language-Hearing Association, January 1995, Sea Island, GA

Campbell L R 1994a Discourse diversity and black English vernacular. In: Creaghead N, Ripich D (eds) School discourse problems, 2nd edn. Singular Publishing, San Diego, CA, pp. 93–131

Campbell L R 1994b Clinical practicum and English proficiency. In: Scott D (ed) Challenges in the expansion of cultural diversity in communication sciences and disorders, Sea Island Multicultural Institute: compilation of papers. American Speech-Language-Hearing Association, Rockville, MD

Campbell L R 1996 Issues in service delivery to African American children. In: Kamhi A G, Pollock K E, Harris J L (eds) Communication development and disorders in African American children: research, assessment, and intervention. Paul H Brookes, Baltimore, pp. 73–93

Creaghead N 1994 Collaborative intervention. In: Creaghead N, Ripich D (eds) School discourse problems, 2nd edn. Singular Publishing, San Diego, CA

Fantini A 1991 Bilingualism: exploring language and culture. In: Malavé L M, Duquette G (eds) Language, culture and cognition. Multilingual Matters, Philadelphia, PA, pp. 110–119

Gallois C, Franklyn-Stokes A, Giles H, Coupland N 1988 Communication accommodation in intercultural encounters. In: Kim YY Gudykunst W (eds) Theories in intercultural communication. Sage Publications, Newbury Park, CA

Gudykunst W B 1991a Effective communication with strangers. In: Bridging differences: effective intergroup communication. Sage Publications, Newbury Park, CA, pp. 23–41

Gudykunst W B 1991b Our expectations of strangers. In: Bridging differences: effective intergroup communication. Sage Publications, Newbury Park, CA, pp. 60–82

Gudykunst W B 1991c Attributing meaning to strangers' behavior. In: Bridging differences: effective intergroup communication. Sage Publications, Newbury Park, CA, pp. 83–100

Gudykunst W B, Ting-Toomey S, Chua E 1988 Intergroup relationships. In: Culture and interpersonal communication. Sage Publications, Newbury Park, CA, pp. 201–217

Gumperz J J 1982 Discourse strategies. Cambridge University Press, New York, NY

Hall E T 1983 The dance of life. Doubleday, New York, NY

Haslett B 1989 Communication and language acquisition within a cultural context. In: Ting-Toomey S, Korzenny F (eds) Language, communication, and culture. Sage Publications, Newbury Park, CA, pp. 19–34

Langdon H 1992 Hispanic children and adults with communication disorders. Aspen Publications, Gaithersburg, VA

Levine R 1984 Properties of culture: an ethnographic view. In: Shweder R, Levine R (eds) Cultural theory. Cambridge University Press, Cambridge, UK

Luterman D M 1991 Counseling communicatively disordered and their families, 2nd edn. Pro-Ed, Austin, TX

Mandelbaum D G (ed) 1949 Selected writings of Edward Sapir. University of California Press, Berkeley, CA

Mulvaney B M 1994 Gender differences in communication: an intercultural experience. [Online] Available HTTP://sun.soci.niu.edu/~weblinks/links/ mulvaney.txt [1996, June 3].

Pennington D L 1985 Intercultural communication. In: Samovar L A, Porter R E (eds) Intercultural communication: a reader, 4th edn. Wadsworth Publishing, Belmont, CA

Ting-Toomey S 1994 Managing intercultural conflicts effectively. In: Samovar L A, Porter R E (eds) Intercultural communication: a reader, 7th edn. Wadsworth Publishing, Belmont, CA, pp. 360–372

Triandis H 1995 Individualism and collectivism. Westview Press, Boulder, CO

Turnbull A, Turnbull H 1986 Family interaction. In: Families, professionals, and exceptionality. Merril Publishing Company, Columbus, OH, pp. 47–66

Vygostksy L S 1962 Thought and language. MIT Press, Cambridge, MA

Wood J T 1994 Gender, communication, and culture. In: Samovar L A, Porter R E (eds) Intercultural communication: a reader, 7th edn. Wadsworth Publishing, Belmont, CA, pp. 155–165

Yum J O 1994 The impact of Confucianism on interpersonal relationships and communication patterns in East Asia. In: Samovar L A, Porter R E (eds) Intercultural communication: a reader, 7th edn. Wadsworth Publishing, Belmont, CA, pp. 75–86

Professional issues

Section 2, 'Professional Issues', explores topics pertinent to the attempt of rehabilitation professionals to become culturally competent practitioners in cross-cultural and international settings.

Chapter 9 outlines a historical perspective of the development of rehabilitation services throughout the industrialized and developing world. Because public policy regarding PWD and rehabilitation has historically been a low priority, Ronnie Leavitt emphasizes new models of care – community based rehabilitation (CBR) – that have proven more successful than rehabilitation services based on the Western 'medical model' in allowing individuals with a disability, especially those who have had few or no services, to lead a more satisfying life. Most rehabilitation therapists have no knowledge of these alternative models or the accompanying strategies to enhance the quality of life of PWD by improving service delivery, providing more equitable opportunities and promoting and protecting their human rights.

Leavitt provides some of the required background material to fully appreciate the practice of cross-cultural rehabilitation and the research that underlies it. She illustrates the context of how rehabilitation services have evolved over time and outlines the numerous challenges facing CBR. The evolution of these models is still in its infancy, yet practitioners will find a familiarity with CBR philosophy and practice valuable as they attempt to meet the needs of the increasingly diverse population of PWD via socially and culturally appropriate models. Although these models have been primarily employed in the developing world, Leavitt suggests that the principles can also be useful within the industrialized world. In any society, successful outcomes generally depend on a 'match' between the culture of the community being serviced and the health personnel or system providing care.

In Chapter 10, Karin Schumacher presents a conceptual model and classification system of 'disablement'. She describes the evolution and application of the International Classification of Impairments, Disabilities and Handicaps (ICIDH), a system that has been endorsed by the World Health Organization (WHO). This system can provide a universal framework for understanding the consequences of disease, injury, and disorder. (The terminology used throughout this book is consistent with that defined by the ICIDH.)

Schumacher gives several examples of how this classification system is being applied in different countries. She introduces the model to many practicing clinicians (more recently, it has been included in the curriculum of some professional schools) and as a resource for researchers and practitioners who wish to more formally compare the concept of disablement across cultures. For example, the ICIDH can be a tool from which measurement instruments can be developed to determine the effectiveness of various conventional and CBR models that are being implemented. Schumacher notes the difficulties in developing a system that can be applied universally as well as the dynamic process of revision that is ongoing.

An important element of rehabilitation is assistive technology, technology that can enhance the life of a PWD by offering easier and more efficient means of task accomplishment, and access to more life opportunities. In almost every instance, health professionals who work internationally in middle- and low-income nations note the considerable difficulties resulting from the unavailability and insuitability of assistive technology, due to multiple economic

and environmental constraints. Technology that is merely transferred from the developed world, even if economically affordable, is often inappropriate, or even useless, in the local environment. For example, Western style wheelchairs are generally unusable in the steep, muddy, rutted terrain that is common in many parts of the world. In Chapter 11, 'Appropriate assistive technology', Jean Anne Zollars and Patricia Ruppelt discuss these issues.

Using multiple examples and descriptions of 'low-tech' adaptive devices, Zollars and Ruppelt introduce rehabilitation professionals to the idea that many creative solutions to problems encountered by the PWD in a low-income setting are possible. They stress the importance of taking into account the personal lifestyle and local environmental realities. The authors also address some of the issues associated with how appropriate assistive technology is designed, tested and produced, keeping in mind that the client should always be a key part of the process. The professional who works in a developed nation, and with clients whose way of life might be different than that of the therapist, or who might have limited funding sources for equipment that is typically quite costly, should also find this chapter instructive. This chapter complements Chapters 24 and 25, which address more specific application of appropriate assistive technology concepts.

Tomlin Paul and Marigold Thorburn, in Chapter 12, discuss basic epidemiological principles and tools as well as considerations in the assessment of disability. This chapter is geared to the professional who is not very familiar with epidemiology (there is considerable variation in what may be taught in the basic curriculum for the range of rehabilitation professionals). It includes an introduction to basic terminology regarding the measurement and determinants of disease and disability, epidemiological study designs, the concept of health status, and implications for rehabilitation professionals.

For those therapists working in a familiar environment, with an array of medical professionals, and in a secondary or tertiary care setting, it might not be necessary to consciously reflect on the distribution and determinants of diseases and disabilities. However, in an unfamiliar setting it may be beneficial – or even a necessity – to learn the incidence, prevalence, and determinants of disability. The occurrence of risk factors and types of disabilities varies by place, time and person; that is, there will be variation in cross-cultural environments. Practitioners must also realize that cultural considerations must play a part in surveillance and screening efforts. Especially in the very poor nations, there may be little or no knowledge of the epidemiology of disability. In fact, many intervention efforts must begin by inaugurating a surveillance system and/or screening programs. Disability prevention and treatment, including the planning and implementation of rehabilitation programming are, in part, dependent upon this knowledge.

The last two chapters in Section 2 concern the process of education. Both apply beyond the particular population being written about.

Sophie Levitt, a British pediatric physical therapist who has worked in many settings, describes the collaborative learning approach (CLA). Although she primarily focuses on CLA for training community level personnel, the principles can be applied in more formal educational systems or in less formal systems such as during a client–therapist interaction. Material that may appear to be 'common sense' is often that which one needs to be reminded to use. Professionals too often lecture or demonstrate skills without taking into consideration the learning styles, abilities, and needs of the learner, which, in fact, may be quite different from those of the teachers. Chapter 13 is of value for professionals who must understand the importance of rethinking their traditional teaching methods, especially when immersed in a cross-cultural setting.

The educational theories underlying the CLA stress active and participatory learning, listening and communication abilities, and the development of human relationships and counseling skills. Levitt describes several learning principles and ways to promote more effective learning, including the art of negotiation. She includes a description of the practical application of the CLA to foster a positive learning climate. This information complements Neufeldt's recommendations for a collaborative approach to service (Ch. 3) and Cornielje and Ferrinho's description of a community rehabilitation facilitator (CRF) training program in South Africa (Ch. 18).

In describing the advantage of a CLA, Levitt cites documentation of the notion that the aims of therapists frequently differ from those of PWD or their families. The need to minimize this occurrence and to make treatment as practical as possible for clients within their own cultural context are themes appearing in many of the later chapters.

In Chapter 14, 'Cross-cultural supervision of students', Richard Ladyshewsky specifically addresses the issues of cultural and language variability when the clinical educator and rehabilitation student come from different cultural backgrounds, as well as the resulting challenges that may emerge. The implications for communication and learning can also be applied to a more global context; that is, these lessons are relevant to other professional roles, population groups, and cross-cultural settings.

Ladyshewsky suggests that it is imperative for clinical educators to be aware of the impact of culture on the performance of the learner (the student). He cites specific examples of culturally determined language style and behaviors for Australian clinical educators and Southeast Asian students, reinforcing the relationships between cultural value orientations and language presented by Brice and Campbell (Ch. 8). The quotations Ladyshewsky present demonstrate how easy it is for miscommunication and conflict to arise. He reminds us that this may be so even when students appear to speak the host language quite well. Learning a foreign language, especially in your home country, may teach you the words of a language but not the cultural context of the language. Additionally, the pressures of 'word stress' and 'wait time' further inhibit an interchange. Also, supervisory techniques, such as the nature and format of feedback, commonly practiced within a Western educational system, may not be the most appropriate in a cross-cultural situation. The individuals participating in an interaction do not intend there to be misunderstanding, yet it is often inevitable. Furthermore, misunderstanding may lead to the clinical educator making inappropriate assumptions about a student's performance.

To achieve cultural competence, cross-cultural sensitivity and the ability to incorporate strategies to enhance the cross-cultural teaching and learning experience will become increasingly necessary as the cultural and language diversity of students continues to grow. Possibly, the collaborative learning approach, as described by Sophie Levitt, could be an additional model to consider in the clinical education setting.

In sum, the diverse group of chapters in Section 2 adds to the relevant knowledge base and leads to the following sections on the practice of rehabilitation in cross-cultural and international settings, and the cross-cultural research examples.

9

The development of rehabilitation services and community based rehabilitation: a historical perspective

Ronnie Leavitt

Despite a range of estimates and some disagreement on the exact numbers of disabled people, it is generally estimated that there are about 450 million persons with a disability (PWD) in the world, or around 10% of the population (Helander et al 1989, PAHO/WHO 1994). The prevalence rate of moderate and severe disability (i.e., those people who are more likely to need rehabilitation) is estimated at 5.2% (Helander 1993). Without improved programs in disability prevention, the absolute numbers and relative proportions of the disabled will grow in the next decades as the world's population increases and medical advances allow for the survival of increased numbers of children under 5 and elderly above the age of 65 who are in a marginal state of health. By the year 2000 it is expected that more than 80% of PWD will live in Third World countries (Marfo & Walker 1986). The World Health Organization (WHO) and The Pan American Health Organization (PAHO) estimate that rehabilitation services for individuals with disabilities in the Third World serve a minute fraction (1–3%) of the total number of those in need (WHO 1981b, Helander et al 1989, PAHO 1994).

The situation for PWD can be improved upon in the 21st century. New models of care are developing that will undoubtedly prove more successful in allowing individuals with a disability to lead a more satisfying life. The purpose of this chapter is to present an overview of the development of rehabilitation services throughout the world, with emphasis on the present situation in developing nations and the concept of community based rehabilitation (CBR).

HISTORICAL OVERVIEW OF HEALTH POLICY AND REHABILITATION INTERVENTIONS

Health care systems have historically existed in some form in all societies. Forms of rehabilitation, in contrast to mechanisms of curing or healing (restoring a sense of normalcy), also have a long history, and allow individuals with disability to be maintained within societies (Tappen 1968, Ackerknect 1971, Granger 1976, Benton et al 1981, Sanders 1986, Leavitt 1992). Hanks & Hanks (1948) hypothesized that the degree to which a society is willing or able to bear the costs incurred in caring for PWD depends upon several interrelating materialistic and cultural factors. Some of these determinants are the relative socioeconomic status of the society (which includes such factors as the number and type of productive units, the need for labor, the amount of economic surplus, and its mode of distribution), the social structure of the society (including whether or not the society is egalitarian or hierarchical, how it defines achievement, and how it values age and sex), the cultural definition of the meaning of the disability (does the symptom of the disability require magical, religious, medical, legal, or other measures?), and the position of the society in relation to the rest of the world. Although there are significant differences in health status and health care systems, including rehabilitation, among contemporary societies, the differences are most extreme between the developed or industrialized societies and the so-called developing or Third World societies. These differences, although influenced by sociocultural practices, primarily reflect the wide economic gap between the two groups, a gap that is widening (UNICEF 1995).

A major impediment to the process of public policy development regarding individuals with a disability is the fact that general health care and rehabilitation for PWD has historically been a very low priority throughout the world (Kaufman & Becker 1986, Groce 1987, Leavitt 1992, PAHO 1993, PAHO 1994). Reasons include:

• The cost–benefit ratio of providing rehabilitation to PWD, which has always been considered poor compared to other health programs.

• There has traditionally been an under-estimation of the potential achievements that a disabled person can accomplish.

• The history of negative attitudes toward persons who are disabled (Leavitt 1992, Westbrook & Pennay 1993). In many societies PWD have been considered to be deviant from the norm, and have been seen to have a social stigma or 'attitude that is deeply discrediting . . . a failing, a shortcoming, a handicap' (Goffman 1963).

• When discrimination limits participation by people with disabilities in various social roles, their plight becomes even more invisible.

• An apparent absence of urgency. Rehabilitation is associated with disease and illness that is, for the most part, neither acute, communicable, nor 'exciting'. The general public will not be at risk, nor will its opposition be mobilized, if rehabilitation services are not given to the populations in need.

• On an individual level, mainstream biomedical practitioners tend to reflect a value orientation that stresses mastery of disease and taking personal credit for recovery. In cases in which an individual has a disability, often very little dramatic curing can occur; in some instances, further loss of function is anticipated. Although a wide array of simple and complex technologies are available, the provision of these services does not ensure dramatic results. Thus, many caregivers find rehabilitation frustrating and often not worthwhile.

• Individuals with disabilities are a disadvantaged minority and, accordingly, have little political influence when lobbying for the opportunity to affect public policy.

When this low priority of care is coupled with a scarcity of resources, limited access to rehabilitation results. Access may be limited by shortages of personnel and facilities. In many countries, geographical impediments and architectural barriers further limit access. Most national development policies stress a concentration of services in urban areas despite the fact that in developing nations a majority of the population may live in rural or peri-urban communities.

The industrialized world

Rehabilitation was originally conceived of in narrow terms, such as giving someone an artificial leg. The USA had no comprehensive programs for PWD prior to World War I, although such programs did exist in Europe (Hazenhyer 1946, Groce 1992). The war-injured from World War II and the polio epidemic in the USA were instrumental forces in the further development of the art and science of rehabilitation. Modern programs consider many more facets of rehabilitation, including psychological, social, educational and vocational services for individuals having a broad range of ills. In some developed nations there is a great demand for services.

Often, however, the most complete set of services exists only in urban areas and only at the hospital or professional level. This system is very expensive and not necessarily conducive to societal integration of the person with a disability. Even community care is based on the premise that services are to be primarily provided by professionals. A mix of in-patient hospital and out-patient and/or home care services is often available, especially in urban areas.

In the last few decades, Western societies have seen an increase in public visibility and empowerment of individuals with a disability, along with a concomitant increase in legislation mandating the rights of the disabled. For example, in the USA the Rehabilitation Act of 1973, calling for civil rights for PWD, Public Law 94-142, the Education for All Handicapped Children Act (1975), and the Americans With Disabilities Act of 1990 are revolutionary in that they are based on the philosophy that in a just society *all* individuals (including PWD) must be accorded equal access and opportunity to pursue their individual goals. The relative newness of these laws implies that the non-physical components of the rehabilitation process (such as guaranteeing PWD the opportunity for education or employment) have begun to develop even later in history than the physical components. This mid-to-late 20th century phenomenon indicates that societies have begun to accept the idea that all persons have a right to a certain level of social well-being. Thus, an analysis of the cost–benefit ratio associated with rehabilitation has begun to consider humanitarian benefits as well as associated economic costs to society.

Nevertheless, even in the most developed societies, an analysis of the literature (Savilios-Rothchild 1970, Bodgen & Biklin 1977, United Nations 1981, Zola 1982, Wright 1983, Goerdt 1984, Nagler 1992) and personal experience lead to the conclusion that public policy, as it presently exists, often fails to function optimally and integrate PWD into the larger society. Although services are generally available, they are arguably not comprehensive enough. In modern times, nations appear ambivalent and vacillate between doing nothing and doing something for individuals with disabling conditions.

The developing world

In the developing world, the delivery of health care services has not completely paralleled that of the more industrialized world. Historically, with the colonization of Asia, Africa, Latin America, and the Caribbean, everything Western, including the medical care systems, received official support. Typically, the health system was centrally controlled at the Ministry of Health. Health services were distributed through urban-based hospitals, with minimal resources left for rural dispensaries. Tertiary and curative care by highly trained personnel were emphasized. National programs were disease-oriented (e.g. malaria, smallpox), without follow-up to ensure further disease prevention and health promotion. Often the hospitals and medical programs were supported by religious or private voluntary organizations. The major human resources were physicians, assisted by nurses and occasional auxiliaries. This system of care is known as the 'Western medical model'. At the same time, traditional systems of medicine, such as care given to persons by a shaman, obeah, espiritisma, and others, were ignored or consciously suppressed (King 1966, Bryant 1969, Gish 1979, Marfo & Walker 1986, PAHO 1993).

During the 1960s and 1970s, developing nations, which were becoming increasingly independent of their colonial ties, prepared national health plans and policies based on the Western medical model while attempting to be less dependent on outside agencies. Paradoxically, these countries experienced relatively few successes in eliminating communicable diseases, controlling rapid population growth, or decreasing food shortages. These factors, along with interrelated environmental realities of Third World nations, such as the majority of people living in rural areas, the enormous presence of poverty, and a general decline in the world economy, have reduced the Western medical model's effectiveness.

Presently, vital health statistics confirm striking differences between the developed and less-developed worlds, both in quantity and quality of care (UNICEF 1995). Although many Third World nations have highly technical medical procedures available, poor or rural populations cannot readily access this sophisticated tertiary care. Many have limited access to even basic primary health care. The disparity in the provision of health care services between lower and upper socioeconomic groups is even more profound in developing countries than in developed countries.

Similarly, PWD living in the developing world experience more difficulty receiving care and integrating into society than those who live in the industrialized world. Although some care has historically been provided at the household or community level, it has been minimal. International rehabilitation programs, such as the World Rehabilitation Fund and Re-

habilitation International, have helped to provide care. However, these programs have largely depended on charitable and religious organizations for administrative and financial support and have reached only a fraction of those in need (Groce 1992). At best, only a few services, for a select few, are provided at major teaching hospitals in the capital cities. Comprehensive and timely rehabilitation services are rarely available due to lack of trained personnel and limited private and public resources. Even the most basic adaptive equipment is usually unavailable. Educational and vocational services are even more of a rarity than physical rehabilitation.

A realization that the conventional Western medical model is inappropriate and unsuccessful in meeting the health needs of a majority of the people in the developing world has led to efforts to develop alternative strategies. A new era has begun within the fields of health and rehabilitation in the Third World. In 1977, the World Health Assembly declared that 'the main target of governments and the WHO in the coming decades should be the attainment by all citizens of the world by the year 2000 of a level of health that will permit them to lead a socially and economically productive life' (WHO & UNICEF 1978, p. 3). In 1978, at the Alma-Ata International Conference on Primary Health Care (PHC), PHC was identified as the means by which this goal could be achieved. The Alma-Ata Declaration defines PHC as 'essential health care based on practical, scientifically sound and socially acceptable methods and technology made universally available to individuals and families in the community through their full participation and at a cost that the community and country can afford' (Helander 1993, p. 38). PHC has as its themes the maximum use of local resources, including trained community health workers and traditional healers; personal and community participation; affordable and accessible care; the integration of prevention, promotion, treatment and rehabilitation; and coordination between the health sector and other related development sectors such as agriculture, housing and education.

Since the 1970s, many nations have initiated major shifts in policy and practice and have explicitly stated that health care is a right to which all citizens are entitled. The principles of PHC are purportedly observed and supported, yet implementation is where the real challenge lies. Since the initiation of a PHC focus, economic conditions in many nations have worsened, impeding or reversing improvements in the delivery of service, and it is feared that Health for All by the Year 2000 (HFA/2000) may not be attainable (Tarimo & Creese 1990, Mesa-Lago 1992).

The content of programs designed to improve primary health services rarely includes a consideration of prevention and treatment of those with disabilities. Perhaps if the philosophies and practices concerning rehabilitation were considered more valuable in developed societies, they would be of more significant concern in the Third World.

COMMUNITY BASED REHABILITATION

Specific to disability prevention and rehabilitation, the WHO has adopted the PHC approach with two main strategies. Because the major causes of impairment in the Third World are considered potentially avoidable, the first strategy is primary prevention. The second strategy is the delivery of rehabilitative community based services with an appropriate system of supervision and referral.

In light of the above, the WHO introduced an innovative approach to prevention and rehabilitation within the less developed countries, known as community based rehabilitation (WHO 1981a, WHO 1984, Smilkstein et al 1984, Helander 1993). CBR is a strategy for enhancing the quality of life of PWD by improving service delivery, providing more equitable opportunities and promoting and protecting their human rights. This policy involves measures taken at the community level to use and build upon the resources of the community. The family of a disabled person is often the most important resource. The supporting personnel in such a

program, who are likely to be local persons with minimal traditional or specialized education, are often referred to as community rehabilitation workers (CRWs). Ideally, the CBR system should be multi-level and multi-sectoral. CBR represents one possible solution to meeting the rehabilitation component of the goal HFA/2000. A meaningful working definition of CBR and alternative models continues to evolve from within the WHO and from individuals working in the field.

The philosophical principles of the CBR approach are equality of rights, solidarity with others who are denied equality, and integration into the mainstream of community life. These require recognizing the capability of PWD to fulfill their human rights and facilitating participation in the social and economic activities of society while maintaining personal dignity. Personal empowerment is a major component of CBR.

CBR based the provision of rehabilitation services on a three-tier referral system:

- a basic home and community level
- intermediate supports
- national, specialized services.

At the community level, CBR involves PWD, their families, and the community workers. It may be a component of an integrated community development program that bases decisions on the will of the community. At the intermediate level the sponsor, i.e. the government or non-governmental organization (NGO), is likely to be involved with the training and technical supervision of community personnel and provide managerial support as well as direct medical interventions when a referral is appropriate. At the national level, it is expected (but certainly not always the case) that the government, in cooperation with the community, will be involved with planning, implementing, coordinating, and evaluating CBR and will provide tertiary care and technical support for some individuals who should then be referred back to the community level as soon as feasible.

Since the development of the CBR concept, its goals have been elaborated and presented in the

1982 United Nations (UN) World Program of Action Concerning Disabled Persons. The UN has taken a leading role in trying to persuade communities to use the CBR approach, whether it be formally linked to the WHO model or to an independent government or non-governmental model (Groce 1992). Field testing of CBR began in 1979 and continues today (Periquet 1984, Jonsson 1994). However, detailed descriptions and/or evaluations of these CBR programs are limited. Numerous community based programs have been adopted throughout many regions of the world; many use the CBR label but lack some of its critical components. A review of the literature supports the notion that these programs take on a variety of forms based on local conditions, existing resources and experience from other development programs, and exist under the auspices of public and private sponsorships. For example, Werner (1983) favors PWD living together in a village setting; Miles (1990) prefers neighborhood centers staffed by community and professional workers; and Thorburn (1994) relies on home visiting by CRWs and the development of parent associations. As the concepts become more widely spread and better understood, more models develop; some remain focused on small projects in rural areas while others consider national programs. Although each has its own particular constraints, and CBR is not a panacea, programs across a variety of cultures in developing and developed nations are being implemented and appear to be accomplishing some of their goals to a considerable degree (Werner 1983, Momm & Koenig 1989, Thorburn & Marfo 1990, O'Toole 1990, Mbise & Kysela 1990, Jaffer & Jaffer 1990, Zaman & Munir 1990, Groce & Zola 1991, Leavitt 1992, Boutros-Ghali 1992, Peat 1993, Finkenflügel 1993, PAHO 1993, Helander 1993, Thorburn 1994, CBR News, Kay & Dunleavy 1996, Peat & Shahani n.d.). (See Chs 15–18, 26–28 for discussion of particular CBR programs.

The challenges confronting CBR

The evolution of the CBR concept has supported the development of promising rehabilitation programs for PWD. Yet, according to Helander (Helander 1993), too many services remain insufficiently planned and many projects are abandoned by donors or governments during times of economic hardship. There remains significant debate over multiple issues relating to CBR and barriers to successful care are still plentiful. The following describes some of these issues and offers some suggestions regarding public policy to enhance the future role of CBR.

Public policy

Leaders, both within the disability rights movement and political arena, must foster reasonable and effective public policy and practice, given the realities of life in developing nations. Naturally, each nation or community will complete its own specific epidemiological and situational analysis before the development of policy. It is also understood that the situation of PWD is an overall function of the fundamental societal processes and current conditions. Significant changes can only occur with modifications of the system as a whole. For example, socioeconomic development (such as a decrease in poverty, and/or increase in community development) would, in itself, undoubtedly improve the status of PWD.

While recognizing the difficult choices regarding the allocation of limited resources, PHC can be viewed as a means to improve the cost–benefit ratio of money spent on PWD. The principles of PHC, such as the importance of early intervention and using low-cost, socially acceptable practices, support the Alma-Ata Declaration of the WHO and provide the foundation for the delivery of rehabilitation services.

Prevention of disability should continue to be stressed. This can only occur in conjunction with other PHC activities, including the provision of clean water, enforced safety regulations, prenatal care, adequate labor and delivery facilities and staffing and development of universal immunization services. Cost–benefit analyses generally support the concept that preventive services serve society best.

The question of whether or not a CBR project should stand alone or be associated with other health or development services continues to be debated. Some believe that rehabilitation services are more likely to succeed if CBR clearly exists as its own PHC program, rather than blended into a more general health care or development program. Most agree that rehabilitation should be 'de-medicalized' as much as possible. An argument in favor of keeping CBR separate is that it must be a 'special' service because there is simply too much unique information for the CRW to learn and convey to the families of individuals with disabilities. As it is, the CRW must function as a special educator, physical therapist, occupational therapist, speech and language pathologist, etc. If the CRW must share this time and energy with health arenas such as family planning or nutrition, the rehabilitation information may be diluted sufficiently to sacrifice its value (this is not to deny, however, that all community level health workers should be aware of a broad array of health impairments, and, in addition, should reinforce each other's teaching and support each other's programs). Alternatively, some argue that CBR should be a component of a full-scale development program that reinforces community participation at all levels and the empowerment of individuals. It is especially prudent for a worker to be multi-skilled in villages that are very isolated or where there is a very limited transportation service.

To enhance the life course for persons who are disabled, a multi-disciplinary commission should be instituted to explore and implement alternative comprehensive policies and programs. All sectors within a nation must be encouraged to work together rather than in isolation, to be advocates, and to continue to educate the public on disability and rehabilitation to improve the prevailing societal attitudes. For example, ministries of education could develop and operate more classrooms for children with physical and mental impairments. When possible, attempts should be made to place children in existing classes to provide the most integrated, least restrictive environment. This would also be the most cost-effective. Long-term institutionalization (for children or adults) will further isolate PWD.

Governments must address the apparent societal reluctance to employ PWD in meaningful, productive employment positions. Public policy should support vocational training and the public sector should set a good example. In the private sector, incentives can be developed, possibly in the form of tax breaks, for enterprises that hire a PWD. Integrating PWD into the workforce becomes both cost-effective and humane by supporting individuals who prefer to become gainfully employed, rather than remain non-productive members of society. The ultimate goal of rehabilitation – that is the ability to play an active role in society with dignity and self-esteem – is thereby more likely to be achieved.

Community participation

Community participation and its concomitant increase in self-reliance are prerequisites for successful community health programs. If a program is initiated from the top down by an outside organization or concerned individuals, the intent should be to turn the program over to the community. However, constraints to this ideal scenario should not be minimized. Bottom-up initiation of a program or program management is often quite difficult. It may be difficult for people to perceive or accept ownership of a self-serving program. Dr Thorburn, the founder and director of CBR in Jamaica and an internationally renowned advocate for children with disabilities, notes the difficulties in securing local government or private funding and recruiting middle-level managers from the community. She emphasizes the central role of family, particularly primary caregivers to children with disabilities, and the development of parents' groups as key to the development of community participation. Additionally, Thorburn (1994) advocates expanding the roles of PWD, to include, for example, decision making and education of others. One must stress the abilities and competence of PWD and increase their responsibilities and rights; that is, CBR should advance a sense of empowerment.

Personal empowerment and community participation are surely linked to improved attitudes among family and community members in order to lessen the degree of stigma toward PWD at the societal level. Thorburn (1994) and others (Thorburn & Marfo 1990) have continually focused on the need for training for parents and the wider community (such as the parent teacher associations) to begin the process of eliminating bias toward PWD. She believes that 'the most critical factor in the development of a program . . . is the attitude of the parents towards the child. From a positive, caring, educating and advocating stance by parents will come positive community attitudes . . . and fulfilling role for disabled people in their own communities' (Thorburn, personal communication, 1995).

Equality and social integration will also be enhanced through direct participation of PWD in local and national political bodies. Additionally, disabled persons and their families must form their own organizations to gain political clout, access to human rights, and the privileges that others in society already have.

Human resources

The development of human resources is one of the most critical factors facing CBR programs. Previously, there was a tendency to overlook the potential to train community based individuals. When developing CRWs, local, relatively unskilled members of the community who are themselves disabled or show concern for individuals with disabilities can be the most appropriate people to be trained in rehabilitation and advocacy principles and techniques. Attention should be paid to the type of training and level of skill development, which has often been noted as a central concern in many community based health programs. Training models are numerous and must fit with the local culture and resources. CRWs are capable of providing intellectual stimulation, exercise regimes, and social interaction. More continuous and compre-

hensive training, integrated with practical real-life examples and supervised experience, generally allow the CRWs to upgrade their level of expertise and problem-solving, which subsequently should improve their clients' status.

At issue is whether CRWs are to be paid employees or volunteers. Helander (1993) notes that it is easier to recruit non-salaried volunteers in Asia, whereas in Africa the tendency is to seek financial compensation. Most CBR volunteers are women. A report in *CBR News* (1994) suggests that assumptions are often made about volunteers. It is, for example, assumed that volunteers are women with extra time, that they are selected by the community, that it is easy for them to work in the community after being trained in CBR, and that they volunteer solely because they want to help others. These assumptions are often inaccurate. At times, a program must begin with people willing to volunteer, with the intention of salaried positions at a later date. In either case, CBR workers can find compensation through appreciation by other people, training that might prove useful for self-satisfaction or future career prospects, or the knowledge that their efforts diminish the dependency of a family member who is disabled. Also, CRWs are most likely to bridge the gap between the community culture and the medical culture.

CBR recognizes that PWD will often need immediate and specialized support services. In fact, as more people are identified as being disabled, specialized support services, both within and outside of institutions, are likely to increase. To this end, the infrastructure must be developed to educate and provide regional training of rehabilitation professionals and to promote the development of rehabilitation institutions or departments within hospitals. Physical therapists, special educators and specialists in vocational rehabilitation are paramount. The development of other allied health professionals in occupational therapy and speech and language pathology must follow because services in these areas of expertise are almost universally absent. Controversy exists regarding the best way to advance the rehabilitation professions within the developing world while still maintaining an emphasis on meeting the needs of the majority of people with disabilities and not just those with access to the limited facilities in the major cities. Similarly, what is the most appropriate educational degree for training specialized professionals? There is a need to balance the country's ability to provide advanced degrees and employment for graduates with the need for knowledge of professional content and the ability to encourage graduated professionals to seek employment in areas of greatest need, that is, in the rural areas and in CBR.

Efforts are needed to increase the retention of already trained professionals. This is currently a serious problem in most developing countries, as many wish to emigrate to countries which offer better salaries or career prospects. Professional development and continuing education can assist by helping personnel remain current and motivated. Often these programs are not available. The use of visiting professionals from industrialized nations is helpful both for developing human resources and for providing continued learning opportunities for those who are providing services. But, as discussed by Kay & Salzman (1994), this role may be fraught with inherent ethical and professional dilemmas, such as defining one's appropriate scope of practice, respecting the concerns of local colleagues yet not forgetting the needs and rights of the many under-served PWD, and being honest about one's motivation or intent in volunteering or working abroad. The permanent use of expatriates is not a solution, and transfer of knowledge and skills to local personnel should be the aim.

In most situations, the educational programs for all of these rehabilitation professionals must be modified to include concepts of PHC/CBR. Medical and allied health educational curricula are usually based on the Western medical model, without consideration of the particular needs of the local population or the alternative strategies that could be implemented to meet these needs. Knowledge of the total national environment should provide health workers with a better understanding of their clients and the need for community based services. For example, traditional health beliefs and practices should be acknowledged as factors affecting PWD. Although historically little information has been available, culture-specific beliefs and behaviors should be directly addressed as potential confounding variables and, when appropriate, as potential means of effecting positive outcomes. Rehabilitation professionals and CRWs must consciously consider such information and have greater insight into this domain (Leavitt 1992, Young & Garro 1982). Although it is predominantly practical factors (such as the availability of services and the cost of care), rather than philosophical issues (such as beliefs about the efficacy of a treatment), which govern the acceptance or rejection of community health programs, cultural-specific models may be highly influential (Fabrega 1974, Kay & Salzman 1994, Helander et al 1983).

The concepts of 'team', interdisciplinary communication and action, and collaboration must be strengthened. When health personnel resources are severely limited, it is even more important for professionals and community workers at every level to understand that all individuals are working for the benefit of PWD; they are all members of the same team. Organizations and professionals should be encouraged to have a more reciprocal relationship at the local level with community based projects. In addition, the relationship between any service provider and those who are the recipients of those services must be based on mutual power and mutual respect.

Rehabilitation technology

Demystification of rehabilitation technology and an emphasis on improved functional capacity are necessary in CBR. To that end, a number of screening tools and simple technologies have been developed, such as the WHO manual *Training in the Community for People With Disabilities* (Helander et al 1989). This manual, which has thus far been translated into over 40 languages, is directed toward the achievement of independence in mobility, self-care, play and schooling opportunities, income-generating opportunities, and the enjoyment of family and social life through the use of local resources. There are 30 training packages, each focused on a particular subject, such as activities for people who have difficulty moving, play activities, prevention of complications, etc. These are complemented by four guides for community members having special tasks within CBR (local supervisors, the community rehabilitation committee, people with disabilities and schoolteachers). It is presumed that basic principles can be used globally, but questions remain, such as how a manual can be culturally and socially relevant within a local context and how best to disseminate the technologies in societies with low literacy.

Alternative technologies must also be developed in the arena of adaptive equipment. Low-cost, culturally and economically appropriate adaptive equipment for PWD should be developed locally whenever possible. Importing highly technical and expensive equipment is both wasteful and impractical. Imported wheelchairs, orthoses, and prostheses, for example, are extremely expensive, and replacement or repair of parts is often impossible. Equipment that is appropriate for one country may not be well suited for the terrain and environmental obstacles in another country. Resource manuals are available that describe how to make simple and low-cost rehabilitation equipment (Helander et al 1983, Werner 1987, Helander et al 1989, Hotchkiss 1985). CBR programs should consider further support in this area by offering workshops directed toward the development, production, and maintenance of appropriate technology (see Chs 11, 24 and 25).

Sustainability of CBR

Difficulties in management also need attention if limited resources are to be maximally utilized. The Pan American Health Organization (PAHO) estimates that 30% of available health resources are wasted (Mesa-Lago 1992). In particular, there is a lack of community mid-level managerial personnel. Public policy must include an expectation of accountability, monitoring of programs, and evaluation of programs (Tarimo & Creese 1990). Regardless of the organizational structure, attainment of program goals can be affected by administrative problems in areas of hiring, establishing role responsibilities, training of community-level workers, and determining who is to receive economic benefits and prestige from the program (WHO 1968, Gartner 1971, Torrey et al 1973, WHO 1987, Yee 1989, Boyce 1994). It is prudent to be cautious of too extensive, and thus impractical, initial programming or too rapid expansion. As suggested by Miles (1990), to facilitate success it is wise to think easy before difficult, children before adults, and limited geographic focus as basic axioms. Flexibility and adaptability are certainly key concepts.

The United Nations is currently evaluating a new draft questionnaire for field testing of some CBR programs. The questionnaire, known as OMAR (A Guide on Operations, Monitoring and Analysis of Results), includes questions on:

- relevance (does the program meet the needs of PWD, the families and communities and does its purpose remain valid and pertinent?)
- effectiveness (did the program meet its objectives in terms of population coverage and benefits for individuals?)
- efficiency (were the available resources used most efficiently?)
- sustainability (will the program continue once external support is withdrawn?)
- impact (what effects has the program had on its institutional, technical, economic, and social settings?) (Jonsson 1994).

Additional quantitative and qualitative research will undoubtedly facilitate the development of ideal, culturally-specific models (Boyce 1994).

As some of the CBR programs begin to celebrate milestones (such as 10 years of service), the issue of future sustainability becomes critical. Sustainability is presumed to depend upon a perceived need, a response from the community indicating a readiness to support the need, and support from outside of the community (Momm & Koenig 1989, UNESCO 1994). Sustainability will likely be enhanced if research and evaluation data are exchanged among CBR programs and adjustments are made accordingly. The International Center for the Advancement of Community Based Rehabilitation is one example of an organization whose mandate is to contribute to this body of knowledge through research and program evaluation (ICACBR 1993). It would also be advantageous if there were increased cooperation among all governmental and non-governmental organizations working on disability-related issues. Helander (1993) argues strongly for increased government involvement initially and a process of decentralization so that the community can increasingly make their own decisions regarding priorities and resource allocation. He suggests that it is no longer acceptable to rely solely on charity and uncoordinated voluntary efforts, especially since donor agencies rarely remain involved for the 'long haul'. In reality, government funding of 'social' programs is often the first to be cut in times of economic austerity.

Determining what cultural factors contribute to success in CBR programs could be most important, if the general premise regarding public policy relating to disabled persons is to be based on a community model. Networking with religious and lay leaders, traditional healers, and educational, health, and social service representatives is useful. Generally speaking, successful outcomes from community health programs depend on a match between the culture of the community being served and the health personnel or system providing care. That is, the cultural approaches of the two groups involved in the interaction must be complementary, and the program organization must be attuned to the environmental realities of the community. This is difficult to attain, and many community programs are hampered by disjunctions in cultural beliefs and behaviors.

Thus, national policy and programming should consider supporting individuals whose major responsibility is to ensure that such a match is developed. For example, the applied medical anthropologist may be an important professional to add to the rehabilitation team.

This person can develop and test theory, gather data, and propose solutions to problems with a focus on cultural explanations of behavior. Furthermore, the anthropologist is often an effective 'culture broker', someone who can help to ensure an ecological, holistic approach by bringing about some communication among various modern and traditional health practitioners or systems and the various peoples in need of service.

CONCLUSION

The last few decades have seen many positive developments with regard to ensuring that PWD live a humane life. Although economic conditions during the 1980s forced a decline in health and education services in many developing countries, PWD are increasingly educated in the regular school system, given vocational training, and receiving physical rehabilitation and appropriate assistive devices to enhance functional outcomes. However, the job of designing and implementing socially and culturally appropriate models of care is far from complete.

Sound public policy must be both pragmatic and humanitarian. In most parts of the world, social processes of urbanization, migration, industrialization, and the expansion of medical knowledge have had a major impact on the care of PWD. Governments, along with organizations of PWD, rehabilitation professionals and donor agencies, especially in Third World countries, must begin to deal with the issues and problems of maintainence and rehabilitation of PWD as this population increases.

To those who argue that rehabilitation is too expensive, pragmatists as well as humanitarians can argue that individual nations and the world community cannot afford not to rehabilitate the persons who are disabled. Left without rehabilitation, they can be a costly drain on society even as they are denied their right to a meaningful life.

The Decade of Disabled Persons (1983–1992) has come and gone. 'Undoubtedly, the major achievement of the Decade was increased public awareness of disability issues among policy makers, planners, politicians, service providers, parents and disabled persons themselves' (Boutros-Gali 1992, p. 4). But the job of ensuring the integration of disabled persons into society has not been completed. As appropriate rehabil-itation programs incorporating CBR principles are advanced both in the developed and developing world, national and international policy makers must seek to join forces with the local community to foster a positive adaptation process for PWD.

REFERENCES

Ackerknect E 1971 Medicine and ethnology: selected essays. Johns Hopkins Press, Baltimore, MD

Benton L et al 1981 Functional electrical stimulation: a practical clinical guide. Rancho Los Amigos Hospital, Downey, CA

Bogden R, Biklin D 1977 Handicapism in social policy. Social Policy Corp, New York

Boutros-Ghali B 1992 Message of the Secretary General: world programme of action opens way to full participation in society. In: Disabled Persons Bulletin, No. 2, Publication 64. United Nations Center for Social Development and Humanitarian Affairs Vienna, Austria

Boyce W 1994 Research and evaluation in CBR: an integrated model for practice. Presented at the Asia Regional Symposium on Research and Evaluation in CBR, Bangalore, India. Dec 5–7

Bryant J 1969 Health and the developing world. Cornell University Press, Ithaca, NY

CBR News AHRTAG – 1–23

CBR News 1994 Newsletter No. 17

Fabrega H 1974 Disease and social behavior. MIT Press, Cambridge, MA

Finkenflügel H 1993 The handicapped community. V. U. University Press, Amsterdam, Netherlands

Gartner A 1971 Paraprofessionals and their performance. Praeger, New York

Gish O 1979 The political economy of PHC and health by the people: a historical exploration. Social Science and Medicine 13: 203–211

Goerdt A 1984 Physical disability in Barbados: a cultural perspective. Unpublished PhD dissertation, New York University

Goffman E 1963 Stigma: notes on the management of spoiled identity. Prentice Hall, Englewood Cliffs, NJ

Granger F B 1976 The development of physiotherapy. Physical Therapy 56(1): 13–21

Groce N 1987 Cross cultural research, current strengths, future. Disabilities Studies Quarterly 7(3): 1–3

Groce N 1992 The U.S. role in international disability activities: a history and look towards the future. A study commissioned by the World Institute on Disability. World Rehabilitation Fund and Rehabilitation International New York, NY

Groce N, Zola I 1991 Multiculturalism, chronic illness, and disability. Pediatrics 5: 1048–1055

Hanks J, Hanks L 1948 The physically handicapped in certain non-occidental societies. Journal of Social Sciences 4: 11–20

Hazenhyer I M 1946 A history of the American Physical Therapy Association. Physiotherapy Review 26: 1

Helander E 1993 Prejudice and dignity: an introduction to CBR. United Nations Development Fund, Publication No. E93-111-B3, Washington, DC

Helander E Mendes P, Nelson G 1983 Training disabled people in the community. WHO, Geneva

Helander E, Mendes P, Nelson G, Goerdt A 1989 Training in the community for PWD. World Health Organization, Geneva

Hotchkiss R 1985 Independence through mobility. Appropriate Technology International, Washington, DC

International Center for Advancement of Community Based Rehabilitation (ICACBR) 1993 Program description. Queen's University, Ontario, Canada

Jaffer R, Jaffer R 1990 The WHO-CBR approach: programme on ideology – some lessons from the CBR experience in Punjab, Pakistan. In: Thorburn M, Marfo K (eds) Practical approaches to childhood disability in developing countries. Project Seredec, Newfoundland and 3D Projects, Jamaica, West Indies, pp. 321–340

Jonsson T 1994 OMAR in rehabilitation: a guide on operations, monitoring, and analysis of results. United Nations Development Program, Interregional Program for Disabled People, Washington, DC

Kaufman S, Becker G 1986 Stroke: health care on the periphery. Social Science and Medicine 22(9): 983–989

Kay E, Salzman A 1994 Volunteer PTs in developing nations. PT Magazine of Physical Therapy 2(10: 52–56

Kay E, Dunleavy K 1996, Community-based rehabilitation: an international model. Pediatric Physical Therapy 8: 117–121

King M 1966 Medical care in developing countries. Oxford University Press, Lusaka

Leavitt R 1992 Disability and rehabilitation in rural Jamaica: an ethnographic study. Fairleigh Dickinson University Press Rutherford, NJ

Marfo K S, Walker B 1986 Childhood disability in developing countries: issues in habilitation and special education. Praeger, New York

Mbise A, Kysela G 1990 Developing appropriate screening and assessment instruments: the case of Tanzania. In:

Thorburn M, Marfo K (eds) Practical approaches to childhood disability in developing countries. Project Seredec, Newfoundland and 3D Projects, Jamaica, West Indies, pp. 263–284

Mesa-Lago C 1992 Health care for the poor in Latin America and the Caribbean. Pan American Health Organization and Inter-American Foundation. PAHO Scientific Publication No. 539 Washington DC

Miles M 1990 The 'community base' in rehabilitation planning: key or gimmick? In: Thorburn M, Marfo K (eds) Practical approaches to childhood disability in developing countries. Project Seredec, Newfoundland and 3D Projects, Jamaica, West Indies, pp. 287–302

Momm K, Koenig A 1989 Disabled Persons Bulletin. Geneva, Switzerland, International Labor Office, No. 1

Nagler M 1992 Perspectives on disability. H Markets Research, Palo Alto, CA

O'Toole B 1990 Community-based rehabilitation: the Guyana evaluation project. In: Thorburn M, Marfo K (eds) Practical approaches to childhood disability in developing countries. Project Seredec, Newfoundland and 3D Projects, Jamaica, West Indies, pp. 341–366

PAHO 1993 Development and strengthening of local health systems in the transformation of national health systems: the rehabilitation services. PAHO/WHO, Washington, DC

PAHO 1994 Health conditions in the Americas. World Health Organization, Washington, DC

PAHO/WHO 1994 Situational analysis of disabilities and rehabilitation in the English speaking Caribbean. World Health Organization, Washington, DC

Peat M 1993 International centre for the advancement of CBR. Queen's University, Kingston, Ontario

Peat M, Shahani M (n.d.) Community based rehabilitation: international perspectives. Queen's University, Kingston, Ontario

Periquet A 1984 Community based rehabilitation services: the experience of Bacolod, Phillipines and the Asia Pacific region. Monograph No. 26. World Rehabilitation Fund, New York

Sanders G 1986 Lower limb amputations: a guide to rehabilitation. F A Davis, Philadelphia, PA

Savilios-Rothchild C 1970 The sociology and social psychology of disability and rehabilitation. Random House, New York

Smilkstein G Mendis P, Sanghavi S, Campbell J B, Kamwendo K 1984 The role of physical therapists in primary care in the developing world. Clinical Management 4(1): 24–27

Tappen F 1968 Massage techniques: a case method approach. Macmillan, New York

Tarimo E, Creese A (eds) 1990 Achieving health for all by the year 2000. WHO, Geneva, Switzerland

Thorburn M 1994 Roles and relationships of CBR services in the community. Presented at the Asia Regional Symposium on Results and Evaluation in CBR, Bangalore, India. December 5–7

Thorburn M, Marfo K 1990 Practical approaches to childhood disability in developing countries: insights from experience and research. Project Seredec, Newfoundland and 3D Projects, Jamaica, West Indies

Torrey F F, Smith D, Wise H 1973 The family health worker revisited: a five year follow-up. American Journal of Public Health 63(1): 71–74

UN 1981 Integration of disabled persons into community life. UN Publication No. E.81.IV.I. UN, New York

UNESCO 1994 CBR: for and with people with disabilities – a joint position paper. International Labor Organization/ UNESCO/WHO, Paris, France

UNICEF 1995 The state of the world's children. UNICEF, New York, NY

Werner D 1983 Project PROJIMO, a village run rehabilitation program for disabled children in western Mexico. Hesperian Foundation, Palo Alto, CA

Werner D 1987 Disabled village children: a guide to community health workers, rehabilitation workers, and families. Hesperian Foundation, Palo Alto, CA

Westbrook V L, Pennay M 1993 Attitudes towards disabilities in multicultural society. Social Science and Medicine 36(5): 615–623

World Health Organization 1968 Training manual of medical assistants and similar personnel. Technical Report Series No. 385. WHO, Geneva

World Health Organization 1981a Disability prevention and rehabilitation. Technical Report Series No. 668. WHO, Geneva

World Health Organization 1981b World health: international year of disabled persons. WHO, Geneva

World Health Organization 1984 World health: rehabilitation for all. WHO, Geneva

World Health Organization 1987 The community health worker: working guide, guidelines for training, guidelines for adaptation. WHO, Geneva

World Health Organization/UNICEF 1978 Report of the international conference on PHC (Alma-Ata, USSR). WHO, Geneva

Wright B 1983 Physical disability: a psychosocial approach. Harper and Row, New York

Yee H 1989 Training of rehabilitation persons in Micronesia. Presented at the Annual American Physical Therapy Association Meeting, Nashville, Tennessee

Young J, Garro L 1982 Variations in the choice of treatment in two Mexican communities. Social Science and Medicine 16: 1453–1465

Zaman S, Munir S 1990 Meeting the challenge of implementing services for handicapped children in Bangladesh. In: Thorburn M, Marfo K, (eds) Practical approaches to childhood disability in developing countries. Project Seredec, Newfoundland and 3D Projects, Jamaica, West Indies, pp. 161–175

Zola I 1982 Missing pieces: a chronicle of living with a disability. Temple University Press, Philadelphia, PA

10

International classification of impairments, disabilities and handicaps (ICIDH): a universal framework

Karin Schumacher

INTRODUCTION

This chapter will introduce the World Health Organization's (WHO) *International Classification of Impairments, Disabilities and Handicaps* (ICIDH) (WHO 1980), a document that has the potential to help with the daunting task of understanding the spectrum of human disablement. It is relevant to all nations and peoples. The ICIDH comprises a conceptual model and an extensive classification of disablement, both of which apply across cultures. 'Disablement' is an umbrella term used in the ICIDH to include three identified experiences, namely impairment, disability and handicap. Discussion will include background and a description of the model, distinction among the three experiences, an overview of the coding (classification) system, and current application examples. In addition, discussion of the ongoing revision process and a brief comparison with other models will be presented, as well as resources for further exploration of these complex topics.

Disablement issues

What is 'disablement'? Is it a state of being? a status? a stereotype? an experience? a dynamic process? A further question is, 'Who defines the value of disablement?' The answers to these questions will be expressed in as many different ways as there are responses. Furthermore, interpretation of these varied responses by others will reveal as many different perspectives again as responders. Should these questions be posed

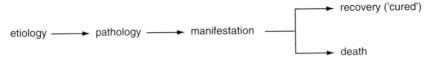

Fig. 10.1 The medical model of disease.

in different cultures, or even to similarly trained rehabilitation workers within one culture, one would still receive a mixture of responses.

Ramifications for health care practice and social policy of using disablement concepts for which there is no universally recognized understanding are enormous and challenging. They can be seen in the disparate array of medical and rehabilitation practices, programs, educational curricula, social policies, and laws throughout the world. In addition to these often positive yet insufficient approaches to disablement issues, there is still lingering – and in some places pervasive – discrimination against those with physical and mental capacities different from the majority.

Within the past 30 years, significant progress has been made in beginning to clarify the consequences of disease, injury and genetic disorder on individuals and on society. This effort has allowed examination of how, why and when intervention may be possible – or desirable – to alter any of these consequences which can limit the quality of life of the individuals experiencing them.

One example of an intervention targeting discrimination against those with disabilities can be found in the USA. In 1992, the United States passed the controversial and revolutionary Americans with Disabilities Act (ADA), with the aim of ensuring equality in all areas of US society, especially in employment and community access. The act and its enforcement continue to be challenged, both in and out of courts of law, but it is widely acknowledged 'to be a start'.

THE ICIDH

Background

The ICIDH is intended to provide a universal framework for understanding the consequences of disease, injury and disorder. From this framework will emerge an improved capacity to compare disablement meaningfully across cultures, from demographic, statistical, social, legal and medico-rehabilitative perspectives. The ICIDH can be seen not only as the 'disablement model', but also as a 'consequence model' (G Swanson, personal communication, 1994), as opposed to the medical model.

The medical model of disease, as shown in Figure 10.1, explains the usual sequence of events in acute ill health as a simple, linear chain from cause to either recovery or death. Until the mid-20 century, most formal systems of health and medical care involved treatment of injuries and infectious diseases, with a goal of full recovery or cure. Those born with congenital deformities either died young or lived out their lives in socially constricted and stigmatic ways (as 'beggars', 'cripples', 'village idiots', 'welfare burdens' . . . and so on) (Leavitt 1992). It was accepted that people with amputations or obvious paralyses could not assume usual family or societal roles and would need to be cared for, if not inhumanely left to suffer 'natural' complications that often led to an early death. Unfortunately, this situation still exists in many parts of the world.

Later in the 20th century, following two world wars, booming population growth, spectacular advances in medical technology, and a steadily increasing life expectancy (at least in the West), the scenario of health care needs began to change. People with infectious diseases were often no longer doomed to die, nor were those with disabling injuries automatically confined to institutions without meaningful work or activity for the rest of their lives. Surgical and pharmaceutical advances increased survival rates, but many of the survivors left with a disability were not guaranteed an acceptable quality of life – the availability of social and financial resources did not match their needs.

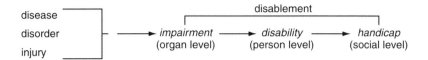

Fig. 10.2   The disablement model. (WHO 1980)

By the middle of the 20th century, there was a clear predominance of chronic disease in the more industrialized societies of the world, and a steadily rising incidence of them in less developed countries. With this evolution came the recognition that WHO's *International Classification of Diseases* (ICD), in use since the late 19th century as a standard disease reference worldwide, was ineffective for chronic conditions, which were characteristically nonfatal yet also not amenable to medical 'cure'. The ICD is based on the medical model, but changing circumstances indicated a need for additional resources to clarify the aftermath of nonfatal episodes, namely a 'consequence model'.

In 1976, the WHO commissioned the development of a companion classification to the ICD which would be devoted to clarifying and classifying the consequences of disease or disorder. A trial document was published in 1980, the *International Classification of Impairments, Disabilities and Handicaps* (ICIDH) (WHO 1980). It has now been translated into 14 languages and distributed around the world. Its usefulness has been tested in areas ranging from statistical data gathering to clinical decision making. The United Nations, including WHO, and many governments are employing the ICIDH in efforts to increase the body of usable knowledge about the disablement process.

Description

There are two major components of the ICIDH. The first is a conceptualization of disablement, and the second is an extensive numerical coding, or taxonomy, of each of its three domains.

As the term is used, disablement comprises three distinct 'planes of experience'. These domains theoretically encompass the spectrum of possible consequences on the life of an individual following a disease, disorder or injury. As defined in the ICIDH, the domains are *impairment*, *disability* and *handicap*. Figure 10.2 depicts the disablement, or consequence, model, as described in the ICIDH.

A. The conceptual model

The planes of experience as defined in the ICIDH are:

1. *Impairment*: 'In the context of health experience, any loss or abnormality of psychological, physiological or anatomical structure or function.' An impairment is objective, observable, measurable and often the basis for a diagnosis. It occurs on an organ/system level. Examples include cardiac arrhythmia, muscle paralysis, joint contracture and absence of a limb.

2. *Disability*: 'In the context of health experience, any restriction or lack (resulting from an impairment) of ability to perform an activity in the manner or within the range considered normal (*sic*) for a human being.' A disability occurs on a whole-person level. Examples include insufficient cardiac endurance to climb steps, inability to walk or dress oneself, and emotional disturbance precluding useful social interaction.

3. *Handicap*: 'In the context of health experience, a disadvantage for a given individual, resulting from an impairment or a disability, that limits or prevents the fulfillment of a role that is normal [*sic*] (depending on age, sex, and social and cultural factors) for that individual.' It occurs on a societal level. Examples include confinement to one's home, a sparse social network and lack of a fulfilling occupation.

Although the original document presented handicap as an experience 'resulting from' an impairment or disability, almost all critics, and even the authors themselves, now describe handicap in terms of an interaction between an individual and his or her environment (Badley 1987, Badley et al 1990). Acknowledgement that handicap causality is external, not internal, is almost universal at this point in the revision process, although there are numerous approaches to describing and coding this interaction (Bolduc 1991, Fougeyrollas 1988, Whiteneck 1992b). Thus, examples more appropriate to the current interpretation of handicap (correlated with the examples of handicap above) include lack of accessible public transportation, negative attitudes toward persons with impairments or disabilities, and discrimination in hiring.

Disablement is a term encompassing all three planes of experience. Table 10.1 lists some examples in terms appropriate to the experience of impairment, disability or handicap. Note that it is not necessary for a disability or a handicap to follow a related impairment, and that each domain can exist by itself. (See Table 10.2 for list of domains.)

A discipline-specific perspective

Within the range of medico-social services, different sectors fit better with one level of consequence than others. Figure 10.3 shows some common disciplines that intersect, either formally or informally, with people experiencing

Table 10.1 Examples of potential planes of experience following disease or disorder, (Schumacher, 1987)

Impairment	Disability	Handicap
C2 spinal lesion	Eating	Self-care/physical independence
Blindness	Seeing	Occupation/economic independence
Hemiplegia	Walking	Mobility
Amelia: 1 toe	(None)	(None)
Eschar (history of burn)	(None)	Social integration
(None) history of mental illness	(None)	Economic independence/ social integration

each plane of disablement. Each sector of society has the potential to prevent or minimize one or more particular experience within the spectrum of disablement. There can be considerable overlap among sectors as they intervene at the three levels.

Not only can there be overlap, but some service sectors have the potential to intervene at all three levels. Public health services are appropriate at each level and especially important in secondary and tertiary disability prevention. Rehabilitation services also encompass all three experiences.

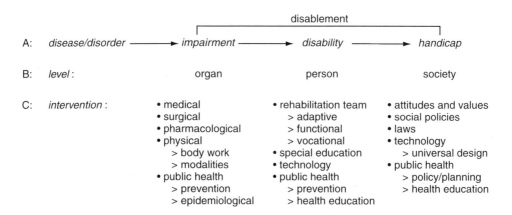

Fig. 10.3 The intervention model.

Evolution of thought

Since 1980, many modifications of the disablement model have been suggested. These include variations of the conceptual framework (new theories on the relationships within disablement), alternative names for the three domains, and major changes in the coding. Exploration of the relationships within disablement by numerous scholars has resulted in a variety of expanded ICIDH models and modified schemas, as well as other conceptual frameworks (Nagi 1991, Pope & Tarlov 1991). Some proponents of new naming feel the word 'handicap' perpetuates a negative stereotype or stigma of persons with impairments or disabilities. None of the variations refute the ICIDH's original premise, that of differentiation between internal characteristics of disablement (involving impairment and disability) and external ones (involving handicap).

Nagi model. The most common alternative model in use today is the Nagi model. Nagi uses the terms *functional limitation* for disability, and *disability* for handicap. Thus, in the Nagi model: pathology → impairment → functional limitation → disability. Functional limitation is of two types: function of an organ or part of the body (for example range of motion of a joint) and functional activities of a person (for example sitting, walking or eating). In this model, the interaction between an individual and the environment is termed a disability; the word handicap is not used.

Although Nagi's original studies on the nature of disability were published in the 1960s, and constituted an acknowledged resource for the authors of the ICIDH, it was not until after publication of the ICIDH that his theories became more widely discussed and debated within the rehabilitation and disability research community (Nagi 1991, Pope & Tarlov 1991, Guccione 1991, Jette 1994, 1989).

Classification. Another difference between the ICIDH and alternative models is the taxonomy or classification of the ICIDH. Only the ICIDH has a coding system to accompany its conceptual model. This advantage allows one to bring the model, at any domain level, into daily health care practice, using any of the ICIDH based survey or clinical instruments currently being tested. It also allows and encourages individuals to develop their own clinical application tools from the raw taxonomy of the three disablement experiences of the ICIDH.

Modified disablement model. Almost all ICIDH scholars at this time agree that disablement does not take place in a linear way and that the three domains can be mutually exclusive. Schumacher's (1987) simple triangular modification of the disablement model, seen in Figure 10.4, demonstrates a basic underlying interrelationship among the three planes more realistically than a linear format. Other modifications emerged in the 1990s.

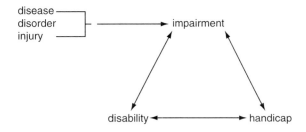

Fig. 10.4   Modified disablement model. (Schumacher 1987)

B. Taxonomy of disablement

The second aspect of the ICIDH is a unique classification system, one for each domain of disablement. As such, the ICIDH belongs to a large family of WHO-endorsed health and medical taxonomies, along with the ICD and others. The organization of the impairment, disability and handicap codes and their use in potential applications of the ICIDH will be briefly described here. To increase understanding, further exploration is recommended through the resources listed at the end of this chapter.

The impairment and disability codes each comprise nine basic 2-digit categories; for ease of reference, these will be referred to as the *I-code* and the *D-code*. Each category can be further subclassified, up to a maximum of 4 (I-code) or 5 (D-code) digits. The handicap section (*H-code*) comprises seven 1-digit categories, or

Table 10.2 Coding categories in ICIDH

Impairment domain (exteriorized)	Disability domain (objectified)	Handicap domain (socialized)
Intellectual	Behavior	Orientation
Other psychological	Communication	Physical independence
Language	Personal care	Mobility
Aural	Locomotor	Occupation
Ocular	Body disposition	Social integration
Visceral	Dexterity	Economic self-sufficiency
Skeletal	Situational	Other
Disfiguring	Particular skill	
Generalized/sensory & other	Other activity restrictions	
(1009 items)	(332 items)	(72 items)

Box 10.1   Characteristics of impairment, disability and handicap (ICIDH)

Impairment characteristics
At the organ/system level
- losses, anomalies or abnormalities
- temporary or permanent, reversible or irreversible
- represents *exteriorization* of a pathological state
- threshold phenomenon (i.e., present or not present; no grading of degree of impairment possible)
  Examples of major and subclassifications:
  a. 24   **impairment of attention**
     24.0 distractibility
     24.6 impairment of alertness
  b. 72   **spastic paralysis of more than one limb**
     72.0 complete spastic paralysis of upper and lower limbs on same side, with involvement of speech
     72.6 complete paralysis of all four limbs

Disability characteristics
At the person level
- result of impairment, or response to it, especially psychologically
- excesses or deficiencies of customarily expected activity performance and behavior
- temporary or permanent, reversible or irreversible
- represents *objectification* of an impairment
  Examples of a major and a subclassification:
  46   **transfer disability**
     46.0 transfer from lying
     46.1 transfer from sitting
- Not a threshold phenomenon; may be rated by degree via two scales within the disability section: level of severity, and outcome prognosis

- Severity rating scale: 10 levels describing amount of human aid or assist by device needed, represented by a fourth digit
  Example of severity rating:
  46.13 sitting transfer – needs assist
- Outcome rating scale – 10 levels describing probable future situation related to improvement or lack of it, represented by a fifth digit
  Example of outcome rating:
  46.131 sitting transfer – needs assist; has improvement potential

Handicap characteristics
At the societal level
- represents interaction between individual and the environment
- discordance between individual's performance and expectations of group of which he or she is a part
- disadvantage imposed by the value attached to an individual's situation or experience
- represents the *socialization* of an impairment or disability
- includes six survival roles in society, or key dimensions in which individuals are expected to be competent (see Table 10.2).
  Within each survival role there are eight levels of competence. Examples
  a. 2   **physical independence handicap:**
     2.1 aided independence
  b. 5   **social integration handicap:**
     5.8 socially isolated

dimensions, that can be further classified with 1 extra digit. Individuals are rated in all seven handicap dimensions to produce a 'handicap profile'. Rules for classification and subclassification are given in the ICIDH document and in other references (WHO 1993, 1980). See Table 10.1 for a list of categories or dimensions in each section.

Characteristics of each experience differ. Box 10.1 gives a brief overview of the characteristics of each experience, and a few code examples, which may assist the reader with this taxonomy.

A helpful resource in learning the ICIDH, understanding the conceptual differences among the planes, and becoming efficient and accurate in coding is available in software. Code-IDH is an automated, interactive training tool currently being used in some places in the USA. A user's manual is available (See Further Resources, p. 123).

Integrating disablement domains in rehabilitation

Rehabilitation professionals have important roles to play at each level of disablement. Figure 10.5 demonstrates the primary approaches that physical, occupational and speech therapists might use to intervene at each level. Traditionally, therapists have been trained to affect the impairment level with varying physical treatments. For example a muscle strain may be treated with heat and massage to relieve pain and promote healing. As the professions matured, training a patient to adapt to and compensate for a permanent impairment or disability became as important a skill for a therapist as providing treatments for impairments. For example a therapist may train a patient to integrate the originally painful 'phantom sensation' of an amputated limb into a helpful sensory clue while learning a new prosthetic gait.

It is only in recent years that the significant roles of rehabilitation therapists have become clearer and more highly valued in issues related to the third domain, handicap. Especially in countries with a shortage of certified, trained therapists, these contributions at a societal level can have a great effect on the lives of persons experiencing disablement, even though many have never had the opportunity to receive individual therapy.

impairment
- alternative medicine
- manual therapies
- neuro-facilitation
- physical modalities
  (electro-, hydro-,
  thermal)
- splinting/taping
- traditional healing
  (indigenous)

disability
- adaptive equipment
- functional training
- patient education
- orthotics
- prosthetics
- technology assistance
  (high or low)
- therapeutic exercise

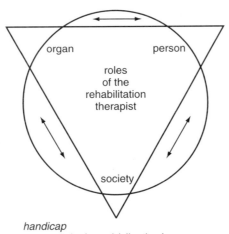

handicap
- community-based (client) advocacy
- practical clinical approaches
  e.g. community-based rehabilitation (CBR)
- consultation to: architecture, business, engineering,
  industry, government
- environmental modification
- public education

Fig. 10.5   Integrating disablement domains in rehabilitation. (Modified from Schumacher 1994)

The public health role of the rehabilitationist is very evident in countries without formal rehabilitation professional training programs and is also taking on increasing importance in countries with established professional training. In the USA, proposed health care reform and managed care systems are forcing more therapists into public advocacy, both to ensure access to rehabilitation services and to work alongside consumer-driven initiatives. These include the international Independent Living Movement (ILM), laws protecting the rights of persons with disabilities, and promotion of 'universal design.' Universal design is architectural or technical design which is suitable for the whole population and which does not draw attention as being accommodating to persons with disabilities (for example a broad, shallow, sloping entrance to a public building).

Application

The ICIDH is a tool from which measurement instruments may be developed according to need. Use of the ICIDH has been international and broad based, cutting across scientific and clinical disciplines in many countries. Fields in which the document has been tested and applied include health care planning, policy and practice, health care statistics, social security, social care and welfare, employment, special education, disability research, rehabilitation evaluation and outcomes. Most of the work in research and application so far has been done in Europe, although there is an increasing amount emerging in North American literature.

Examples in which the ICIDH has been used in the rehabilitation field are many:

• The United Nations (UN) began collecting international data on the incidence and prevalence of impairments and disabilities in the 1980s after developing a survey instrument based on the ICIDH (Chamie 1989). The resulting database compares disability statistics across and within countries. The data have been used in some countries as a basis for developing new and more relevant rehabilitation policy. A code book and user's guide is available (see Further Resources, p. 123).

• Registration of persons with disabilities using the ICIDH codes has been carried out in at least eight European countries: Austria, Belgium, France, the UK, Luxembourg, the Netherlands, Spain and West Germany. Comparison of country statistics on disablement has been difficult in the past due to the lack of registration systems by most countries (the USA and Canada included) and the absence of common terms and definitions related to disablement.

• Whiteneck et al (1992a) developed the Craig Handicap Assessment and Reporting Technique (CHART), at Craig Rehabilitation Hospital in Denver, Colorado, USA, primarily for patients with spinal cord injury. Based on the ICIDH, it provides a profile of a person's present interaction with the environment, given his or her impairments and disabilities, thus clarifying the likely external societal impact (handicap) on the individual.

• Nieuwenhuijsen et al (1991) developed and researched modified methods of assessment of older people with blindness using the severity scale in the disability section of the ICIDH.

• For one major private USA insurer, payment for rehabilitation therapies (occupational, physical, respiratory, speech, cardiac) is based on the disability codes of the ICIDH (Swanson 1993, Blue Cross of California, 1990).

• In rehabilitation training, some physical therapy schools are including the ICIDH concepts in curricula; they have been incorporated into the Dutch schools since the 1980s.

• Schumacher (1992) described the use of the concepts to teach student therapists assessment and treatment approaches to stroke patients.

• Nieuwenhuijsen, et al (1996) used the ICIDH in a study of prevention of office work-related pain and functional difficulties. They concluded the ICIDH can be a useful tool in rehabilitation clinical decision making.

• The US Department of Education has begun to use the ICIDH to back-code disabilities related to special education, using data from several national surveys (WESTAT 1993).

• The provincial government of Quebec, Canada, had integrated the ICIDH into public policy by 1987, naming its project *On Equal Terms*. The intent of this policy was to eliminate the disadvantage (handicap) experienced by persons with disabilities living in Quebec, and equalize opportunity for all citizens.

• The US government formally supported WHO's effort to promote and study the ICIDH in 1993 when WHO named the National Center for Health Statistics (NCHS), a federal agency, as the official US liaison for the ICIDH. Prior to that time, several researchers and rehabilitationists in the USA had already applied the ICIDH to their work: special education, visually impaired students (Frey 1988); occupational therapy, personal care (Nieuwenhuijsen 1985); physical therapy, documentation (Schumacher 1987).

In 1999, the newest of the WHO classifications, the ICIDH, remains largely unknown in the USA rehabilitation community, despite a steadily growing number of presentations and published papers. The Nagi model and the 1993 Institute of Medicine model of disablement (Pope and Tarlov, 1991) have received more conceptual support in the USA physical therapy research literature (Guccione 1991, Jette 1989). In other parts of the world, rehabilitation practitioners may find that their colleagues are more familiar with the ICIDH, and even more, are using the concepts and terms of impairment, disability and handicap in consistent, reliable ways.

Limitations and revision of the ICIDH

It would be misleading to discuss the ICIDH as it is now without emphasizing the dynamic process of revision that has been an evolving international project for more than 15 years. In the 1980s, health care policy experts, medical and rehabilitation practitioners, and social science researchers began to critically examine aspects of the ICIDH that were unclear, inconsistent or in disagreement with established values within the disability community. These discussions and papers emphasized the need for revision, and were the beginning of an extensive body of literature about the ICIDH that now totals more than 1500 items.

Among the problems are the following:

• There are inconsistencies in the codes, which are not seen as complete or always in the appropriate place in the taxonomy. The impairment code is missing some items, and some groupings are not as useful as they could be. For example, there is no separate section in the I-code for the nervous system; rather motor control is listed in the 'musculo-skeletal impairment', and sensory impairment is in the last impairment category, 'other'.

• The distinction between impairment and disability is not clear to some, for there are multiple levels of 'function'. One can describe cellular function within an organ, function of the organ itself, function of a body system of which the organ is a part, or functioning of the whole human being. For example, in a person with cerebral palsy, there can be impaired tone, which affects the function of muscle tissue, while disabled grasping or dressing affect whole-person activity functioning. Thus, impairments are usually related to 'functions' at a physiological or anatomical level, while disabilities relate to 'functions' of the whole human being, or substantial units or parts thereof.

• Another example relates to a person with an absent limb. The 'function' of an amputated upper limb can be described in either musculo-skeletal terms (impairment) or in human activity terms (disability), depending on the intent of the descriptor. A prosthetist will be concerned with the impaired bio-mechanical leverage which must be compensated for, while an occupational therapist will be more concerned with the feeding disability the person will need to overcome, with or without a prosthesis. However, it is fair to state that one cannot come to a good understanding of the ICIDH concepts by simply knowing their definitions; one must read thoroughly the discussions and descriptions of the concepts and their interactions within the whole model before presenting thoughtful criticism.

• Another concern of critics is some overlap between the *International Classification of Diseases* (ICD-10) and the impairment code of the ICIDH. However, this overlap can be seen as a useful bridge for understanding how acute conditions can lead to chronic conditions and resultant experiences of disablement. The ICD and the ICIDH are intended to be used as companion resources and references.

• The handicap concept has been criticized by those who interpret the ICIDH's original description as too internally based, that is, too focused on the individual instead of the environment with which he or she interacts. The original linear form of the model (Fig. 10.2) leads one to infer that handicap is a result of impairment and disability, something that the model actually disputes if one studies the codes as they are written. The handicap section is likely to be the one most extensively revised. In anticipation, the Quebec Committee of the Canadian Society for the ICIDH has proposed a detailed classification of environmental factors (Whiteneck & Fougeyrollas 1995).

• Titles of the ICIDH subsections have come under steady attack for being negative by nature, viz. 'dis-abilities' and 'handicap', both words connoting the idea of absence or abnormality. Revision proposals gaining popularity include changing the second classification from one of 'disabilities' to one of 'abilities'. The third classification, rather than being one of 'handicap' or 'disadvantage' would be called what it actually describes, that is, the level of an individual's participation in society. The Canadian Society for the ICIDH has taken the lead in proposing major changes to the H-code, including its name, definition and purpose.

In the Netherlands, the ICIDH has been used extensively in physical rehabilitation; the Dutch have proposed a major revision of the D-code (WCC 1995).

The Dutch Collaborating Center for the ICIDH (WCC) was the first government-supported agency to collect and reference the rapidly growing body of ICIDH literature in a comprehensive manner (WCC *List of References in Relation to the ICIDH*, 1992; for address see Further Resources, p. 123; regular updates available). WCC is an international leader in the study and application of the ICIDH, and it continues to enjoy strong support from the Dutch government.

Collaborating centers

In 1993, the ICIDH was re-published with a modified foreword, and is no longer bearing the 'trial basis' qualification. At that time, WHO also approved three collaborating centers for the ICIDH, in addition to the existing Dutch Center, in order to organize and streamline the revision process, and to allow as much international participation as can be accommodated. These three collaborating centers are located in France, North America (combined Canada and USA) and Sweden (see Further Resources, p. 123).

WHO has divided the revision into three focus areas, delegating primary responsibilities to each collaborating center as described below. The French collaborative center is the focal point for revision of the impairment section, the Dutch center is focused on the disability section and the North American center is working on revising the handicap section. Each center is responsible for gathering input and developing consensus both on conceptual aspects of the model and on specific recommendations for code changes.

In addition, a special collaborative center, the Nordic Center in Sweden, was established by WHO to explicitly examine and compare the ICD-10 to the ICIDH, especially to the I-code.

Special issues that need further development, such as ICIDH's applicability to children, mental health, sensory and perceptual problems, and movement/mobility functions, are also assigned by WHO to the collaborative centers (France: sensation, perception and communication; Netherlands: mobility; North America: mental health, behavior and development). Input related to these issues is still sought from users of the ICIDH. Comments and questions may be sent to the respective collaborative centers (see Further Resources p. 123).

WHO has also established a sequence of yearly international meetings related to specific revision topics. Through these multidisciplinary conferences each year, and ongoing communication among all those involved, the process moves slowly toward the goal of publishing *ICIDH II.*

CONCLUSION: A VISION FOR THE FUTURE

This chapter has introduced a universal model of disablement, applicable across all cultures and social systems. Its focus is on the common characteristics of human functioning in society, and its potential is very promising.

At this time, the global community of disability rights activists, rehabilitation professionals and research scholars is far from consensus about where this exciting and creative process will lead. But, at the very least, stimulation of thought in this arena has led to actively challenging long-held assumptions that have shaped the culture of disability in this world. Deeper understanding of disablement can lead only to increased respect for the vastness and beauty of human variability. As a result, the human spirit is raised, releasing energy and creativity to advance the quality of life for all humanity.

ADDENDUM

WHO's ICIDH revision process is ongoing, through the work of the four international collaboration centers. The current version, *ICIDH-2: International Classification of Impairments, Activities and Participation,* known as the ICIDH-2 Beta-1 Draft, was field tested during 1997 and early 1998 in Canada, the Netherlands, the United Kingdom and the USA.

The basic model of the ICIDH remains intact, but several significant changes were made for the field trial draft. First, the section on 'Disabilities' was changed to 'Activities' and the 'Handicaps' section was changed to 'Participation.' Both new terms are considered neutral and avoid negative connotations of the previously used terms, which was a primary criticism of the ICIDH. Negative circumstances within each of the renamed domains are now denoted by 'activity limitations' and 'participation restrictions' respectively.

Second, a new section was added, 'Contextual Factors,' to further qualify all three of the original domains. Contextual factors comprise two areas, 'environmental factors,' considered to be external to the individual, and 'personal factors,' considered to be intrinsic to the individual. Interaction with both groups of factors determines the level of 'participation' (formerly 'handicap') an individual experiences.

Finally, changes are being made to the codes in each of the three domains, including additions, deletions and modification of current categories. Publication of ICIDH-II (the acronym will remain the same for ease of reference) is now targeted for the year 2001.

FURTHER RESOURCES

ICIDH Collaborating Centers
FRANCE
Annick Deveau PhD
Director, CTNERHI
236 bis, rue de Tolbiac
75013 Paris, France

NETHERLANDS
Maryke W. de Kleijn-de-Vrankrijker PhD
WHO Collaborating Center for the ICIDH National Institute of Public Health and the Environment (RIVM)
P.O. Box 1
3720 BA Bilthoven
The Netherlands

NORTH AMERICA
Gerry E. Hendershot PhD
Deputy Director for Science
Division of Health Interview Statistics, NCHS
6525 Belcrest Road, Room 850
Hyattsville, Maryland 20782 USA

SWEDEN
Anna Christina Nilsson MD
Department of Social Medicine
University Hospital
S-751-85 Uppsala, Sweden

To purchase ICIDH
1. World Health Organization (WHO)
   20, Avenue Appia
   Ch-1211 Geneva 27
   Switzerland

2. USA WHO Publications Center
   49 Sheridan Ave.
   Albany, New York, 12210 USA

Newsletter/Network
ICIDH and Environmental factors International Network

Canadian Society for the ICIDH
P.O. Box 225
Lac St Charles, Quebec
G3G 3C1 Canada

Software
Code-IDH, including training manual, available from:
Swanson and Company
2734 E. Broadway, Suite 7
Long Beach, California 90803 USA
Telephone: 800-984-8489;
Facsimile: 310-439-2059

REFERENCES

Badley E M 1987 The ICIDH: format, application in different settings and distinction between disability and handicap. International Disability Studies 9:(3) 122–125

Badley E M, Tennant A, Wood P H N 1990 The assessment of physical independence handicap: experience in a community disablement survey. International Disability Studies 12(2): 47–53

Blue Cross of California. 1990 Classification of out-patient services: economic aspects. June

Chamie M 1989 Survey design strategies for the study of disability. World Health Statistics Quarterly 42(3): 122–140

Fougeyrollas P 1988 Research project on the third level of the ICIDH: the handicap. Quebec Committee on the ICIDH Bulletin 1(2): 20–22

Frey W E 1988 Functional outcome: assessment and evaluation. In: Delisa J A (ed) Rehabilitation medicine principles and practice. Lippincott, Philadelphia

Guccione A A 1991 Physical therapy diagnosis and the relationship between impairments and function. Physical Therapy 71(7): 499–504

ICIDH-2: International Classification of Impairments, Activities and Participation. A manual of dimensions of disablement and Health. 1997 Beta-1 draft for field trials. World Health Organization. Geneva

Jette A M 1989 Diagnosis and classification by physical therapists: a special communication. Physical Therapy 69(11): 967–969

Leavitt R L 1992 Disability and rehabilitation in rural Jamaica: an ethnographic study. Associated University Presses, Cranbury, NJ

Nagi S Z 1991 Disability concepts revisited; implications for prevention. In: Pope A M, Tarlov A R (eds) Disability in America: toward a national agenda for prevention. National Academy Press, Washington, DC

Nieuwenhuijsen E R 1985 The international classification of impairments, disabilities and handicaps: a method of determining personal care needs for the severely physically disabled. University of Michigan School of Public Health, Ann Arbor

Nieuwenhuijsen E R, Frey W E, Crews J E 1991 Measuring small gains using the ICIDH severity of disability scale: assessment practice among older people who are blind. International Disability Studies 13(2): 29–33

Nieuwenhuijsen E, Marcoux B, Krause V 1996. The 12 golden tips for office workers. Center for Occupational Rehabilitation and Health. The University of Michigan Health System. Ann Arbor

On Equal Terms 1987. The social integration of handicapped persons. A challenge for everyone. Office des personnes

handicappes du Quebec. Quebec City, Canada. (Also available in French.)

Pope A M, Tarlov A R (eds) 1991 Disability in America: toward a national agenda for prevention. Report of a study undertaken by the committee on a national agenda for the prevention of disabilities. Institute of Medicine, Division of Health Promotion and Disease Prevention. National Academy Press, Washington, DC

Schumacher K 1987 The international classification of impairments, disabilities and handicaps (ICIDH): relevance to physical therapy and rehabilitation. In: Proceedings of the XI World Congress of Physical Therapy, Book II. Link Printing, Sydney

Schumacher K 1992 Classification of stroke problems and the use of standard terminology in persons with stroke. American Physical Therapy Association, Alexandra, Virginia. Neurology Report 15: 4–8

Schumacher K. 1994 Integrating disablement domains in rehabilitation. In: Training Manual for the International Classification of Impairments, Disabilities and Handicaps. US Department of Health and Human Services. Public Health Service. National Center for Health Statistics (NCHS), Rockville, Maryland USA

Swanson G 1993 The value of ICIDH codes in describing the benefit of therapy services. Swanson and Associates. Long Beach, California USA (Unpublished paper).

WCC 1995 Proposal for adaptation of the classification of (dis)abilities of the ICIDH. WCC/Collaborating Center for the ICIDH, Zoetermeer, Netherlands

WESTAT 1993 Draft report on extant datasets and disability classifications. US Department of Education Contract No. HS92035001. WESTAT, Rockville, MD

Whiteneck G G, Fougeyrollas P 1995 Environmental factors and ICIDH. Task force position paper. NAC-CSICIDH-QCICIDH Meeting. Quebec City, September 22

Whiteneck G G, Charlifue S W, Gerhart K A et al 1992a Guide for use of the CHART: Craig handicap assessment and reporting technique. Craig Rehabilitation Hospital, Denver, Colorado USA

Whiteneck G G, Charlifue S W, Gerhart K A et al 1992b Quantifying handicap: a new measure of long term rehabilitation outcomes. Archives of Physical Medicine and Rehabilitation 73: 519–526

World Health Organization 1980 International classification of impairments, disabilities and handicaps. WHO, Geneva, Switzerland

World Health Organization 1993 International classification of impairment, disabilities and handicaps. (ICIDH) WHO, Geneva, Switzerland

11

Appropriate assistive technology

Jean Anne Zollars
Patricia Ruppelt

Throughout the history of humankind technology has influenced, guided and enhanced our lives from the invention of the wheel to automobiles and computers. For people with disabilities (PWD), assistive technology, or technology designed to enhance the life of PWD, can have a critical role in helping to accomplish tasks and access more life opportunities when physical impairments prevent them from doing so. The use of assistive technology is often the first step towards personal freedom. It can foster independence in everyday personal and community functional activities, or, at minimum, can mean that less assistance from another person is required. Assistive technology for a PWD includes tools to improve access to family and community participation, or to improve mobility, dexterity, communication, and basic bodily functions such as breathing, eating and elimination. In addition, as PWD continue to make political changes to gain access to basic human rights, such as equal opportunities to employment, they must become increasingly visible and vocal in their communities. Assistive technology such as a wheelchair may be a requirement for getting out of the house and into the community. Only then can individuals join with others to organize in support of their rights.

Assistive technology always needs to be appropriately designed or chosen to meet the consumer's unique needs. Appropriate technology, whether it be in developed or developing countries, implies the use of inventive know-how to address problems of everyday life with equipment and techniques that work well in the context of the available local, community and personal resources, the person's functional needs, environment, culture, and lifestyle. Appropriate assistive technology may be very 'high-tech', using computers or expensive and difficult to manufacture materials, or 'low-tech', using more basic, readily available, less costly materials. Technology for PWD must be individualized; technology appropriate to one culture or person may not be appropriate to another.

Technology, if truly designed and distributed appropriately, is much more than just a piece of equipment – it is an ongoing creative and collaborative problem-solving process between those using the equipment and people who design and produce it. This can help to ensure the equipment's functional relevance and its continued usefulness. The more people allow themselves to journey into the complexities and possibilities of the evaluative and design process, the more appropriate the end product is likely to be for the person who needs it. This demands a spirit of curiosity, coupled with a desire to learn, expand, and challenge one's own creative problem-solving skills.

Some community based rehabilitation (CBR) programs and organizations of PWD believe that the provision of adaptive equipment reinforces the top-down, disempowering medical model of rehabilitation. They prefer to emphasize the social side of rehabilitation, such as education, jobs and skills training. In contrast, David Werner, in *Nothing About Us Without Us* (Werner 1998), comments that many programs for PWD in poor countries and communities *under*-emphasize the importance of the technological side of rehabilitation and that the lack of low-cost, appropriate mobility aids and assistive equipment is a major barrier to social integration – including schooling, jobs, and self-reliant living. These authors believe that programs must incorporate both appropriate assistive technology and the social aspect of rehabilitation. Neither alone is adequate; each enhances the other.

HOW PEOPLE GET WHAT THEY NEED

It is estimated that tens of millions of people in the world need some form of assistive technology, such as a wheelchair for mobility, but do not have any. A common response to the lack of available equipment in developing countries is for the developed world to send second-hand equipment like old and heavy wheelchairs, walkers, crutches, or braces. Although some of these devices, or parts of them, can be used, they only reach a fraction of PWD and most often the cast-off equipment is in perpetual need of repair. More typically, the equipment ends up in a storage room or heaped on top of a junk pile (Figs 11.1, 11.2). People living in the rough environmental conditions found through-

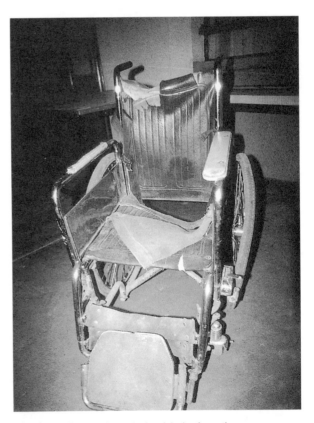

Fig. 11.1 Donated used wheelchairs from the industrialized world can be an inappropriate and unsafe solution to the pressing need for mobility in most of the world. Photo courtesy: Ralf Hotchkiss.

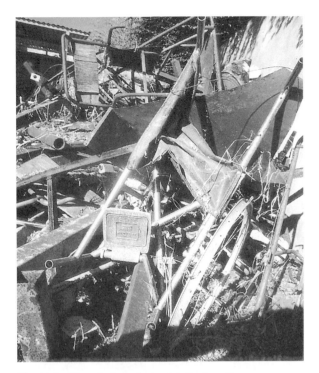

Fig. 11.2 Exported used wheelchairs from the industrialized world are often junked upon receipt since they are inappropriate for use in rough terrain and nearly impossible to repair. Photo courtesy: Ralf Hotchkiss.

out most of the world require mobility equipment that is far more durable and repairable than an old hand-me-down from the USA or Europe. A heavy, oversized wheelchair with thin tires will be difficult to push anywhere outside of a hospital hallway. Moreover, a poorly fitting seating system can cause pain and new postural problems. Orthoses not fit for an individual can further hinder the ability to walk, instead of enhancing independence.

In some situations, a PWD, or a friend or family member, will problem-solve a situation and come up with a solution. In developing countries, PWD have few role models or rehabilitation scripts to follow. In order to survive and to participate in family and community life, creativity and ingenuity are required in every aspect of life, including technological solutions. Ralf Hotchkiss, wheelchair rider and inventor, describes some differences between the problem-solving approaches in the industrialized

world in contrast to the developing world. 'When consumers in industrialized countries must solve technological problems they generally (1) look for ready-made solutions, (2) rely on "experts", or (3) seek a newer, advanced model . . . that will do the job. [In] under developed countries . . . they must show exceptional persistence and ingenuity to solve everyday problems. In the process, grass-roots inventors have come up with novel means of improving the lives of people with disabilities' (Hotchkiss 1998, p. 123).

Especially in the developing world, where financial constraints are considerable, the invention of low-tech equipment is especially important. For instance, building parallel bars or crutches from bamboo or tree branches is common (Fig. 11.3). In addition to using specially

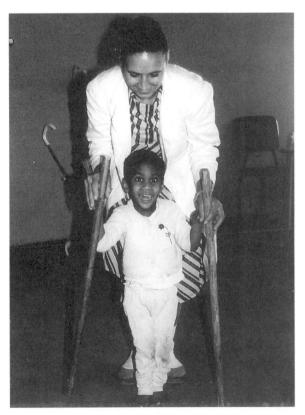

Fig. 11.3 An orphaned child in Ethiopia, who lives in the hospital, crawled on the floor until the use of wooden sticks/'Bobath poles' for mobility was suggested. Photo courtesy: Ronnie Leavitt.

designed wheelchairs, there are several common low-tech approaches for mobility. These can include such things as scooter boards, backpacks for carrying children with disabilities and use of horses or burros. Kelvin Frank, a 24-year-old man from Guyana, used two pillows for mobility after his spinal cord injury. Since dragging himself on the floor would result in skin breakdown, he would leap-frog on the floor from one pillow to another. Usually, a PWD has few choices, and the creative solution can be quite practical. Sometimes, ideal alternatives do present themselves. For example, after some time, Kelvin received a wheelchair produced in Trinidad and started local wheelchair production in his region. He recently traveled to San Francisco State University, USA, where he has learned basic wheelchair building.

CONSIDERATIONS FOR APPROPRIATE TECHNOLOGY

The person's functional requirements

Understanding the client's needs can be challenging, especially across cultures. It may seem obvious that the first step before acquiring technology is precisely understanding why the person needs a piece of technology. However, well-intentional therapists, engineers, or PWD often tend to jump to a solution before thoroughly looking at the problem or considering the client's goals.

The following story is from *Nothing About Us Without Us* (Werner 1998):

Mira, in rural Bangladesh, became paraplegic (paralyzed from waist down) as a result of fighting between religious groups in her village. In the hospital, a social worker gave her a[n imported] wheelchair from Wheels of Fortune. On the hospital floors, Mira learned to move about in her chair. But on returning to her village, she had problems. Traditionally, cooking was done at floor level on a cooking pot called a chula. Everyone ate sitting cross-legged on the floor. In her wheelchair, Mira was separated from her kitchen work and from the family at mealtime. For a while she sat in her chair without working; others served her food onto a board across the armrests. But Mira wanted to fit in better and to contribute more to family life. So she stopped using

her wheelchair and began dragging herself around the dirt floor on her hands and backside. Maybe it was not the best solution, she thought. (It could cause severe and infected pressure sores.) But it was better than the isolation of sitting in her wheelchair.

An answer to the need of village women like Mira was found at the Center for Rehabilitation of the Paralyzed in Dhaka, Bangladesh. The center is staffed and run mostly by spinal cord injured persons who seek solution to their own and other disabled persons' needs. They designed a 'low-rider' wheelchair or trolley to meet village women's need to cook and eat at ground level. First they created several working models. Then, in response to feedback and suggestions and different spinal cord injured villagers, they adapted and modified the design. The trolley can even be used as a toilet. (Werner 1998, p. 15) (Figs. 11.4, 11.5)

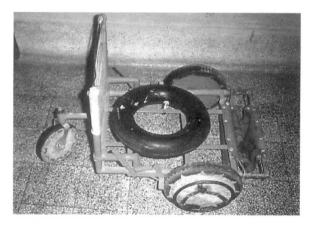

Fig. 11.4 A metal-frame, wood-wheel trolley in Bangladesh. The rubber tube serves as a cushion and also as a toilet seat. Photo courtesy: D. Werner.

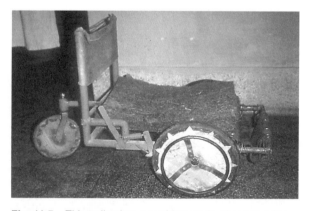

Fig. 11.5 This trolley has a cushion made of coconut fiber coated with rubber. Firm but spongy, it helps prevent pressure sores. Photo courtesy: D. Werner.

Another example of considering functional needs within a person's particular cultural context involves an appropriate prosthetic design for people in Asia. P. K. Sethi, orthopedist and prosthetic designer, realized the failure of the copied Western-model prosthetic foot being issued to his Indian clients with amputations. He observed that after some time people went back to using crutches without a prosthesis. Sethi attributed this to the discrepancy between chair-sitting cultures and floor-sitting cultures. With the design of the Jaipur foot, 'pre-eminence was given to the design of the prosthetic footpiece which could permit our people to walk barefoot, squat or sit cross-legged on the floor and allow comfortable navigation over our rugged rural landscape' (Sethi 1995). The Jaipur foot has revolutionized appropriate prosthetics production worldwide (see Ch. 24).

Environment and climate

Appropriate adaptive devices cannot be designed without consideration of the physical environment in which they will be used. To have independent mobility, via a wheelchair, to move about the house and outside on a porch, is wonderful for children or adults who previously have not been able to get past their bed. However, most of the world is still physically inaccessible to wheelchairs, strollers and bicycles. Wheelchairs may seem to be the most appropriate mode of mobility for people in cities and towns but, more often than not, even within cities, the roads are impassable, rutty or steep. Other mobility devices may better allow people, especially in rural areas, to leave their homes. In Bolivia, a wheelchair designer built a modified backpack with a postural support to carry a child with a disability on the paths. In the mountains of El Salvador, a horse provides a young man with paraplegia the mobility and freedom he needs to live his life again. In other environments, people with paraplegia are encouraged to learn to stand and walk short distances with braces, because wheelchair access is close to impossible.

If one considers the physical environment,

using equipment donated from developed countries is once again not a satisfactory solution. For instance, transferring a US sports wheelchair design, intended to be manufactured from lightweight metals, to Tanzania is inappropriate. The materials available in Tanzania are heavy metal, such as steel. Because of the rainy climate and rough, sandy terrain, a chair that is too heavy will soon suffer any number of problems – frozen bearings, a failed frame – resulting in very limited mobility for the rider. Understanding environmental conditions is essential to a successful intervention.

The design of a low technology wheelchair seat cushion also demonstrates the need to take into account varying environmental constraints for wheelchair riders, as well as personal preferences and functional needs. Therapists, engineers and technicians with an interest in appropriate technology have investigated several kinds of cushions to help prevent the life-threatening problem of pressure sores. Across the globe, people use a variety of available materials to decrease pressure when they sit. Cushions made of cardboard, foam, beans and rice, or bicycle inner tubes are some of the solutions to the critical need for pressure relief.

Once again, however, some solutions are inappropriate in certain environments. In 1995, Michael Heinrich, a seating designer and engineer, and Jean Anne Zollars, a physical therapist, gave seminars in El Salvador on pressure sores and cushions. During a seminar, one very active wheelchair user who works as a street musician smiled at the idea of the cardboard cushion (which incidentally is excellent for decreasing pressure under the significant bony prominences). He stated: 'Forget that cushion when the rains come, because when they come, they are here instantly, and wherever you are you are drenched. That cushion would be destroyed.' Leaving town the next day on the bus during a monsoon rain, Heinrich and Zollars saw the street musician drenched, pushing himself home in his wheelchair. For his personal environment, cardboard would not be an ideal material for his seat cushion. He certainly knew better than the expatriate 'experts'.

Siberian wheelchair riders have very different climatic concerns. Some of the foams used on pressure cushions tend to freeze up like an ice block. Sheepskin and down feathers are more useful materials in the harsh Siberian climate. Nicaraguans, on the other hand, prefer any air-inflated rubber cushion to foams. The foams increase the heat and sweating under their buttocks. For many PWD urine leakage is a common problem, so in any case cushions that are easy to clean are essential.

Aesthetics

Even though a device may be wonderfully functional for a person, if it is plain ugly it will be rejected. Self-image and beauty are important to everyone in different ways. One organization, Motivation, based in England, pays particular attention to aesthetics. Made up of therapists, engineers and designers, Motivation has sponsored wheelchair workshops in developing countries since 1991 to establish production and distribution systems for low-cost wheelchairs. In 1994, they decided to focus on special seating for children with disabilities. The designers, who had previously only worked on adult wheelchairs, noticed that with most Western seating systems for children, the seating systems were big and bulky so that one's attention was first drawn to the equipment instead of the child. Thus, a goal has become to see the beauty of the child, and have the child feel good about him or herself within the seating system. Keeping a keen eye on aesthetics, but not letting go of function, they have contributed greatly to the design of seating and mobility systems, not only in poorer countries, but worldwide.

Kylie Inwood, an occupational therapist working with the special seating team of Motivation, relates a story of Kamile, a Lithuanian child with cerebral palsy. Kylie met Kamile (aged 2) in 1992. She described Kamile as a terrified, quiet and withdrawn child, becoming very anxious whenever anyone wanted to take her from her mother's arms.

Through the integration of therapy and assistive devices, Kamile gained more confidence and independence. Being very conscious of how she looked, she chose her daily hairstyles and clothes.

Motivation provided Kamile with a MOTI, which is a seating system within a wheeled base. Kamile's mother related the following story about how the MOTI changed their lives. One day the whole family went out for a walk together (it is still rare in Lithuania to go out of the house with a child who has a disability). Suddenly her mother was struck by a strong feeling and thought – this is 'normal', it is OK. We are a family, and we are together. For a long time, a simple walk had not been possible. In the chairs Kamile has had in the past, she had not been comfortable and had been hidden by the chair – slumped down and lost. In the MOTI she looks great, sits quite well, and it is easy for her brother to push her. She continues to gain in confidence and independence (Figs. 11.6a, 11.6b).

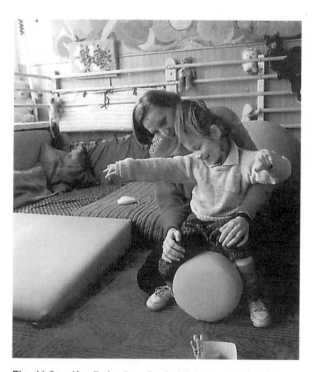

Fig. 11.6a Kamile having physical therapy, working on balance and posture. Photo courtesy: Kylie Inwood.

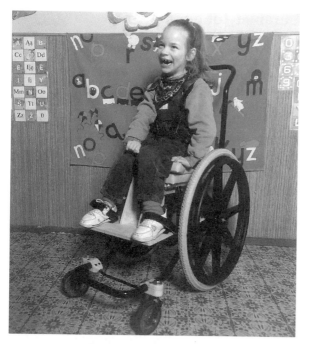

Fig. 11.6b Kamile at Motivation. Photo courtesy: Kylie Inwood.

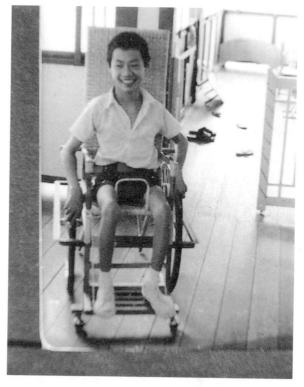

Fig. 11.7 Child in wheelchair made of rattan. Photo courtesy: Jean Anne Zollars.

Available materials

One of the biggest problems encountered in rehabilitation technology in developing countries is the lack of high-strength, low-cost, manufacturable materials. In response to this, there is a concerted effort by many individuals to come up with low-cost innovative gadgets made of all kinds of materials – sticks, mud, sawdust, beans, plastic buckets, bamboo, paper (see Ch. 25) and more. Sometimes these materials are referred to as 'low-tech'.

However, just because the technology is low-cost or fabricated from local materials it does not necessarily mean that it is appropriate. As noted above, technology, high or low cost, is useless unless it meets the needs of the individual, is safe, durable, and repairable. A case in point is using rattan. While working in Malaysia at the Spastic Children's Association of Johor Bahru, author Jean Anne Zollars was impressed by the effective use of rattan for building walkers and crutches, parallel bars, potty chairs, and seating systems (Fig. 11.7). For children who

were unable to walk, technicians built the rattan chairs with additional postural supports to help the children sit up. The rattan was comfortable to sit in and allowed air flow, a necessity in a hot, humid climate. However, rattan did not survive outside when it was raining and was prone to insect infestation. Sometimes a compromise is necessary.

Another example of a simple technology using locally available materials is that of a device to measure sitting pressure. This device also exemplifies how a local innovation can be used as a means to test the usefulness of another piece of low-tech equipment (in this case wheelchair cushions). In North America sophisticated pressure gauges can be used to evaluate sitting pressure, but, in most countries, no comparable device is available to evaluate the effectiveness of locally produced cushions. Answering this challenge, Heinrich began developing a low-tech pressure monitor, an idea

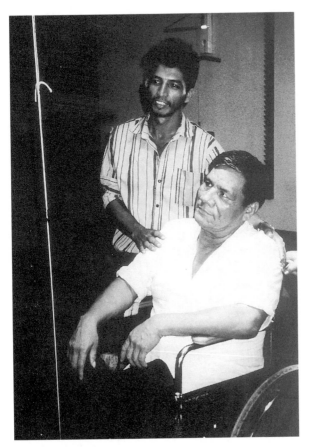

Fig. 11.8   A person with a disability can judge the pressure on his buttocks with this 'low-tech' pressure monitor. Photo courtesy: Jean Anne Zollars.

Durability of equipment

The longevity of a piece of equipment or a device is another important consideration in choice of materials and design. This is especially so in low-income environments where buying equipment is a great economic sacrifice. Repairs can be costly and difficult. There might not be available replacement parts and/or a person to repair the equipment locally. How long a piece of equipment will be useful is determined by the strength of the materials used, how it is assembled, and whether it adjusts for changes in the individual's size and functional ability. This issue is especially apparent with children.

The therapists and carpenter at Centro de Invalideces Multiples in San Salvador, El Salvador, have devised simple and effective methods to make growth adjustments for seat-

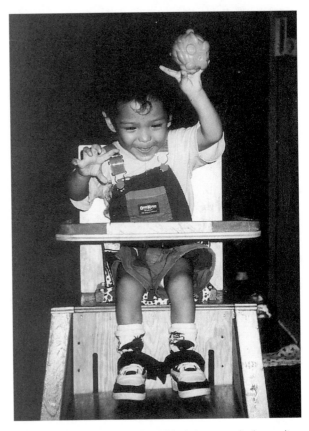

Fig. 11.9a   This seat is adjustable to increase its longevity for this child. Photo courtesy: Jean Anne Zollars.

first conceived during a brainstorming session at the 1991 annual meeting of the Rehabilitation Engineering Society of North America (RESNA). Heinrich suggested using a balloon filled with colored water connected to clear plastic tubing. The tubing is calibrated to correspond to pressure measurements. The balloon is placed underneath a bony prominence (under the buttocks in sitting) and the water rises through the tube depending on the intensity of the pressure in that area (Fig. 11.8). Thus, areas of dangerously high pressure can be detected and the seat cushion can be modified accordingly (see Werner 1998 for a complete description of this device). In this way, environmentally appropriate grass roots solutions to this problem can be properly evaluated for effectiveness.

ing systems. For example, they have developed footrests that can lower when the legs grow longer, backrests that can move backwards and be rebolted into place, and hip supports made out of layers of cardboard so that a layer can be taken off when the child's hips widen (Figs. 11.9a, 11.9b).

At Los Pipitos, a school and therapeutic program for children in Managua, Nicaragua, they have found it more efficient and less costly to have a seat-lending program. If a child grows out of a wooden seat, the family brings it back and exchanges it for another one that fits better. The concept of a children's wheelchair lending program is also being developed in Hong Kong, at Prince of Wales Hospital in conjunction with local universities. Los Pipitos has also experimented with the use of paper technology to fabricate seating systems. This is a wonderful application since it is inexpensive and can accommodate changes and growth easily (see Ch. 25).

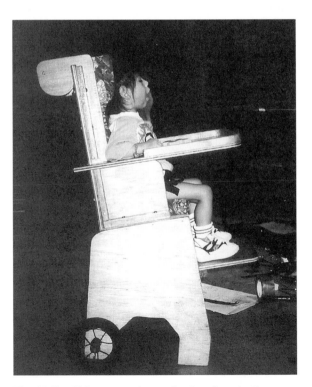

Fig. 11.9b Using appropriate technology for adaptive seating. Photo courtesy: Jean Anne Zollars.

PRODUCING APPROPRIATE TECHNOLOGY
Testing and redesigning

The design and distribution of appropriate rehabilitation technology requires in-depth evaluation of consumer need, locally available materials and manufacturing techniques. Once a design or prototype has been developed, it is imperative to have consumers use and test the product to evaluate its effectiveness, durability and functionality. The consumer and designer can then modify the device as needed. This part of the process often occurs informally. The most elegant solution to a technical problem comes after much reworking and collaboration. Once a prototype is developed a reliable system of production is decided upon.

Mass production vs. small scale production

Within international rehabilitation circles there is a tension between those who propose central mass-production of adaptive devices, such as wheelchairs, and those who believe that technology is usually more appropriate if manufactured locally or regionally, so that the consumer remains a member of the production process. In Hotchkiss (1985), E. F. Schumacher (1973) discusses this difference of outlook, which reverberates beyond the rehabilitation field: 'The system of mass production . . . presupposes that you are already rich, for a great deal of capital investment is needed to establish one single workplace. The system of production by the masses mobilizes the priceless resources which are possessed by all human beings, their clever brains and skillful hands, and supports them with first class tools, and the training/instruction to fully utilize these resources.' In either case, production solutions are often suggested by 'experts' from other countries working with a particular project. If the 'expert' leaves without training local consumers to continue the work, the project will more likely have a poor long-term prognosis (see Ch. 24).

The debate regarding the best model of production is likely to continue and a variety of production models will surely develop depending on local conditions. Depending on the type of production used (customized, small, medium, or large scale), a distribution network must then be established. Evaluation of a project's long term sustainability is important.

MODEL PROGRAMS PROVIDING APPROPRIATE ADAPTIVE TECHNOLOGY

There are many models of design and delivery of equipment today that rely on collaboration between a consumer, designers and builders of equipment. Most typically, access to equipment can be a top-down process, as can all aspects of rehabilitation. In the traditional medical model, professionals such as therapists, doctors or rehabilitation technology providers, work with a PWD to determine the equipment to be provided. The professional is seen as an expert who knows what is best, often encouraging passivity from the person in need of equipment. This model is not ideal.

In contrast, with a client-centered approach, the client and family are at the center of the problem-solving and decision-making process. The client is the team leader in the selection and design of equipment and the medical and equipment professionals are seen as knowledgeable consultants. No one knows more about living with a disability than the client herself. In the case of a child with a disability, the parents and teachers know how the child responds and interacts at home, which is often very different from the child's behavior at a medical clinic. Client-centered, collaborative approaches are becoming more common.

The Whirlwind wheelchair. The genesis of the Whirlwind wheelchair (Figs. 11.10, 11.11a, 11.11b) is an example of cross-national collaboration between wheelchair riders and builders. It is designed for use and production in the developing world. The Whirlwind is relatively lightweight, built to be ridden over rough terrain, is made of materials such as steel tubing,

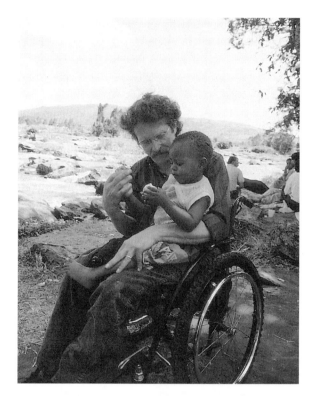

Fig. 11.10   Ralf Hotchkiss, riding a Whirlwind wheelchair, takes a break during wheelchair building training in Nairobi, Kenya. Photo courtesy: Jan Sing.

found in most places in the world, and can be repaired by a local blacksmith. The evolution of the Whirlwind design has been a cooperative process that began in Nicaragua in 1980 during

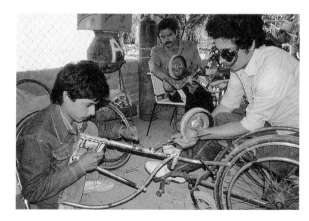

Fig. 11.11a   Building a Whirlwind wheelchair at Proyecto Projimo, Ajoya, Mexico. Photo courtesy: Ralf Hotchkiss.

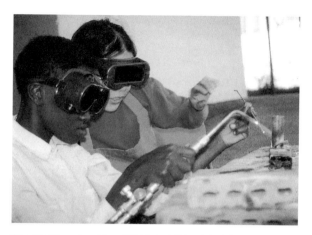

Fig. 11.11b Jan Sing, Whirlwind Wheelchair International trainer, teaches welding to Rafael Muturi of Kenya. Photo courtesy: Ralf Hotchkiss.

a visit by Ralf Hotchkiss. A group of four teenagers, who had been sharing one second-hand wheelchair, began making modifications to the homemade chair Hotchkiss was riding. Since 1980 the Whirlwind design has continued to improve with innovations from the people who ride and build it. A jumpseat was added by Peninah Mutinda of Nairobi, Kenya. This second, flat seat enabled her to sit near the floor in her wheelchair to take care of her daughter. Visiting Chinese wheelchair builders added a hole to the jumpseat to allow for latrine use. The wide, flexible front caster was modified from a common Zimbabwean pushcart wheel that Hotchkiss spotted during a visit in 1988. This caster, made of formed retread rubber, is now made in wheelchair shops in India, Thailand, Mexico and Fiji, where the design has continued to improve. Today the 'Zimbabwe wheel' caster, commercially unavailable in industrialized countries, offers cross-terrain mobility and dependability.

PROJIMO (Program of Rehabilitation Organized by Disabled Youth of Western Mexico) is an internationally recognized model community organized and run by PWD since 1981. Today, it is made up of people with and without disabilities, working together to address the concerns of its members. PROJIMO is located in Ajoya, a village of 1000 inhabitants in the mountains of western Mexico. It is a village-based rehabilitation center, where PWD and their families learn skills for survival and assist in the fabrication of adaptive equipment including orthoses, prostheses, wheelchairs and seating systems. The project is successful in providing adaptive equipment to those in need using a client-centered approach. Over the years, the participants in PROJIMO have had a lot of training from rehabilitation professionals and leaders in the field of disability who visit for short periods of time. David Werner has worked as a facilitator and advisor to PROJIMO since its inception. *Nothing About Us Without Us* (Werner 1998) and *Disabled Village Children* (Werner 1987), two highly recommended books for information on appropriate assistive technology, are based on ideas and experiences from PROJIMO.

CEPRI (Centro de Promocion de la Rehabilitacion Integral, located in Managua, Nicaragua, is another example of an organization of PWD working together to provide technical and educational support to their community, in part regarding appropriate assistive technology. Globally, CEPRI has contributed in many ways – one way has been through the education of other people with spinal cord injuries. They have developed and carried out educational programs on issues ranging from wheelchair repair to pressure sores to sexuality and have developed a manual on spinal cord injury survival. (The manual, written in Spanish, is clear, easy to read, and illustrated with cartoon-like characters.) Nicaraguan wheelchair riders-mechanics in organizations allied with CEPRI have been instrumental in the innovative designs of the Whirlwind wheelchair and pressure cushion designs noted above (for more information on CEPRI, see Ch. 16).

CONCLUSION

Appropriate assistive technology is often the first step towards independence for PWD. For technology to be truly appropriate the PWD must be the center of the team. Awareness and investigation of the requirements of individual clients is paramount, no matter where across the globe one is working. The process of evaluating the person's needs and designing technology can be very exciting to be involved in. For the process to be successful, the team must be open to new possibilities and avenues for creativity and they must listen to each other. In this way, local or international collaboration can be exceptionally rich and fertile.

Note: We wish to thank Ralf Hotchkiss for his collaboration on this chapter.

FURTHER READING

CEPRI 1995 Manual of self care after a spinal cord injury. CEPRI, Nicaragua. *Only available in Spanish. Order from: CEPRI, Nica Box 243, PO Box 52-7444, Miami, Fl 33152 ($15.00 + $4.00 shipping).*

Packer B 1995 A manual: appropriate paper-based technology (APT). Intermediate Technology Publications, London. *Order from: Intermediate Technology Publications, Ltd. 103–105 Southampton Row, London WC1B 4HH, UK.*

Hotchkiss R 1985 Independence through mobility. Appropriate Technology International, Washington, DC. *Order from: Whirlwind Wheelchair International, San Francisco State University, Department of Engineering, 15400 Holloway, San Francisco, CA 94132.*

Werner D 1998 Nothing about us without us.* HealthWrights, Palo Alto, CA. *Order from: HealthWrights, P.O. Box 1344, Palo Alto, CA 94302, USA. *Exceptional resource – also contains additional reference resource books, teaching aids and international groups working with disability and technology.*

Werner D 1987 Disabled village children: a guide for community health workers, rehabilitation workers and families. HealthWrights, Palo Alto, CA. *Order from: HealthWrights, P.O. Box 1344, Palo Alto, CA 94302, USA.*

Zollars J A 1996 Special seating: an illustrated guide. Otto Bock, Minneapolis, MN. *Order from: Otto Bock Orthopedic Industry, Inc., 3000 Xenium lane, Minneapolis, MN 55441, USA.*

PROJECTS AND PROGRAMS

Appropriate Health Resources and Technologies Action Group (AHRTAG) Farringdon Point, 29–35 Farringdon Road, London EC1M 3JB, UK. Tel: (44-171) 242 0606. *Contact: Ann Robins, Disability and Rehabilitation Unit. Information and resources on rehabilitation in developing countries.*

Handicap International, Home Office, 18 rue de Gerland, 69007 Lyon, France. Tel: (933 47) 861-1737. *Contact: Jean-Baptiste Richardier. Orthopedic and rehabilitation equipment and designs.*

HealthWrights, P.O. Box 1344, Palo Alto, CA 94302, USA, e-mail: healthwrights@igc.apc.org. *Contact: David Werner. Development and publication of educational materials for community based health care and rehabilitation. Works with PRO-JIMO.*

Hesperian Foundation, 1919 Addison Street, Suite 304, Berkeley, CA 94704, USA. Tel: (510)-845-4507, FAX (510) 845-0539, e-mail: hesperianfdn@igc.apc.org. *Publication of educational materials for international health and rehabilitation.*

Motivation UK Office, Brockley Academy, Brockley Lane, Backwell, Bristol BS19 3AQ, UK. Tel: (44-1275) 464 012; FAX: (1275) 464 019. *Works with projects in developing countries focusing on design, education, development and production of wheeled mobility devices and seating systems.*

People Potential, Plum Cottage, Hattingley Road, Medstead, Alton, Hampshire, GU34 5NQ, UK. Tel. or FAX: (44-1420) 563 741. *Contact: Kennett Westmacott. Design of aids for people with disabilities, training in low-cost production of rehabilitation aids, including APT.*

Whirlwind Wheelchair International, San Francisco State University, Department of Engineering, 15400 Holloway, San Francisco, CA 94132, USA. Tel: (415) 338-6277. *Contact: Ralf Hotchkiss or Peter Pfaelzer. World-wide network of wheelchair designers and builders. Hands-on courses in wheelchair building in many countries.*

REFERENCES

Hotchkiss R 1985 Independence through mobility. Appropriate Technology International, Washington, DC

Hotchkiss R 1998 Reinventing the wheelchair. In: Medical and Health Annual, Encyclopedia Britannica, Chicago D. p. 123

Schumacher E F 1975 Small is beautiful. First Perennial Library, New York NY

Sethi P K 1995 The Jaipur experience. In: Report of International Society for Prosthetics and Orthotics Consensus Conference, Copenhagen, Denmark p. 89

Werner D 1987 Disabled village children: a guide for community health workers, rehabilitation workers and families. HealthWrights, Palo Alto, CA

Werner D 1998 Nothing about us without us. HealthWrights, Palo Alto, CA

12

Epidemiological considerations in the assessment of disability

Tomlin J. Paul
Marigold Thorburn

INTRODUCTION

This chapter will provide a theoretical framework for understanding issues related to the epidemiology of disability, including a description of basic epidemiological principles and tools. This will be useful for rehabilitation and health professionals who will be working in diverse and sometimes unfamiliar settings where they are expected to have a knowledge about the incidence and prevalence of disease and disability and also assist in decision making about rehabilitation programming.

Epidemiology, a basic discipline of public health, has applications to both individual and population based medicine. It is defined as the study of the distribution and determinants of disease and injuries in human populations (Mausner & Kramer 1985). This appreciation of distribution and determinants will help in understanding disease from a population perspective. Of course, the concept of epidemiology can be applied to health problems and issues in a more general sense, such as normal growth, and development and is therefore not only disease-specific.

Epidemiological tools and concepts are useful in describing and analyzing the outcomes of exposures to various risk factors. These factors vary widely in different settings. For rehabilitation professionals, a sound grasp of epidemiology's tools and approaches is crucial to meaningful analyses of disease and disability in different environments.

Distribution

The distribution of disease or health problems can be viewed in relation to the epidemiological variables of time, place and person. Put another way, with respect to disease, epidemiologists ask the questions when, where, and who. This basic framework is useful in describing events in communities such as the trends over time for disabilities of different types or the distribution of disability by country or region. Disability occurrence can be broken down by person characteristics such as age, sex, educational status, ethnic grouping, and so on. This is at the heart of what is called descriptive epidemiology, that is, describing what exists in the community or population.

Measurement issues

Being a scientific discipline, epidemiology has measurement tools that it uses to describe basic distribution and determinants and to assist in the analysis of disease occurrence in populations. These basic measurement indices are rate, proportion and ratio. These fairly straightforward measures are critical to understanding epidemiology.

Rate

Rate is represented by the formula $x/y \times k$ where x represents the number of events occurring in a community over a particular time, y the number of individuals at risk of this event, and k is a constant that helps to express the rate against a constant population base. For example, in a community with a population of 10 000, if 50 cases of hearing disability are found, then the rate of hearing disability in the population can be calculated as:

$$\frac{50}{10\,000} \times 1000$$

This works out to 5 per 1000. The constant – in this case 1000 – is necessary to expressing the rate. One cannot say a rate of 5; the population base is not clear. This rate of hearing disability may be compared with another community that has only 10 cases and a population of 1000. In

this second case, the rate will be 10 per 1000 – i.e. $\frac{10}{1000} \times 1000$.

Note that the problem cannot be described with respect to rates until the occurrences have been related to the population at risk. The concept of a population at risk is important. Sometimes rates are calculated using populations that are not truly representative of the population at risk. For instance, in calculating the crude birth rate the total population is used (men and women). This is clearly crude.

A number of types of rates can be used to measure morbidity and mortality. Common examples are the incidence rate and the prevalence rate. The *incidence rate* looks at the number of new cases of disease in a population, while *prevalence* looks at all the cases (old and new) occurring in a population. Incidence gives a useful measure of risk or the probability of getting the condition if exposure to a particular factor takes place. Of course incidence of new cases will contribute to the prevalence pool. The prevalence rate is useful for health planners who need to estimate the burden of disease in a community. For instance, in planning services for children who are mentally retarded one would be interested in the prevalence of the condition.

The prevalence of a condition relates directly to its incidence and duration (Mausner & Kramer 1985). Because of this definition, prevalence statistics can be deceiving. When medical care successfully prolongs survival, prevalence will rise without an increase in incidence. Gruenberg (1977) speaks of 'The Failure of Success', noting a marked increase in the prevalence of mental retardation and other disabilities resulting from the use of medications and medical technology to prolong the life of children born with congenital defects and life threatening conditions.

The prevalence of childhood disability in the International Epidemiological Study on Childhood Disabilities (IESCD), a large scale study conducted in Clarendon Parish, Jamaica, revealed an overall prevalence rate of 93.9 per 1000 children for all types of disability and a rate of serious disability of 24.9 per 1000 children aged 2–9 years (Paul et al 1992). Such prevalence indicators are important in assessing the presence of disability in a population and in helping to plan services. Arising from work done in Jamaica, Thorburn et al (1992a) estimate a shortfall of 39 000 places for community based rehabilitation in Jamaica. Prevalence measures of disability in this study have therefore contributed to a greater awareness of the real need for services.

Proportion

The measure of a proportion is expressed by the formula x/y where x is a part of y. For example in a group of 100 children, if 10 are disabled then the proportion of disabled is $10/100$ or 10%.

Ratio

With the ratio, the measure x/y is such that x is not part of y. Groups with two distinct characteristics are being compared. The concept of a ratio is well known in epidemiology. The male–female ratio, for instance, is commonly used.

Measurement methodology

Measurement is an important issue in epidemiology. One needs, however, to be clear about what is being measured and the validity of the measurements. In the area of disability, the literature is replete with discussions pertinent to definitions attempting to clarify the differences between impairment, disability and handicap and also the criteria for assessing disability. An attempt has been made by the World Health Organization (WHO 1980) to clarify and gain consensus on this situation through 'The International Classification of Impairments, Disabilities and Handicaps (ICIDH) (see Ch. 10).

Furthermore, without measures of the prevalence of disability and handicap, it is not possible to plan interventions rationally or system-

atically. In particular, information in developing countries is lacking, but it is especially hard to make comparisons when methodologies differ considerably between studies (Thorburn 1990).

Determinants

The determinants of disease refer to the factors that relate to the development and cause of the condition. This major aspect of epidemiological work forms the basis of disease and disability prevention.

Disability provides a useful point of reference for looking at causation. Studies have shown that people's perception of disability causation does in fact spread over a wide spectrum. The epidemiological triad of disease causation illustrates the link between host (humans), agent, and environment existing in a dynamic equilibrium. Changes such as host susceptibility, virulence of the agent, and the quality of the environment will all play a role in the determination of disease. This model is more applicable for conditions that are infectious or have a clearly defined agent. It becomes more difficult to apply where the etiology is related to a socioenvironmental set of factors.

The development of disability, for example, is a complex phenomenon involving a multitude of factors. These factors can be called risk factors, that is, factors associated with the disease. Radiation, for instance, is a risk factor for fetal teratogenesis and consequent congenital defects and disabilities. In the same way, inappropriate parenting environments can be risk factors for certain sociobehavioral impairments or dysfunction. Risk factors can be environmental, related to inherited characteristics, or related to personal behavior and lifestyle. It is important to determine if a risk factor is simply a marker for the disease or a determinant that can be manipulated to decrease the chances of the condition occurring.

One of the underpinnings of epidemiology is that disease is not randomly distributed among human beings (Basch 1990). The prevalence or occurrence of risk factors varies by place, time, and person. As such, rehabilitation and health professionals can expect variations in disease/disability occurrence based on these variables.

Variations in the presence of certain elements and minerals in soil, for instance, contribute to wide variations in the prevalence of diseases such as goiter and cretinism. Iodine deficiency is common in high mountain areas where rainfall leaches minerals from the soil, so much so that northern Pakistan, India, Nepal and Bhutan constitute the 'Himalayan goiter belt' (Basch 1990). In such areas, cretinism highlighted by mental retardation and associated deaf-mutism and stunting of growth are endemic.

Other conditions, such as chronic lead and arsenic poisoning, iron deficiency anemia, and chronic fluorosis, all relate to local conditions, sometimes interplaying with cultural beliefs, practices, and health-seeking behavior. Distinct climatic factors can also play a role in disability/disease occurrence. For instance, the relationship between the occurrence of rickets and low vitamin D production and lack of sunlight is well known. This was a condition of the poor in industrial cities of England and Europe and is now seen in some countries of the Middle East where, for cultural and religious reasons, women are always completely covered or remain indoors (Basch 1990). In moving from one environment to another, rehabilitation professionals can expect to find patterns of disability and disease reflective of local conditions and cultural and ethnic dimensions.

Climatic conditions can also predispose people to the presence of certain vectors, such as mosquitoes, that carry diseases like malaria, dengue and yellow fever. Some major vector-borne and zoonotic diseases of humans are shown in Table 12.1 (Basch 1990), highlighting the widespread geographical distribution.

The genetic makeup of the host can also vary tremendously within and between populations. A large number of diseases are known to be under direct genetic control, but much work needs to be done to clarify the extent to which hereditary factors influence susceptibility. Table 12.2 shows some disorders for which there is an inherited factor (Basch 1990). Sickle cell disease, for instance, has a genetic factor distributed in a broad band across Africa south of the Sahara and north of the Zambesi and Kunene rivers. The gene is thought to have been introduced into the Western hemisphere through the slave trade. Some investigators argue that this disease has persisted because of the partial protection conferred by the trait against infection with malignant tertian malaria. This is an interesting interaction of ethnic host, vector, and climatic factors and illustrates the variation in the range of determinants affecting disease and disability in cross-cultural settings.

STUDY DESIGN

Epidemiology seeks to answer questions about the distribution and determinants of disease and disability through the use of descriptive and analytic study designs.

Descriptive studies

Descriptive studies are very common and more easily done. They usually aim to collect data on situations that exist at present or have occurred in the past. For example, a study seeking to determine the age and sex distribution of disability in a population and one that assesses parents' attitudes toward children with disabilities are both descriptive.

Descriptive studies usually follow the standard research process, including the development of aims and objectives and appropriate measuring instruments and they help to generate hypotheses relating to variables being studied. For instance, a descriptive study might reveal a higher prevalence of mental retardation among children of women who smoke during pregnancy. The hypothesis emerging here is that cigarette smoking might play a role in causing mental retardation. Testing this hypothesis calls for another type of epidemiological investigation called an analytical study.

Analytical studies

Analytical studies are generally of two varieties – prospective and retrospective. Prospective

Table 12.1 Some major vector-borne and zoonotic diseases of humans (Basch 1990)

Disease	Mode	Animals usually involved	Vector	Distribution
Yellow fever	V	Monkeys, marsupials	*Aedes* mosquitoes	Africa, Central & S. America
Viral encephalitis	V	Rodents, birds, horses, monkeys	Mosquitoes or ticks	Many types: temperate and tropical areas
Dengue	V	Humans	*Aedes* mosquitoes	Pacific, S.E. Asia, Caribbean, S. America
Rabies	D	Dogs, wild mammals		Cosmopolitan
Influenza	D, I	Swine, birds		Cosmopolitan
Typhus	V	Rodents	Lice	Africa, Asia, Central & S. America, Balkans
Murine typhus	V	Rodents	Fleas	Cosmopolitan
Scrub typhus	V	Rodents	Mites	Asia, S. Asia, N. Australia
Q fever	D, I	Cattle, sheep, goats, birds		Cosmopolitan
Spotted fevers	V	Rodents, other mammals	Ticks	Several types: Australia, N. & S. America, Africa, India
Psittacosis	D, I	Birds		Cosmopolitan
Anthrax	D, I	Cattle, goats, horses swine		E. Mediterranean, Asia, Caribbean, Latin America
Brucellosis	D, I, M	Cattle, goats, sheep		Cosmopolitan
Plague	D, V, I	Rodents	Fleas	Widespread
Lyme disease	V	Deer, rodents	Ticks	N. America, Europe
Relapsing fever	V	Rodents	Ticks or lice	Asia, Africa, Mid-East, S. America, Europe
Tuberculosis	D, M	Humans, cattle, goats, cats, dogs, swine		Cosmopolitan
Leishmaniasis	V	Dogs, wild animals	Sand flies	Asia, India, Africa, Central & S. America
Malaria	V	Humans	*Anopheles* mosquitoes	Mainly in tropics
Chagas disease	V	Small mammals, dogs	Triatomid bugs	Central & S. America
Sleeping sickness	V	Large mammals, cattle	Tsetse flies	Tropical Africa
Filariasis	V	Primates, cats, dogs	Mosquitoes	Widespread in tropics
Trichinosis	E	Swine, bear		Widespread in temperate areas
Hydatid disease	E	Sheep, dogs		E. Mediterranean, New Zealand, S. America, Europe, California
Tapeworms	E	Cattle, swine, dogs		Cosmopolitan
Schistosomiasis	V	Humans, cattle, rodents, swine, primates	Snails	Asia, Africa, Mid-East, Caribbean, S. America

Abbreviations:
D Direct   E Eating (ingestion)   I Inhalation
M Milk   V Vector-borne

Table 12.2   The ethnicity of disease: some simply inherited disorders (McCusick, 1973)

Ethnic group	Relatively high frequency	Relatively low frequency
Ashkenazi Jews	Familial dysautonomia Pentosuria Tay–Sachs disease	Phenylketonuria
Mediterranean peoples (Italians, Greeks, Sephardic Jews)	Thalassemia (mainly β) G6PD deficiency, Mediterranean type Familial Mediterranean fever	Cystic fibrosis
Africans	Hemoglobinopathies especially Hb S Hb C, α- and β-thalassemia, persistent Hb F G6PD deficiency, African type Adult lactase deficiency	Cystic fibrosis Hemophilia Phenylketonuria Wilson's disease E_{1a} (pseudocholinesterase deficiency) Pi^z (α_1 antitrypsin deficiency)
Japanese (Koreans)	Acatalasia Oguchi's disease Dyschromatosis universalis hereditaria	
Chinese	α-thalassemia G6PD deficiency, Chinese type Adult lactase deficiency	
Armenians	Familial Mediterranean fever	G6PD deficiency
Finns	Congenital nephrosis	Phenylketonuria Krabbe's disease
Norwegians	Cholestasis-lymphedema	
Eskimos	E_1^s (pseudocholinesterase deficiency)	

studies, sometimes called cohort studies, involve studying a cohort or a group of individuals with a common experience or exposure. The classical retrospective study is the case-control study. Analytical studies are usually concerned with identifying or measuring the effects of risk factors or focus on the health effects of specific exposures (Last 1988).

Prospective studies can determine the incidence of disease in different exposure situations. For instance, by comparing a cohort of children with sickle cell disease with a cohort of non-affected children, researchers can determine the incidence of disability in both groups and come up with a measure called the relative risk. The relative risk is the incidence rate of the disease or condition in the group exposed divided by the incidence in the unexposed group. If disabil-

ity incidence is 10 per 1000 in the sickle cell group and 5 per 1000 in the normal or unexposed group, the relative risk for disability with respect to sickle cell is 10/5 or 2. A relative risk greater than 1 usually indicates that the exposure factor plays a role in the development of the condition. The relative risk is the critical measure for the etiologic significance of a factor in disease (Mausner & Kramer 1985).

Case-control or retrospective studies compare a group of cases or individuals who have the disease with controls or individuals without the disease. The occurrence of the risk factor(s) is examined in both groups and then compared. If the risk factor is significant, it should be more prevalent in the group of cases. Usually controls are chosen to match the group of cases except for the variable that is thought to be of significance. For instance, in examining the role of perinatal asphyxia in cerebral palsy (CP), a group of children with CP (cases) and also a group of children without CP (controls) are identified. The controls have to look like the cases with respect to variables such as age, gender, maternal age, and length of pregnancy. This eliminates the influence of variables that could play a role in the expression of this disease. An assessment is then made of each group for perinatal asphyxia exposure and the differences compared. Usually a determination is made of a factor called the odds ratio, which compares the odds of getting the disease in those exposed with that of those not exposed to the risk factor. For conditions with low prevalence, the odds ratio approximates the relative risk.

The intervention study is another type of epidemiological study. The researcher actually makes decisions about conditions of exposure. For instance, to examine the impact of early stimulation on low birth-weight babies, a group of such children could be assigned to an early stimulation program and another group to a basic program with little or no stimulation. After an appropriate period, the outcomes are measured and compared. There are always ethical issues to be considered in this kind of design.

Proving causation

Although two factors may be statistically associated, they do not necessarily have a causal relationship. For example, even if an association between perinatal asphyxia and CP is found, it cannot be concluded that the former causes the latter. One needs to look further at certain factors, beginning with the strength of association – this being measured by the relative risk. The higher the strength of the association, the more likely the relationship is causal. One would therefore expect to find much higher rates of CP in children with a perinatal asphyxia experience than in those without. Second, the consistency of the association needs to be examined. Does the relationship hold true under different circumstances and when tested with varying methodologies? Third, what is the specificity of the association? If only one factor is implicated in a causal model, the relationship with the outcome factor will be highly specific. Problems associated with disabilities and handicaps may have a number of factors interacting that, by themselves, are not specific for that condition. For example, a complex condition such as CP can be caused by a wide variety of agents and factors including anoxia, neonatal jaundice, infection or prematurity and may result, according to which part of the central nervous system is affected, in a variety of impairments – motor, speech, intellectual, etc. Fourth is the temporality of the relationship: is it certain that the exposure variable precedes the outcome? Prospective or cohort studies may answer this more clearly than retrospective studies. For instance, does perinatal asphyxia precede CP or could it be the other way around? Fifth, what is the coherence of the relationship? Does it make good scientific sense? And sixth, in some situations, a dose–response relationship might be established.

All these factors warrant careful consideration in an evaluation of causation. They may not be completely fulfilled in all situations, but when they are considered and present, they increase the likelihood of a causal relationship. Cause and effect cannot be taken for granted or treated lightly.

Surveillance

Within the discipline of epidemiology, surveillance plays a role in monitoring the status of disease and health concerns in the community. Disease surveillance can be defined as the scrutiny of all aspects of occurrence and spread of disease that are pertinent to effective control (Last 1988). A surveillance effort is systematic and consists of collecting, collating, analyzing and interpreting relevant data, and disseminating it to relevant individuals and authorities.

The benefits of a surveillance system rest largely with the idea of early detection at the population level so that appropriate interventions can occur. But a number of other benefits emerge from the system. These include understanding the natural history of disease, making decisions with respect to priorities, evaluating programs, and understanding trends and patterns for diseases in a community.

Surveillance systems are fairly well developed for conditions such as measles and influenza but less well defined and implemented for chronic diseases and disabilities. Yet if one looks at disability as an outcome of disease and socioeconomic conditions, then monitoring disability patterns and trends can provide very useful insights into populations.

Sources of data for disease surveillance vary from formal health facilities and laboratories to morbidity and mortality reports. With respect to monitoring and quantifying disabilities in the population Thorburn et al (1991) identify six methods: monitoring clinic referrals, performing developmental screening on all babies, inserting questions on disability in a census, developing a registry, asking key informants, and doing a house-to-house screening survey. Each of these has relative costs and benefits.

Screening

Screening is an important part of epidemiology and public health work that comes largely under the umbrella of secondary prevention which represents the strategies aimed at early detection and prompt treatment. Screening can be defined as the detection of preclinical disease using a relatively simple test. The screening assessment is usually presumptuous and as such a more definitive evaluation is usually done to confirm the presence of the condition. Screening programs can be set up for detecting disease (e.g. coronary artery disease) or risk factors for that disease (e.g. hypercholesterolemia). On a practical basis, screening is often used as a means to ensure early detection and prompt treatment.

A number of prerequisites should be considered before implementing a screening program. Perhaps the most critical is whether there are diagnostic and intervention services in place to deal with individuals identified to be in need. This is an ethical issue. For example, should screening for mental retardation be done in the absence of follow-up services for such children or individuals?

Other important considerations in the development of screening programs are that: the natural history of the condition should be understood, there should be a suitable diagnostic test, and the screening should not be just a one shot activity.

A suitable screening test should be safe, acceptable to those being screened and to those using it, reliable and valid and have a good cost–benefit ratio. In developing a new screening instrument, the technique being developed is usually measured up against a 'gold-standard' or diagnostic test.

A screening instrument must be able to detect people with the condition in the population (sensitivity) and, secondly, be able to identify individuals without the disease or condition (specificity). Practically speaking, a test that is not very sensitive will miss a large proportion of individuals who have the disease and falsely label them negative. A test that is not very specific will not identify all of the normal individuals and will falsely label some of them as positive.

The ten question screen. A lot has been written about the experience with the ten question (TQ) screen in the identification of childhood disability. The International Epidemiological Study on Childhood Disabilities (IESCD) (Durkin et al 1990) was a major international collaborative effort to address the need for simplified screening instruments that could be used by non-professionals in disability detection. It followed an earlier pilot study in 1981, the International Pilot Study of Severe Childhood Disability (IPSSCD) (Belmont 1984) in which the TQ screen was tested for severe mental retardation and found to be sensitive in identifying cases. The TQ had good specificity but poor positive predictive value, the latter having to do with the low prevalence of the condition in the community. In the IESCD the TQ was used to screen for six disabilities (Durkin et al 1990).

The addition of probes improved the positive predictive value of the screen but decreased the sensitivity. In the Jamaican component of the IESCD, it was concluded that to maintain the good sensitivity and to minimize false positives, it would be necessary to add other, objective screens of vision and hearing to positive TQ cases (Thorburn et al 1992b). This is in contrast to Bangladesh and Pakistan where sensitivity for these sensory disabilities was poor (Durkin et al 1994). The use of the TQ has been extensively documented in Schuurman (1995).

The process of screening as a means of gaining insights into prevalence could be considered in terms of the efficiency and effectiveness of the process itself. Screening tests may be simple and have good sensitivity and specificity, but setting up screening programs, either in an integrated fashion or as distinct programs, involves serious resource considerations. Proper planning is therefore necessary.

HEALTH STATUS

The discrete approaches and tools discussed above provide information of a descriptive and analytical nature that is important for decision making in implementing and evaluating public health and rehabilitation programs. However, epidemiology must also concern itself with the question of the health status of the population. In the same way that the rehabilitation therapist and health professional are concerned with the health status of the individual patient and make assessments with particular indicators in mind, so, too, indicators that are population – or group – based must be devised.

The search for objective measures of health status of a population is an ongoing tradition of public health. Infant mortality and the mean expectation of life at birth are widely accepted as valid indicators of health status. On the other hand, enmeshed in the literature but still of very little practical use, is the suggestion that disability can be used as an indicator of health status.

Health indicators – definitions

A health indicator is defined by Last (1988) as a variable susceptible to direct measurement that reflects the state of health of persons in a community. The attempt to move away from disease-oriented definitions to functional and holistic appreciations in fact makes measurement more difficult. Disease is the outcome of a variety of factors and represents one end point in an abnormal homeostatic process. However, diseases produce states of abnormal functioning, whether transient or permanent, that have implications for productivity and social adaptation.

From a functional perspective, disability assessment is an appropriate contributor to the measurement of the health status of a population, particularly as measures such as infant mortality rates have declined and begun to level off. It is not that health gains no longer occur but rather that improvement may be more in terms of quality of life than in mortality transformations. Sinha (1988) argues that the increased survival of children is not matched by meaningful enough changes in strategies for preventing disability or rehabilitating affected persons. This anomaly perhaps relates to a false sense of security that health gains are satisfactory or that enough achievements have been made. In effect, mortality based indicators may be losing their information utility.

Does disability prevalence stand up to scrutiny as an appropriate health indicator? Hansluwka (1985) argues that 'one of the problems with a disability-based indicator of the health status of the population is the doubts one has to entertain whether disability is a single, one-dimensional phenomenon which can be measured in an objective way across the world.' Progress is being made on this front, though somewhat slowly. The IESCD survey instruments for measuring disability were designed to achieve comparability across countries (Durkin et al 1990). Disability could therefore live up to the scrutiny of international comparisons if methodological issues are clearly agreed upon and followed.

Changing patterns of disease and disability

An examination of broad or long-term patterns can be quite revealing for a population and provide useful information on the transformations in health status and general conditions of living.

The way in which disease patterns have changed over time is referred to as the epidemiological transition. This concept was formulated in an effort to provide a comprehensive approach to the dynamics of the mortality–fertility transition, with emphasis on changing patterns of health and disease. A number of variables affect this transition, including social, economic, and demographic factors.

The transition accompanies the economic change from low per-capita income to high per-capita income and in effect is the transition from high mortality and high fertility to low mortality and low fertility (Omran 1974). In early phases, there are large burdens of infectious diseases accounting for the major causes of death. In the last phase of the transition, human-made and degenerative diseases are the principal causes of death.

In another example, life expectancy, which is an indicator of a country's health status, has increased significantly in the past 4–5 decades in developing countries, but significant health challenges remain. Child mortality rates in developing countries are about 10 times higher

Table 12.3   Population, economic indicators, and progress in health by demographic region, 1975–90 (from World Development Report 1993 by World Bank. © 1993 by the International Bank for Reconstruction and Development/The World Bank used by permission of Oxford University Press, Inc.)

Region	Population, 1990 (millions)	Deaths, 1990 (millions)	Income per capita Dollars 1990	Income per capita Growth rate, 1975–90 (percent per year)	Child mortality 1975	Child mortality 1990	Life expectancy at birth (years) 1975	Life expectancy at birth (years) 1990
Sub-Saharan Africa	510	7.9	510	−1.0	212	175	48	52
India	850	9.3	360	2.5	195	127	53	58
China	1134	8.9	370	7.4	85	43	56	69
Other Asia and islands	683	5.5	1320	4.6	135	97	56	62
Latin America and the Caribbean	444	3.0	2190	−0.1	104	60	62	70
Middle Eastern crescent	503	4.4	1720	−1.3	174	111	52	61
Formerly socialist economies of Europe (FSE)	346	3.8	2850	0.5	36	22	70	72
Established market economies (EME)	798	7.1	19 900	2.2	21	11	73	76
Demographically developing group[a]	4123	39.1	900	3.0	152	106	56	63
FSE and EME	1144	10.9	14 690	1.7	25	15	72	75
World	5267	50.0	4000	1.2	135	96	60	65

Note: Child mortality is the probability of dying between birth and age 5, expressed per 1000 live births; life expectancy at birth is the average number of years a person would expect to live at the prevailing age-specific mortality rates.
a. The countries of the demographic regions Sub-Saharan Africa, India, China, Other Asia and islands, Latin America and Caribbean, and Middle Eastern crescent.

than in established market economies. So although health has improved, even in the poorest of countries, the pace of progress is uneven. Table 12.3 provides a summary of regional progress in mortality reduction between 1975 and 1990 (World Bank 1993).

Premature mortality is one aspect of the analysis, but a substantial portion of the burden of disease consists of disability arising from a variety of sources. The World Bank and the WHO have devised a measure to assess the global burden of disease (GBD). This has been done by combining (a) losses from premature death and (b) loss of healthy life resulting from disability. The GBD is measured in units of disability-adjusted life years (DALYs). Worldwide

in 1990, 1.36 billion DALYs were lost. In the developing world, 67% of all DALY loss was due to premature death and 33% to disability; in established market economies the proportions were 55% and 45% respectively (World Bank 1993). This analysis reveals the impact of disability on the population's health status more clearly than does the use of basic prevalence figures. One should note that as countries become more developed and gain greater control over infectious diseases and premature death, the impact of disability is shown more readily.

In doing any inter-country comparisons, one needs to look not only at the absolute determinations of DALYs but also the rate per population to account for population size. Rates will

Table 12.4 Distribution of DALY loss by cause and demographic region, 1990 ((from World Development Report 1993 by World Bank. © 1993 by the International Bank for Reconstruction and Development/The World Bank used by permission of Oxford University Press, Inc.)

Cause	World	Sub-Saharan Africa	India	China	Other Asia and islands	Latin America and the Caribbean	Middle Eastern crescent	Formerly socialist economies of Europe	Established market economies
Population (millions)	5267	510	850	1134	683	444	503	346	798
Communicable diseases	45.8	71.3	50.5	25.3	48.5	42.2	51.0	8.6	9.7
Tuberculosis	3.4	4.7	3.7	2.9	5.1	2.5	2.8	0.6	0.2
STDs and HIV	3.8	8.8	2.7	1.7	1.5	6.6	0.7	1.2	3.4
Diarrhea	7.3	10.4	9.6	2.1	8.3	5.7	10.7	0.4	0.3
Vaccine-preventable childhood infections	5.0	9.6	6.7	0.9	4.5	1.6	6.0	0.1	0.1
Malaria	2.6	10.8	0.3	•	1.4	0.4	0.2	•	•
Worm infections	1.8	1.8	0.9	3.4	3.4	2.5	0.4	•	•
Respiratory infections	9.0	10.8	10.9	6.4	11.1	6.2	11.5	2.6	2.6
Maternal causes	2.2	2.7	2.7	1.2	2.5	1.7	2.9	0.8	0.6
Perinatal causes	7.3	7.1	9.1	5.2	7.4	9.1	10.9	2.4	2.2
Other	3.5	4.6	4.0	1.4	3.3	5.8	4.9	0.6	0.5
Noncommunicable diseases	42.2	19.4	40.4	58.0	40.1	42.8	36.0	74.8	78.4
Cancer	5.8	1.5	4.1	9.2	4.4	5.2	3.4	14.8	19.1
Nutritional deficiencies	3.9	2.8	6.2	3.3	4.6	4.6	3.7	1.4	1.7
Neuropsychiatric disease	6.8	3.3	6.1	8.0	7.0	8.0	5.6	11.1	15.0
Cerebrovascular disease	3.2	1.5	2.1	6.3	2.1	2.6	2.4	8.9	5.3
Ischemic heart disease	3.1	0.4	2.8	2.1	3.5	2.7	1.8	13.7	10.0
Pulmonary obstruction	1.3	0.2	0.6	5.5	0.5	0.7	0.5	1.6	1.7
Other	18.0	9.7	18.5	23.6	17.9	19.1	18.7	23.4	25.6
Injuries	11.9	9.3	9.1	16.7	11.3	15.0	13.0	16.6	11.9
Motor vehicle	2.3	1.3	1.1	2.3	2.3	5.7	3.3	3.7	3.5
Intentional	3.7	4.2	1.2	5.1	3.2	4.3	5.2	4.8	4.0
Other	5.9	3.9	6.8	9.3	5.8	5.0	4.6	8.1	4.3
Total	100.0	100.0	100.0	100.0	100.0	100.0	100.0	100.0	100.0
Millions of DALYs	1362	293	292	201	177	103	144	58	94
Equivalent infant deaths (millions)	42.0	9.0	9.0	6.2	5.5	3.2	4.4	1.8	2.9
DALYs per 1000 population	259	575	344	178	260	233	286	168	117

• Less than 0.05 percent.
Note: DALY, disability-adjusted life year; STD, sexually transmitted disease; HIV, human immunodeficiency virus.

have to be standardized to allow for age and sex distribution differences. Table 12.4 shows the distribution of DALY loss by cause and demographic region. Here the differences emerging with development are clear. Sub-Saharan Africa, for example, has a rate of DALYs per 1000 almost five times greater than that of established market economies.

Inferences from the epidemiological transition

Depending on a country's stage in the transition, the emerging disability profile will vary. A country that is undergoing heavy burdens of infectious diseases and problems related to low socioeconomic status will have a disability prevalence related to the dominant diseases (such as poliomyelitis, other infections and malnutrition). For example, motor, hearing and

visual disabilities will be seen commonly in children, and where life expectancy is low, disabilities in adults related to chronic lifestyle conditions will not be very frequent (Thorburn 1990). This will have implications for service planning, and must be examined closely in relation to the wide range of determinants discussed earlier in this chapter.

In the the Jamaican part of the IESCD, the prevalence of different disability types in children aged 2–9 years was quite revealing. The following rates for different disabilities were obtained: cognitive, 81/1000; speech, 14/1000; visual, 11/1000; hearing, 9/1000; motor, 4/1000 and seizure, 2/1000 (Paul et al 1992). The particular diagnoses associated with these disabilities are worth considering (Table 12.5). In this study, the major problem associated with motor disability was cerebral palsy. Deafness from post-infective causes accounted for only 19% of cases

Table 12.5 Medical diagnoses in disabled children, by type of disability (Paul et al 1992)

Type of disability	No. of children	Diagnosis	Frequency (%)
Motor	17	Cerebral palsy	70.6
		Musculo-skeletal deformity	17.6
		Ackee poisoning	5.9
		Other	5.9
Hearing	26	(Undetermined)	50.0
		Congenital/hereditary	23.0
		Post-infective	19.2
		Other	7.7
Visual	35	Refractive error	80.0
		Cataracts	5.7
		Undetermined	5.7
		Cerebral palsy	2.9
		Corneal opacity	2.9
		Retinal pigment disorder	2.9
Speech	48	Hearing impairment (unknown cause)	33.3
		Delayed development	33.3
		Articulation disorder	8.3
		Cerebral palsy	6.3
		Down syndrome	2.1
		Toxic encephalopathy (ackee poisoning)	2.1
		Severe mental retardation	2.1
		Other	12.5
Seizure	9	Idiopathic epilepsy	55.6
		Meningitis	22.2
		Febrile seizure	11.1
		Cerebral palsy	11.1

of hearing disability, and meningitis and febrile seizures did not feature as the main causes of seizure disability. This relates well to the changing patterns of disease experienced in the last 2–3 decades in Jamaica due to the virtual elimination of poliomyelitis and the reduction of malnutrition and measles as life-threatening conditions.

Further analysis of disability prevalence along gender, ethnic and social-class variables can be instructive and help in gaining a clearer epidemiological assessment of the problem of disability.

Implications for rehabilitation professionals

Except for the large group of mild learning disabilities that are thought to be of sociocultural origin, the vast majority of disabilities are due to a small group of factors that either inhibit or distort normal development, causing disease or injury by damaging the structure and/or function of the organ or body system. The severity of the disability will be expressed according to the degree to which normal structure and function is affected.

For most disabilities, the main organs and systems affected are the brain, limbs, trunk, eyes, middle and inner ears, and organs of speech. Complexity in cause and effect is due to the fact that several disabilities can be caused by one factor (e.g. hearing loss due to congenital rubella) and several different factors can be responsible for one disability. However, it is probably a good rule that a knowledge of the disease conditions prevalent in a society should make it possible to deduce the types and patterns of disability in that society or community.

For example, if it is known that diabetes and hypertension are prevalent in an area (such as in the Caribbean), it can be expected that the main disabilities in the over 40 age group will be visual due to damage to the eyes, loss of limbs (and therefore movement) due to diabetes, and speech and moving disabilities due to strokes. Or, as in the Western hemisphere, where poliomyelitis has been eradicated, physical disabilities of the type that are caused by polio will not be seen in children under the age of 4 years. In other words, an informed decision about where and how to start a rehabilitation program can be made without doing a survey and provoking expectations that cannot be fulfilled.

More and more rehabilitation and health professionals are going to work in diverse environments with differing geographic and socioeconomic variables influencing health status and disability rates. An understanding of epidemiology and epidemiological principles will enable them to develop more appropriate and effective prevention and treatment programs.

FURTHER READING

Last J M 1988 A dictionary of epidemiology, 2nd edn. Oxford University Press, Oxford
Mausner J S, Kramer S, 1985 Epidemiology – an introductory text, 2nd edn 1985. W B Saunders, Philadelphia

Robinson D (ed) 1985 Epidemiology and the community control of disease in warm climate countries. Medicine in the tropics, 2nd edn. Churchill Livingstone, Edinburgh

REFERENCES

Basch P F 1990 Textbook of international health. Oxford University Press, New York pp. 100–133

Belmont L 1984 Final report of the international pilot study of severe childhood disability. Gertrude Sergievsky Center, Columbia University, New York

Durkin M S, Davidson L L, Hasan M, Khan N, Thorburn M J, Zaman S 1990 Screening for childhood disabilities in community settings. In: Thorburn M J, Marfo K (eds) Practical approaches to childhood disability in developing countries. 3D Projects, 14 Monk Street, Spanish Town, Jamaica, pp. 179–198

Durkin M S, Davidson L L, Desai P et al 1994 Validity of the ten questions screen for childhood disability: results from population based studies from Bangladesh, Jamaica and Pakistan. Epidemiology 5: 283–289

Gruenberg E M 1977 The failure of success. Milbank Memorial Fund Quarterly 55: 3

Hansluwka H E 1985 Measuring the health of populations, indicators and interpretations. Social Science and Medicine 20: 1207–1224

Last J M 1988 A dictionary of epidemiology, 2nd edn. Oxford University Press, New York

McCusick V A 1973 Ethnic distribution of disease in non-Jews. Israel Journal of Medical Sciences 9: 1375–1382

Mausner J S, Kramer S 1985 Epidemiology – An introductory text, 2nd edn. W B Saunders, Philadelphia

Omran A R 1974 Community medicine in developing countries. Springer, New York

Paul T J, Desai P, Thorburn M J 1992 The prevalence of childhood disability and related medical diagnoses in Clarendon, Jamaica. West Indian Medical Journal 41(8): 8–11

Schuurman M I M (ed) 1995 Assessment of childhood disabilities in developing countries. Proceedings of a workshop at the XIth ILSMH World Congress, Delhi, 1994. Bishop Bekkers Institute, Utrecht, Netherlands

Sinha D 1988 Children of the Caribbean, 1945–1984. CFNI, PAHO/WHO, Kingston, Jamaica pp. 211–212

Thorburn M J 1990 Childhood disability in developing countries: basic issues. In: Thorburn M J, Marfo K (eds) Practical approaches to childhood disability in developing countries, 2nd edn. 3D Projects, 14 Monk St, Spanish Town, Jamaica, pp. 26–27

Thorburn M J, Desai P, Durkin M 1991 A comparison of the efficacy of the key informant and community survey methods in the identification of childhood disability in Jamaica. Annals of Epidemiology 3: 255–261

Thorburn M J, Desai P, Paul T J (1992a) Service needs of children with disabilities. Int. Journal of Rehabilitation Research 15: 31–38

Thorburn M J, Desai P, Paul T J, Malcolm L, Durkin M S, Davidson L L (1992b) Identification of childhood disability in Jamaica: evaluation of the ten question screen. Int. Journal of Rehabilitation Research 15: 262–270

WHO 1980 The International Classification of Impairments, Disabilities and Handicaps. World Health Organization, Geneva

World Bank 1993 World Development Report 1993. Investing in health. Oxford University Press, New York

13

The collaborative learning approach in community based rehabilitation

Sophie Levitt

INTRODUCTION

Personnel training is crucial to the effectiveness of any rehabilitation project. Not only do personnel need to master a general body of knowledge and learn what is expected of them, but they in turn must also teach and advise others (patients, caretakers, colleagues) in the course of their work. Thus, it is essential to examine which teaching approach should be given priority. This chapter describes the collaborative learning approach (CLA), a teaching approach that is suggested for rehabilitation personnel, particularly community rehabilitation workers. The CLA has evolved from many years of practical teaching experience with physical therapists, occupational therapists, speech therapists, and others involved with people with disabilities (PWD) and has been adapted for project leaders of community based rehabilitation (CBR). These adaptations, made both in the classroom and in the field, were devised between 1985 and 1993 for people who attend the CBR courses and the Master of Science courses in mother and child health at the Institute of Child Health, University of London, where I was the guest lecturer for the module on motor problems.

Traditional teaching approaches

In a traditional educational environment, the teacher sets the aims of the course, gives lectures and demonstrations and assesses the progress of the rehabilitation workers (RW).

There is often little time for questions and discussion. The teacher wishes to give as much expertise as possible in the short time available. The teacher may be on a short-term visit, or the course participants' daily work may prohibit long periods of absence.

Even if the teacher invites discussion, there may be little response. Students may be unsure of their own knowledge and skills, while the teacher is assumed to be an expert. A teacher's expertise will certainly impress the students, but it can also make them feel inadequate and anxious. They may not feel confident enough to challenge a presentation that is not relevant to their work in their local community or in their local culture. Students' anxiety interferes with their learning, and the teacher will be disappointed that all her work cannot be carried on in her absence.

Teachers and the RW work energetically in such a course, and later in the field, to carry the whole burden of the rehabilitation program. The content of the course teaches RW to take full responsibility for assessments, aims, selection and utilization of methods, and evaluation of progress of PWD. However, in practice, both teachers and RW are often overwhelmed by the numbers of people needing rehabilitation, the inaccessibility of those living too far away to benefit from specialists in a rehabilitation center, shortages of trained staff at centers and in the field, and financial constraints on PWD and their families that prevent regular rehabilitation sessions. All of these practical difficulties are particularly extreme in poorer developing countries.

RWs who are overworked and frustrated may find they have neither time nor patience to listen to the concerns of PWD and their families, leading, unfortunately, to work that is not always relevant or felt to be important by the people who need help. Nevertheless, families are often impressed by the skills and the expert knowledge of RW and want to believe that they will be able to help. This can often result in PWD and their families feeling inadequate and heavily dependent on the RW, which adds to any existing anxiety caused by incurable impairment and the negative attitudes toward disability in a particular society or culture. Anxiety may even become so severe that it prevents the learning of new ideas and practical suggestions given by the RW.

In an alternative yet still traditional model, in addition to giving lectures, the teacher devises more practical work for the students. However, the RW are still trained to use structured protocols for evaluation and treatment. Although the RW understand the need to instruct families in a home program, they remain responsible for all assessments and treatment plans, and for selecting the methods to be shown to family members. This may leave little room for hearing what PWD or their families perceive as their own problems (which may be unrelated to the professionals' diagnoses) or for listening to ways in which PWD have come up with their own solutions. Such lack of communication clearly is not ideal; as studies by Chiou & Burnett (1985) and Rosenbaum et al (1992) have shown, the rehabilitation aims of therapists differ from those of patients or of parents of children with disabilities in their own culture. PWD often feel too vulnerable or unwilling to upset the professional by asserting what they find to be best for themselves in their own lives and experience. Professionals therefore remain ignorant of valuable data that could improve their programs. This is especially likely to happen in cross-cultural rehabilitation.

In some instances, when the course participants go to work in the field they can be confronted by the goals of families and PWD who make unrealistic demands for cures or magical results. Their choice of goals may be contraindicated for a particular impairment, inappropriate for the self-esteem of the PWD, or inappropriate for the available resources in the community. On the other hand, many PWD and their close families set very modest goals, or none at all, because of low self-esteem, cultural attitudes, or social isolation and emotional stress. Or perhaps they do not know that more progress can be expected. Even when a rehabilitation worker tells them more progress is possible, their despair and stress may result in their refusal to cooperate.

Another concern with traditional teaching approaches is that the course participants may sometimes be unrealistic in what they want for their education. They may want to hear lectures on therapy methods rather than spend time on practicing those methods under supervision, or they may want over-simplified knowledge without time for reflection. They may also be reluctant to explore their own negative attitudes toward disabilities.

THE COLLABORATIVE LEARNING APPROACH

The collaborative learning approach (CLA) incorporates the expert knowledge and skills required for the RW, but the teacher of these skills recognizes that she is not the most expert on knowing what particular problems exist for her students or for the people they are trained to help. Sharing of skills takes place. There is a genuine interest and consideration of what students or PWD and their families want for their daily lives. As these wants, and how to achieve them, are explored in a collaborative style, everyone becomes more willing to pool ideas and skills. The teacher asks the students what they want to learn and what problems they encounter in their work. The students appreciate her concern for them and become more amenable to the idea that they need to discover what clients and their caretakers want to achieve. Both teacher and course participants respond by carrying out what they are asked to do, adapting their special expertise to match with what clients and caretakers want. Unrealistic expectations are dealt with by education and negotiation.

The teacher is not only a resource for acquiring knowledge and skills. Her teaching approach also serves as a model for the course participants to follow when they subsequently teach their own staff and other health and community workers involved with PWD. The RW, or local expert, will need to instruct, advise, and show PWD and their families desirable treatment programs and rehabilitation regimes in the most effective way. Personal experience has led to incorporating these educational ideas into the clinical relationship with children with neurological disability and with their parent or caretaker (Levitt 1995, Levitt 1994, Levitt 1991, Levitt & Goldschmied 1990). The RW at the courses will tend to teach new skills and transmit information in the way in which they were taught.

The CLA places great emphasis on positive personal relationships among everyone involved so that all participants in a learning encounter are committed to a successful outcome. Everyone is respected for their views, sensitivities, and capacities. Recognition is also given to the fact that people who face new challenges are often unsure and need to build up their confidence.

Both in training courses and in working with PWD, a framework is used that follows a sequence of learning opportunities. Individuals need to:

- identify what they want to accomplish or learn
- discover what knowledge and skills are needed for these wants
- recognize what they already know and can do
- find out what they still need to know and achieve
- participate in selecting and using training methods
- participate in the evaluation of progress.

Learning theories

The educational theories underlying the CLA are drawn from the adult education, social work, and psychology disciplines. They knit together separate strands, such as active and participatory learning, listening and communication abilities, and the development of human relationships and counseling skills (Levitt 1995, 1994, 1991, 1987, 1976). Particularly important are the views of Rogers (1983, 1961) on human behavior and the learning process, which evolved from his studies of adults in psychotherapy. He sought to create a student-generated curriculum together with a teacher or leader who 'facilitates' learning. This 'facilitator' needs to develop particular qualities so that 'whole person' learning is promoted, both in the students and the teacher. Knowles (1984, 1975) suggests models for enabling adults to learn in small supportive groups. Titchen (1987) and French et al (1994), among others in health education, recommend similar student-generated courses.

Drawing on these models to facilitate the link between theory and practice, it is essential to recognize several learning principles:

- People are more motivated to learn what they have chosen to accomplish.
- People find it easier to learn what relates to their familiar experiences and prior knowledge.
- Prior knowledge and abilities need to be acknowledged and clarified so that new ideas and skills can be built upon these assets.
- Praise of what is achieved, no matter how small, must accompany suggestions for specific improvements or corrections to maintain motivation in the learners.
- People respond best to genuine approval of both their efforts and achievements.

However, external praise is less significant than people's own recognition of what they manage to achieve.

These learning principles not only help the course participants or the PWD to achieve a functional task, but also help learning to change the context of developing interpersonal relationships. The principles enable individuals to change their ideas, behavior, and attitudes. The teacher too learns to give up old assumptions and alter her behavior. Professional and personal development are enhanced.

Learning to change

It is possible to enable people to change if they understand the benefits to be obtained – that they will achieve more, develop their interests, and feel more satisfaction in their daily lives. Altering the traditional structure in which information is received stimulates acceptance of new ideas. Working with others who are changing and supportive of this experience is helpful. People will often take risks together if they feel safe in the atmosphere created by collaborative work. The inspiration of small successes also facilitates change.

Although a teacher may have her own style and preference for specific ways of teaching, she needs to be flexible enough to use a variety of methods. Leavitt (1996) points out that in some cultures the transmission of knowledge relies on a traditional lecture with few questions and little discussion. But adult learners need a variety of teaching methods for effective learning. In the context of the CLA, many methods are used, although only in response to what course participants reveal they need for their situation. Therefore, a teacher who prepares lectures before getting to know course participants will not necessarily use them. Instead, short talks in response to the participants' questions will make the students more willing and able to absorb what they have wanted to learn. The teacher is thus enabling each person to learn in a variety of ways that may not have been experienced before. The atmosphere generated by the tutor in a CLA modifies and changes the traditional ways.

Although a CLA is conducive to accepting new ideas, individual course members or family members may still find that their prior knowledge and ways of coping with their lives is in too much opposition to the new ideas – their set views and mental framework lead them to reject the information offered. However, these people can learn to make some surprising changes if some of their fellow students or other family members or friends support them, are patient with their rate of learning, and reinforce the advantages of some of the new ideas for their lives. The teacher needs to be understanding of cultural ideas in a particular area and try to relate her ideas to them. For example, a teacher will find out about other collaborative activities that are culturally accepted and present the collaborative work in rehabilitation as a similar venture.

There may also be differences of opinion among participants in a course or as a result of study visits and lectures by other visiting experts. The teacher needs to show negotiating abilities with her participants for them to accept ideas and practical skills that they have found personally or culturally difficult and been unwilling to use. Provided the teacher is genuinely interested, individuals may reconsider these ideas in discussions.

Conflict of views can become most evident when the teacher knows it is for the safety and best interest of a PWD to follow the suggestions offered. In some cases, participants may be faced with contradictory views; this is a wonderful opportunity for a teacher to help participants learn that a *difference* of views need not be a *conflict* of views but rather options for solving problems. The teacher helps the participants learn negotiating abilities through their own experiences in the course so that they can see how these abilities may be applied in work with families who have different perspectives from themselves. Negotiation may occur by:

- Reaching a consensus by finding the common ground.
- Shelving ideas for future use.
- Alternating practical ideas to see which works best.
- Having one party step down for a while (such generosity is often rewarded by the other party doing the same on another occasion).
- Sometimes, no agreement can be reached. The option then is for everyone to agree to focus their energies on those things they do agree on.

When course participants or families are learning to change, they may also find themselves facing their own negative attitudes toward disability. Negative attitudes of the RW, the family of the PWD, or the community at large may interfere with recovery and progress. Any rehabilitation course must therefore address this issue. The participants need to become aware of any negative attitudes that still persist in their minds and in their behavior so that there is no reinforcement of discrimination against those with a disability. The CLA encourages an open discussion of these issues.

It is of particular value that PWD are included in rehabilitation courses both as students and as teachers. Course participants can then experience professional and social contact on an equal basis, rather than only consider PWD as their dependent patients. In social situations, trainee RW learn about any social and environmental barriers faced by their colleagues. Participants also gain information and experience on what a PWD can achieve, given the correct pace of learning and appropriate training. The demonstration and practical experience of doing joint assessments with PWD and their families provides such information throughout a period of rehabilitation. There needs to be discussion and demonstration of how a PWD and family members decide which of the teacher's skills they are willing to use. There needs to be evidence of respect for each person's view and contribution. The responsibility of carrying out the rehabilitation program is distributed among a number of people so that one person (usually a woman) is not burdened with the home program. This is best done if these skills form part of what is familiar to everyone. For example, functional rehabilitation, including correcting postural positions for function, can be incorporated into multiple daily life activities involving different caretakers whenever possible.

Learning skills used in rehabilitation

Most of the practical demonstrations involve enabling a family member or the PWD to carry out familiar tasks of self-care, play, or household chores and mobility. At the community level, one needs to function in school or at work, or in play groups and other social activities. It is therefore ideal to use a place in the community for a rehabilitation course. This allows the course participants to practice what they are learning with people from their own culture in culturally appropriate ways. This supplements the practical skill training in a course when participants work with one another.

In some cultures, the participants prefer to learn a task as a whole. In others, learning is better when the task is analyzed into activities and sequences for a task (Ebrahim et al 1988). Physical therapists are often particularly adept at teaching motor tasks in step-by-step sequences. The teacher must discover which approach is preferred.

Most learners appreciate demonstrations. For example, in various countries, skills are taught by parents to children according to their stage of understanding. This 'learning by doing' or apprenticeship model is common in natural life situations as well as in the educational and work environment. The learner first watches and then assists the skilled and experienced person. The learner's assistance is minimal at first but increases with time until the skill is learned. After the course, a less experienced staff member can work with someone who attended a course and so become more knowledgeable and experienced, applying the apprenticeship model in the daily work situation.

The teacher does not isolate skill learning from all other learning involving attitudes and communication with this teaching style. Examples of one-to-one teaching take place in a course when a more experienced participant shows a skill to a less experienced participant. That colleague learns it but also gives feedback on the way in which she was taught. Special skills that are unfamiliar in a culture are only taught once participants or families have gained some confidence in achieving a familiar task.

PRACTICAL APPLICATION IN A COURSE

Introducing the course

The teacher begins the course by welcoming the participants and showing a warm and friendly interest in them. This personal interest can best develop if the group is small (perhaps 16–20 students). The teacher explains that together they will be formulating the program for their course using a collaborative learning model, noting that all of them have both life and work experiences they can draw on for their learning experiences. The participants are invited to introduce themselves.

The participants and teacher sit in a circle to convey respect for each person present and so that everyone can see their colleagues. Each person turns to a partner in order to listen to her account of who she is, what expectations she holds for the course, and what her special professional and non-professional interests are. Partners introduce each other to the group after checking what should remain private, allowing everyone to begin to know each other. The teacher acknowledges some of the students' interests and shows how they can relate to the course. This gives them confidence that they know something and that they are capable of learning new or unfamiliar ideas. For example, if some participants say they are parents, the teacher refers to the value of observing their children's development. In this way, students increase their understanding of stages of achievement, pace of learning, and the natural curiosity of a child which is tempered with caution when attempting new skills.

To create a positive learning climate that encourages the learning of new skills, ideas, behavior, and attitudes, the teacher presents a set of ground rules:

- Each person is respected for his or her views and contribution.
- Attentive listening with no interruption is expected so that different views can be understood.
- No one has to say or do anything that they feel is too much for them.
- Laughter and fun can help people to learn better, but this must never be at anyone's expense.
- Each person's individual pace of learning is respected.
- Mistakes are acceptable and often useful to help understand what can be improved upon and why better performance or behavior is desirable.
- Agreements to do something will be made together and followed up. Renegotiation can occur.

Such rules may be unfamiliar and keeping them can be a learning experience in itself. The teacher must be a good role model.

Defining the learning needs

The tutor invites the participants to form sub-groups of 3–6 people to discuss what they want to learn in the course that would assist them in their daily professional lives. The sub-group must determine its priorities according to its members' daily work. After a short time, they are expected to assemble a list of headings or phrases representing these priorities. These are presented to the larger group and written on a flip-chart. As priorities are pooled, the teacher enables the students to clarify which are best grouped together and which they feel are quite different. Everyone participates in arranging the priorities into a list of coherent study themes or main topics.

Sub-groups offer an easier way to air thoughts and feelings with a few colleagues compared to speaking before a large group of people. In some countries, it can also overcome reticence to participating in discussions arising from a wish not to offend a visitor or cultural taboos on appearing boastful. The teacher needs to hear what her students think and how they solve problems so that she knows at what level to teach. The use of a questionnaire to find out such information is not useful: it can be even more unfamiliar than discussion in some cultures. Moreover, questionnaires rarely supply enough of the information needed by a teacher, and students tend to ask for what they believe the teacher wants. Sub-groups offer the participants experience in discussion and in clarifying their problems and needs.

The list of the participants' priorities or study themes becomes the primary expectations for the course. These themes are kept pinned on a board for all to check throughout the course. The teacher will regularly refer back to it to ensure that the learning needs it expresses are being met. The participants are told to retain their other learning wishes in case there is time for them. It is also possible that these may be addressed during sessions on the primary themes.

Examples of study themes include child or adult self-care activities, communication problems, mobility methods, play activities, equipment, behavior problems, specific impairments and their causes and treatment techniques, as well as concerns relating to work and organizations, referral decisions and administrative problems.

The teacher expects the sub-groups to reform to determine which skills and what knowledge they need to accomplish their study themes. Each sub-group takes one or two themes, and underlines what it already knows and can do. This shows the group's members what they still need to learn and achieve. Depending on the study theme, the sub-group may or may not recognize what they still need to know. The teacher periodically welcomes general feedback from the whole group to gauge how the participants are working and whether they need more time for discussion. This has to be planned within the constraints of the course.

During feedback, the teacher clarifies and adds to each group presentation. She will link ideas, showing how one theme may include part of another. There may be solutions to one problem that can also serve to help solve other problems in other study themes. For example, a sub-group working on training of feeding skills may list a number of components that need to be understood, including body position, postural control, the use of vision, hearing and the other senses, communication, and understanding how to actually feed. The teacher can add any missing components and may link these components with those for other self-care activities.

These components, needed for everyday life, have been labeled 'basic abilities'. The tutor can link 'basic abilities' with assessments of the stages of achievement of abilities. This prepares the course participants for learning the skills needed to achieve the abilities at the appropriate stages for each individual PWD. As the basic abilities are studied within familiar daily life activities, the customary way such activities are carried out emerges. The teacher will therefore gain important knowledge relevant to the culture in which she is working. There is also the opportunity for a teacher to develop the notion that human relationships are integrated into all bodily care by health workers and family members. (This approach is more fully discussed in Levitt (1994). Daily life activities are central to rehabilitation, and cultural adaptations can be made in different places.)

When courses need to be short because of time constraints and expense, integrating study themes allows more information for learning than if topics are taught separately. Using a whole approach with 'basic abilities' has helped bring together a number of the learning wishes of participants in courses internationally (Levitt 1991).

Learning style options

The participants inform the teacher of customary ways of learning in their community (such as story-telling, puppet shows, rhymes, songs, and learning games). These may be used in the course or in the practical work with children or adults with disabilities. Participants can present case histories from their daily work. These may have been prepared before the course. The group and the teacher validate the useful content in the case history. The teacher can also draw out ideas for the rest of the group and offer additional suggestions. The group can make constructive suggestions, particularly when these relate to their local culture.

It is important to hear what participants feel about the teaching style. Some will feel uneasy because they are used to being passive while a teacher feeds them all of the facts. Others become excited by the new experiences and encourage the rest of the group. If a participant is uneasy, she should be gently approached rather than allowed to become sullen or resentful and thus affect the atmosphere in the group.

Throughout the course, the teacher links new ideas with the prior knowledge of the participants as this emerges during the sessions. The teacher must observe the group to see whether she needs to slow the pace of the course, improve her explanations, or possibly use some more traditional teaching methods.

At the same time, the participants are learning how to articulate their experiences in the sub-groups. The teacher's attentive and respectful listening enables them to gain confidence. The course format and the ground rules enable people to modify their customary behavior as far as they feel they can manage.

The sub-groups can also be used in a variety of other ways. They can

- Choose a skill to practice on one another.
- Research an idea and prepare a talk for the group. Participants with special skills or knowledge present it to the group.
- Further divide into partners who can then practice therapy and counseling skills and collaborative teaching skills. Partners may prefer to present their skills to another two than to the whole group.
- Foster role playing. The sub-group willing to carry out an enactment in front of the group needs to know that a person plays the role of someone else in the presentations. Playing one's own role may be embarrassing in front of colleagues. A tutor might play the role of a course participant and learn from that viewpoint.

Teaching and learning materials

It is valuable to use a variety of teaching materials and field trips (see Box 13.1). These need to be considered in terms of what suits the culture and preferences of the course participants. Innovative ideas will be stimulated in a teacher who is responsive to her students. The options listed in Box 13.1 should be considered.

Evaluation of the course

There are two overlapping areas for evaluation: assessment of the participants' learning, and their evaluation of the course itself. Traditionally tests and examinations assess the participants. This causes anxiety and often places the teacher

---

Box 13.1 Teaching and learning resources

- *Training packages and resource guides.* An increasing number of such materials are particularly relevant to developing countries (see Further Resources list at the end of the chapter). However, it can be a valuable learning experience for course participants to make their own teaching materials. This enhances group interaction and reinforces the notion of learning by doing. Materials may or may not be given to individuals to take home with them.
- *Charts.* In some cultures participants need to be taught how to read charts or graphs. They may want to learn to make their own.
- *Illustrations.* It is wise to discuss the cultural relevance of drawings. Therapists' stylized drawings or match-stick figures may be confusing and rarely show detail of body parts. It is best to draw whole bodies, which will also demonstrate correct positions and patterns of movement. Extraneous information and background is confusing. People in the drawing need to look like those in the community and be wearing culturally appropriate clothing. Pleasant facial expressions with some shading give an encouraging message. The emotional or social interaction between the person teaching a procedure and the one learning it should convey a positive relationship.

Arrows indicating direction and movement are rarely understood, while a sequence of a comic type may be clearer in some cultures.
- *Videos and slide shows.* Videos are often quite advantageous and are becoming more popular as a teaching tool. They can show new ideas and approaches in action and provide a 'picture' of how things are done. Videos can sometimes be dubbed into the local language and are easily copied. However, electricity or televisions may not be available.
- *Hand-outs.* These need to be short and clear and summarize what arises in a course. They must be in the proper language and use culturally appropriate pictures. Although teachers may prepare these beforehand, the hand-outs may not all be relevant and more will need to be composed during the course.
- *Field trips.* These are valuable for learning relevant practices within the community. Hospitals, play groups, schools, and other community projects are visited. Preparatory discussion and checklists help the participants make the most of any visit. The tutor can focus on specific information from visits when they are subsequently discussed.

---

in a position of power, which the CLA wants to avoid. Alternative assessment approaches include:

- Peer assessment. One participant records what a colleague can do (but *not* what she cannot do).
- Self-assessment. A participant keeps a private checklist of what she hopes to learn and what she has learned by the end of the course. A participant may have prepared a case study before the course; she can it read after the course, assessing how it has changed and what additional practical ideas have been gained.
- Each participant can personally check whether the skills and knowledge earlier identified as study topics have been learned. Together the group can assess whether they would like more information about specific skills and knowledge.
- Each participant is invited to say what she found most useful, what was enjoyable, and what will be used immediately upon returning to work. The participant may indicate what is missing from the course and what more she

would like to have had for future courses. This information can be written anonymously. The tutor can turn this discussion into a teaching session.

- Questionnaires rarely obtain all the relevant information but may give a general overview of the level of success. (Cohen & Manion 1989). Items on an anonymous questionnaire can rate the level of teaching, type of teaching, and particular teaching methods such as practicals, videos, slides and visits. Specific sessions and guest lectures may be rated, as can the physical environment for comfortable concentrated learning. A section for comments on questionnaires may be the most useful.

More difficult to measure or record are the growth in self-confidence, the ability to relate more sensitively to colleagues and PWD, the creative strategies in solving problems, and improved communication skills. As Thorburn (1990) emphasizes, the personality and behavior of a RW is of more importance than a large amount of technical expertise. These assets are perceived to grow in everyone involved in CLA.

CONCLUSION

A CLA is suggested for the education of RW in training courses and in their field work as well as when educating groups of relatives or parents and others involved with disabilities in a community. This style of education is especially suited for a multi-cultural situation. Cultural differences, either between a teacher and the RW or between the RW and her clients, are inevitably addressed within the context of the CLA. The CLA may certainly also have relevance for the education of rehabilitation professionals.

Throughout the course, parallels are drawn between the CLA and the similar collaborative work in the field with PWD and their families. Teachers and RW gain essential information about each family's child-caring patterns, health beliefs and attitudes. In a collaborative relationship, local RW and PWD and their families can discover ways of interpreting their culture so that rehabilitation is appropriately developed for themselves.

The CLA needs to be adapted to a particular project and to each area of the world. It is left to the individual teacher and RW to adapt and adopt what they find relevant to each situation. Some workers gradually use more and more of this approach according to how comfortable they feel with changing their previous ways of working. It is only through experiential learning that the theories and practice can be understood in both courses and fieldwork. The CLA cannot easily be taught in lectures or it can become a rigid blueprint or recipe that is not dynamic and prevents growth and development in different cross-cultural situations as well as in the same culture.

As teachers and RWs develop this style of work in their own ways they will find themselves becoming more creative and their work more rewarding. The individual PWD and family members discover more of their strengths and resources and grow in self-confidence as they function within a positive personal and social context. Everyone involved becomes more innovative in solving problems and in their thinking.

FURTHER RESOURCES

Organizations providing training guides and resources for rehabilitation in developing countries:
AHRTAG (Appropriate Health Resources and Technologies Action Group, now known as Healthlink), Farringdon Point, 29 Farringdon Road, London, EC1M 3JB, UK. *AHRTAG publishes 'CBR News' and produces booklets on disability and community based rehabilitation.*
Cheshire Homes for Eastern Region, 515 Q Jalan Hashim, 11200 Tanjung Bunga, Penang, Malaysia. 'A better life for all' (8 videos and accompanying workbooks).
Institute of Child Health (ICH), 30 Guilford Street, London WC1N 1EH, UK.
International Centre for the Advancement of Community Based Rehabilitation (ICACBR), Queen's University, Kingston, Ontario, Canada K7L 3N6.
Mental Health Center, Peshawar, North West Frontier Province, Pakistan. Miles C 1990 Special education for mentally handicapped pupils. Miles C 1988 Speech, language and communication with the special child.
HealthWrights P.O. Box 1344 Palo Alto, California CA 94302 USA. Werner D 1987 Disabled Village Children: A Guide for Community Health Workers, RW and Families. Werner D., Bower B 1982. Helping health workers learn. Werner D 1997 Nothing about us without us: developing innovative technologies for by and with disabled persons.
UNESCO, 7 Place de Fontenoy, Paris 75700, France. Ugandan Task Force on Educating Communities about Disability 1991 Guides for special education.
World Health Organization, 1211, Geneva, Switzerland. WHO 1989 Training in the community for PWD. WHO 1993 Promoting the development of young children with cerebral palsy – a guide for midlevel RW.
Zimcare Trust, P.O. Boz 90, Belvedere, Harare, Zimbabwe. Zimcare Trust 1985 Home-based learning programs for children with learning difficulties.

REFERENCES

Chiou L L, Burnett C N 1985 Values of activities of daily living: Physical Therapy 65: 901

Cohen L, Manion L 1989 Research methods in education, 3rd edn. Routledge, London

Ebrahim G J, Ahmed A W, Khan A A 1988 Maternal and child health in practice: training modules for middle level workers. Macmillan, London

French S, Neville S, Laing J 1994 Teaching and learning. Butterworth-Heinemann, Oxford

Knowles M 1975 Self-directed learning: a guide for learners and teachers. Association Press, New York

Knowles M 1984 The adult learner: a neglected species, 3rd edn. Gulf, Houston

Leavitt R 1996 Physical therapy in a different culture. Physiotherapy Theory and Practice 12: 113

Levitt S 1976 Helping the handicapped child at village level. In: The disabled in developing countries: proceedings of a symposium at Oriel College, Oxford. Commonwealth Foundation Occasional Paper XLI, London

Levitt S 1987 We can play and move. Appropriate Health Resources and Technologies Action Group, London

Levitt S 1991 International therapy workshops and patient-centred physiotherapy. In: Proceedings of the 11th international congress of the WCPT, London, p. 283

Levitt S 1994 Basic abilities – a whole approach: a developmental guide for children with disabilities Souvenir Press, London

Levitt S 1995 Treatment of cerebral palsy and motor delay, 3rd edn. Blackwell Science, Oxford

Levitt S, Goldschmied E 1990 As we teach, so we treat. Physiotherapy Theory and Practice 6: 227

Rogers C 1961 On becoming a person. Houghton Mifflin, Boston, Mass

Rogers C 1983 Freedom to learn for the 80s. Charles E Merrill, Columbus, Ohio

Rosenbaum P L, King S M, Cadman D T 1992 Measuring processes of care-giving to physically disabled children and their families: identifying relevant components of care. Developmental Medicine and Child Neurology 34: 103

Thorburn M J 1990 Practical aspects of programme development: prevention and early intervention at the community level. In: Thorburn M J, Marfo K (eds) Practical approaches to childhood disability in developing countries: insights from experience and research. Memorial University, St John's, Newfoundland

Titchen A 1987 Design and implementation of a problem-based continuing education programme. Physiotherapy 73: 318–323

14

Cross-cultural supervision of students

Richard Ladyshewsky

INTRODUCTION

Supervision of students by health professionals is not a new phenomenon in the rehabilitation professions. Methods for executing this supervision, from a Western perspective, are well referenced in the clinical education literature. But does the clinical supervision process change when the learner comes from a different culture or language background? Should this learner be treated the same as all the other 'local' learners, or should the student's cultural background be taken into consideration when evaluating performance? Answers to these questions are not so readily available.

Clinical educators who have the responsibility for observing and evaluating students from diverse cultural or language backgrounds need to be aware of challenges that may surface during the clinical learning process. Without a good understanding of the issues in cross-cultural supervision, clinical educators may lose some of their effectiveness as teachers and may even make inaccurate conclusions about the student's clinical competence.

This chapter will present information on making the clinical learning experience more culturally sensitive when the clinical educator and student are from different cultural and language backgrounds. The first part of the chapter deals with cultural issues, with the second focusing on language and communication issues. The third part outlines some of the specific challenges for the clinical educator, and the fourth deals with cross-cultural clinical teaching strategies.

Many of the insights within the chapter are derived from work conducted at Curtin University of Technology in Perth, Western Australia. Because of the university's proximity to Southeast Asia, a large number of students from this region come to Australia to study, making the environment rich with cross-cultural teaching and supervision examples.

While every attempt has been made to include generic examples, it is important to understand that the author is limited by his own cultural influences and experiences in reporting on the subject. The chapter is also influenced to a large degree by the experiences of Southeast Asian Chinese students from a non-English-speaking background within an English-speaking, Westernized culture; the quotations given in the chapter reflect this context. Further, the information presented here is not definitive; cultures, and individuals within cultures, are not homogeneous groups (Mullins et al 1995).

THE INFLUENCE OF CULTURE IN CROSS-CULTURAL CLINICAL SUPERVISION

The extent to which a student from a different culture may experience difficulty in their clinical education experience largely depends upon the amount of time spent in the new culture. Zhang (1995), for example, noted that new immigrants who have resided in the USA for a few years and first generation Asian-Americans differed in their ability to cope with learning challenges. Those who had spent more time in the host country tended to have better coping and learning skills.

The literature also provides a general description of some of the issues overseas students face when studying abroad, although these are not necessarily specific to health care programs (Kennedy 1995, Ballard & Clanchy 1991). It is notable that overseas students are more likely than local students to experience problems (Mullins et al 1995). Phenomenographic or qualitative studies of students' approaches to learning are cited in the literature but tend to

concentrate on students in Westernized, mostly English-speaking countries, principally Australia and the UK, and the Scandinavian countries (Kember & Gow 1990). Because phenomenology is the study of phenomena within a culture or context, these studies have a Western bias.

Samuelowicz (1987) indicates that some of the difficulties faced by overseas students are coping with the educational system and cultural adjustments to life in a new country. Ballard & Clanchy (1991) also describe the difficulties students experience when studying abroad. They state that many of the problems stem from the culture of learning that is embedded with context-specific values unique to the host country. It is important, therefore, that clinical educators be aware of the impact of culture on learner performance (Ballard & Clanchy 1991).

Waller (1993) found that understanding the foreign environment is a significant struggle for students from Southeast Asia studying in English-speaking Western cultures. A large part of this relates to the different expectations learners have of their educational experiences. Ballard & Clanchy (1991) describe how cultural traditions influence peoples' attitudes to the acquisition and interpretation of knowledge. They state that in a Confucian, Buddhist, Hindu, or Islamic society, the essence of scholarship is the ability to cite quotations from the sacred writings, the sayings of the sages, and the words of leading scholars. The influence of religion and traditional education structures in Asia reinforce cultural learning traditions by emphasizing memory work and passivity (Yee 1989, Walker 1993). This point is illustrated by Kember & Gow (1990), who evaluated the learning approaches of students in Hong Kong. They found that the students have a narrow, systematic, step-by-step orientation to learning that was influenced in part by their cultural traditions of learning and also by their ability to speak English. These learning traditions are quite different from Western approaches, which emphasize critical analysis, fluidity of knowledge, and constant revision. The impact of cultural learning traditions, therefore, is also a variable.

Cultural norms that determine how one should behave in public situations can also influence the teaching and learning experience. Shih (1988), for example, describes cultural influences on the behavior of Asians and Westerners. Asian behavior is influenced to a large degree by Confucianist principles, which emphasize group approval and harmony. This may explain why some Asian students take a relatively passive role in their learning for fear of offending their teacher and being disrespectful. In contrast, Western culture emphasizes the preservation of one's individuality within the group. Thus, challenging a teacher's ideas and demonstrating inquisitiveness are valued learner attributes. With these contrasting teaching and learning expectations it would be easy for clinical educators to assume that the Asian students are lazy, uninterested or lacking specific knowledge. The students, on the other hand, may assume that clinical educators are uninterested, racist, or ignorant of what to do because the teachers do not offer the correct advice or direction. Other cultures would have different behavioral approaches influenced to a large degree by their religion, national history and political systems. These cultural differences will have a direct influence on how learners deal with their day-to-day learning challenges.

Zhang (1995) also comments upon social identity and the linkage to family among Asian students. Inadequate performance often brings shame to the student and his family. The desire to 'save face' may explain why some Southeast Asian students are averse to taking risks during clinical practice, preferring to be guided through their clinical learning experience to ensure success. Another potential influence is the role of women in an Islamic culture. An Islamic female studying in a Westernized educational system may have responsibilities to her family or partner that supersede her clinical learning responsibilities to a much greater degree than those of a Westernized, Protestant female student in a similar situation.

Lack of understanding of these cross-cultural differences can lead to conflict in clinical education. A Westernized clinical educator would typically expect a student to take responsibility for his own learning and to be self-evaluative and questioning of all practices. In contrast, an Asian student would prefer to be guided by the instructor so that no mistakes occur. Samuelowicz (1987) found that international students studying in Western educational systems often have difficulty switching roles from being a passive recipient in the process to being an active participant. These same students also have difficulty questioning and developing critical views on the subject matter under discussion.

The other cultural issue that will have an important influence on students' clinical learning performance is their awareness of local cultural practices and stories. Successful performance in an organization such as a hospital or health care clinic requires students to have some understanding of local cultural practices and language. For most of these students, their time has been spent studying content and learning how to cope within the culture of the educational system. Many have not prepared themselves adequately for the cultural experience of working within a health care agency with the local population. Because of this lack of preparation, these students are at a considerable disadvantage when compared to their local peers. The following examples illustrate how this lack of cultural history and awareness can influence the students' clinical practice success.

1. *Southeast Asian student studying in Australia*: I was doing a placement in psycho-geriatrics. I was supposed to determine the patient's level of orientation by talking about current and past events, for example, prime ministers, facts about World War Two. How am I supposed to know all about Australian culture and history? It puts you at a real disadvantage as you don't know how to communicate around a common issue with your patients because you come from a different culture.

2. *Southeast Asian student*: I ask superficial questions [of the patient] or don't get too involved into the discussion because I don't have the background.

Helping students from diverse cultural backgrounds to become more familiar with the local culture before their clinical practicums is a big challenge. Numerous rehabilitation education programs place the bulk of their clinical practice towards the latter half of the curriculum – after the students have completed all of their basic science and clinical subjects. The clinical placement can suddenly become quite an overwhelming experience if students from different cultural or language backgrounds have not made any attempt to become more familiar with local cultural traditions or manners early in their study.

THE INFLUENCE OF LANGUAGE AND COMMUNICATION IN CROSS-CULTURAL CLINICAL SUPERVISION

While a learner's ability to adequately speak the local language in the health care setting is important, it does not explain all of the special considerations in a cross-cultural supervision experience. Students who speak English quite well may still have difficulties during clinical practice if they come from a different culture. For example, a Japanese student who has learned to speak English in Japan does not necessarily understand the culture of England, Canada, or Australia. Bisong (1995) illustrates this point by stating that a Nigerian variety of English has emerged that expresses Nigerian culture. In other words, the ability of Nigerian people to speak English has not made them less Nigerian or more British. When learning a new language, therefore, particularly when it is learned in one's own country, the individual does not lose his cultural identity. If someone has learned to speak English, for example, the additional language skill he has acquired merely provides him with the means to learn about life and culture in predominantly English-speaking societies.

Students may also find that their lack of fluency in speaking the local language can interfere with their ability to successfully manage a case. Clinical educators need to be aware of these difficulties so that they do not make assumptions about students' abilities in the area of case management. One of the communication obstacles for students from a different language background is word stress. Ballard & Clanchy (1991) call this language panic. Word stress results from speakers who do not speak the language of conversation fluently have difficulty producing the correct words at a pace appropriate to the conversation. Samuelowicz (1987) states that international students often have difficulty formulating complex ideas in a foreign language and doing so at a rapid speed.

The speed of the conversation is another factor that influences the expression of knowledge. In some cultures, it may be appropriate to communicate very slowly. This would be indicative of thoughtful deliberation. In other cultures, a faster communication pace may be the norm. Because of word stress and the expected pace of conversation, clinical teachers have to realize that it may take more time for a student whose first language differs from that of the host country to answer a question. Allowing the student more time provides the supervisor with a better opportunity to assess the student's underlying knowledge base. The clinical educator may otherwise make inappropriate assumptions about the student's knowledge when in fact the problem may be word stress:

3. *Southeast Asian student*: In Singapore and Malaysia we have better English training and a reasonable command of English. We think in English but our choice of words is the most difficult and the source of most misunderstanding. Peers from Australia have a much wider word choice for each particular situation whereas mine is very limited. Peers have so many words to describe pain, for example. . . . This creates the impression in your supervisors that you are not very good. If I spoke in Mandarin I could describe pain in many more subtle ways.

Whereas word stress relates to the difficulties students have when trying to identify a word that best describes what they are attempting to articulate, 'wait time' relates to the time needed to communicate. Wait time can be defined as the time gaps that occur between individuals when communicating (Hall 1992). When a learner from a different language background is asked a question, the following mental processes may occur. First, the learner hears the question and translates it into his own language. Second, he thinks of an answer in his own language. Third, he translates the answer back into the host language. Fourth, he has to think about how to structure the answer appropriately using correct conversational grammar. Fifth, he has to articulate the response. This mental processing can add a considerable amount of time to the question/answer response cycle. Consider the following example, observed by the author. It illustrates the concepts of word stress and wait time and the impression that a supervisor may have of the student's underlying knowledge.

During a Master of Science candidacy presentation, a student from Thailand gave a very eloquent presentation. Her word usage, pace, and articulation were good, and it was obvious that the student had put a lot of energy into preparing her presentation. During the question and answer period, however, the student struggled to find the correct words to the answers. Perhaps being aware of the need to respond to the question in an appropriate time frame, the answer that the student finally provided was brief, hard to understand, brusque, incomplete, and unstructured. Had the student perhaps been given additional time to think of the answer, her response might have been more complete. The end result of the exercise was that nobody asked any more questions because it was obvious that the student was struggling. To the culturally insensitive observer, the manner of the student's response would be indicative of a poor student.

These word stress and wait time frustrations have been clearly articulated by students:

4. *Southeast Asian student*: I found I was having difficulty coming up with the correct words during problem solving sessions with my supervisor. This made me quite anxious. The supervisor was stereotyping me as having insufficient knowledge but the real issue was that it took longer for me to process information and come up with the correct words to express the thought.

5. *Southeast Asian student*: When I speak to a supervisor, I always think twice or three times before I speak – I want to choose the correct words to avoid misunderstanding.

6. *Southeast Asian student*: I find I know a lot more than what we are given credit. Part of the difficulty stems from my ability to express myself clearly in English. The oral examination, for example, demands that you respond to a question then and there! I feel that I know the answer, I just can't put it together on the spot.

7. *Southeast Asian student*: It is hard discussing things with the supervisor because it is harder to express theoretical views – it is another level of English language proficiency. I am just not at the same level as the Australian student. Sometimes you are perceived as lacking knowledge and problem solving ability.

The word stress and wait time phenomena can also inhibit the student–patient interaction. Students and patients may become frustrated during the treatment session because neither party can fully understand the other. Students may miss important information regarding the patient's medical–social status. Misinterpretation of instructions may occur. This interferes with the students' ability to develop a rapport with their clients.

With the combined pressures of word stress, wait time and the need to converse in a manner befitting local cultural customs, students are often at a loss to express themselves appropriately. The quality of the communication may also sound rude or brusque to the patient. What typically comes out of the student's mouth is a 'last ditch' effort to get the message across. Because of this pressure, the instructions or comments to the patient are brief, clipped, staccato in nature, and appear to be lacking any empathy. Because the expression of empathy during conversation is in many ways a cultural phenomenon, it may be difficult for a student from a different culture to express this emotion adequately. Communication with the patient, therefore, may appear cold and clinical even though the student may care deeply about his patient.

Examples of these communication phenomena are described by both clinical educators and students.

8. *Clinical educator*: Quite often the students choose the wrong words or only have a limited set. If they hear a word being used they often will use it [with a patient] even though it may not be appropriate or contextually correct.

9. *Southeast Asian student*: I feel like I am always using the same words to reinforce behavior. I notice how other Australian students and therapists show their appreciation and motivate patients – it seems so natural and well communicated. I am very conscious

of what I am about to say and it sounds like I am saying the same thing over and over again – probably to the point where it sounds insincere.

10. *Clinical educator*: Communication with the local English speaking population is a big problem [for the Southeast Asian students]. . . . Transferring the technical terms acquired during study to lay language in English is very difficult. . . . I think about how I manage patients who don't speak English and it helps me to understand the difficulties these students are experiencing.

11. *Clinical educator*: It takes longer to develop rapport with patients, this relates to the communication difficulties. . . . the [Southeast Asian] students are spending so much time listening, thinking, translating, etc. . . . It becomes difficult for the patients to develop rapport. The student, because they are anxious and busy thinking, often comes across as very blunt – this further cuts off rapport.

12. *Clinical educator*: What words do you say to people to demonstrate that you have empathy – this is difficult for the [Southeast Asian] students.

13. *Clinical educator*: The [Southeast Asian] student's language sounds clipped, the accent sounds brusque or rude and this puts the patient off – even though the student is trying hard. Statements are too brusque and staccato.

The stress of not understanding the local culture, the myriad of communication and language issues, and the pressure to perform to an adequate professional standard are but a sample of the challenges that a student from a different cultural and language background may face during a clinical placement. The impact of this stress on a student's self-esteem may be so great that it interferes with his performance and integration into the local culture.

14. *Southeast Asian student*: When I don't understand something I won't ask them [the clinical educator] to repeat it more than three times because I don't want to feel stupid.

15. *Southeast Asian student*: I don't understand what they are talking about, particularly the jokes – I miss everything and I don't know what is going on. It puts you off and you feel pretty low. You decide not to participate because you feel useless and helpless.

It is not surprising that students from different cultural and language backgrounds find solace within their own community. Mullins (1991) and Mullins et al (1995) revealed very low levels of interaction between local and international students. If clinical educators and local student populations are not aware of the international students' feelings of isolation and inadequacy, it is unlikely that this latter group will thrive in the environment. Nor will this group seek further opportunities for learning about local culture and language.

While it is easy to suggest to the international students that they increase their participation in local cultural activities, it is dependent upon members of the community to embrace and welcome these newcomers. Mullins et al (1995) found that the local (Australian) students tended to stay in their own groups and did not seem to need any new friends.

CHALLENGES FOR THE CLINICAL EDUCATOR

The cultural and language influences cited above are largely from the student perspective. This highlights the fact that if no attempt is made to understand the various cultural and language nuances, the clinical educator is in danger of making inappropriate assumptions about a learner's performance which may lead to conflict and misunderstanding. These assumptions (highlighted in the following contrasting quotations by both educators and students) were evident in cross-cultural supervision experiences at Curtin University of Technology, Perth, Western Australia.

16a. *Clinical Educator*: The students [from Southeast Asia] manipulate the situation – they don't expose their problems – they don't always give you the full picture.

16b. *Southeast Asian student*: Supervisors expect us to bring forward our own ideas whereas we believe that valuing input from others is more important. . . . We were not encouraged to ask questions during our education [in Southeast Asia] whereas in Australia students are expected to be more independent and active in their learning.

17a. *Clinical educator*: The [Southeast Asian] students' problem solving abilities seem very poor. We teach Australian students to be very independent whereas this doesn't appear to be the case with these students.

17b. *Southeast Asian student*: One's own ideas are not as important as what the actual facts are or what is accurate. Rather than take the wrong course of action – it is more appropriate to hear the information from an expert so that the course of action is correct.

18a. *Clinical educator*: The [Southeast Asian] students don't appear to personalize the problems as their own – they throw it back at you. Since you identified the problem you must solve it for them. It is not your typical adult learning situation – you are here to tell them what to do.

18b. *Southeast Asian student*: It is impolite to be assertive or aggressive with your supervisor. You are taught in school [in Southeast Asia] not to talk to your teacher directly. You can disagree but only to a certain level. Because professional behavior is such an important part of your evaluation, if you act in a bad manner you will get low marks.

The implementation of supervisory techniques that are commonplace within a Western educational system may not necessarily work for the clinical educator when applied to a student from a different language and cultural background. The use of feedback is one example. In Western society, feedback is central to adult learning theory. Adults need feedback to learn about their strengths and weaknesses to build both confidence and future learning (Ladyshewsky 1995). Without feedback, adult learners become anxious and concerned and cannot determine where to direct their learning energies.

However, the nature and format of feedback across cultures is likely to have a lot of variation. Students from non-Western cultures learning in a Western environment may find the Westerner's approach to feedback threatening or offensive. Positive feedback would be welcomed, but anything negative could result in a loss of face and feelings of shame. Students may therefore ignore the negative feedback or constantly ask the clinical educator what to do next so they don't make any errors – thus avoiding negative criticism.

19. *Clinical educator*: Feedback is a problem – giving both positive and negative feedback, which is what we consider appropriate in Western culture, doesn't necessarily work [with the Southeast Asian students]. Anything negative is considered a failure – all they [Southeast Asian students] see is the failure – they take negative criticism much more seriously.

The discourse structure of providing feedback may also vary between cultures. In Western culture, clinical educators typically preface critical feedback with something positive. By doing so, the negative comments don't appear as harsh. Western clinical educators, when giving feedback, would also start with the most important items first and end with the least important items. In some cultures, where individuals are more assertive, they may go straight to the negative feedback since this directness is not considered offensive. In Southeast Asia, individuals tend not to be assertive and are generally considered to be more indirect. Scollon & Wong-Scollon (1995) also state that the most important points in a Southeast Asian discourse structure are emphasized at the end of a conversation. Giving feedback in the order of priority, according to the Western model, would therefore lead to great misunderstanding between the clinical educator and the Southeast Asian student. Once again, it would be easy for the clinical educator to make assumptions about the student not following through on the feedback.

The development of cultural sensitivity on the clinical educator's part is also important. Mullins et al (1995) found that international students studying in Australia were more likely to rate 'fair treatment' by the clinical educator as poor, in comparison to local students. Trying to gain an informal understanding of the background culture of the students will make the learning experience more productive for all concerned. Cross-cultural sensitivity in the supervision process will become increasingly important in light of the growing cultural and language diversity of student populations around the world. Asking the students how they went about learning in their own country is a useful starting point and may help the clinical educator to understand why students are behaving or performing in a certain manner.

STRATEGIES TO ENHANCE THE CROSS-CULTURAL TEACHING AND LEARNING EXPERIENCE

Millwater and Yarrow (1992) offer 14 recommendations for preparing students who travel overseas for an educational experience. Some of these, which relate to clinical education, are:

- encourage earlier contact with host agencies so that three or more communications can take place to facilitate planning
- research the language and habits of the overseas cultures so that these can be integrated into the teaching preparations
- have students and clinical educators share their cultural experiences
- discuss the 'context' of the students' practicum so the customs can be more fully understood
- formalize the pre-planning sessions to outline expectations
- plan for an experience of adequate length, taking into account the increased time requirements in a cross-cultural experience.

Ballard & Clanchy (1991) also offer several suggestions to educators to assist them in helping students adapt to local cultural learning expectations. These are:

- recognize the cultural roots of what may at first appear perverse or simply inadequate learning habits
- explain to students, in ways that might seem excessively didactic and explicit for local students, the styles of learning which are more appropriate in the local culture
- build the appropriate behavior into daily teaching practices.

Strategies to minimize the students' cultural isolation need to be implemented early in the students' training. Encouraging students to access local information sources will provide them with a lot of cultural learning. Newspapers, radio, and television all offer a window into the local culture. Participation in the local culture, outside of the program of study and the students' immediate cultural group, is also useful. A part-time job or volunteerism can do a lot in terms of promoting the students' abilities to participate in local dialogue. It will also help students to gain a greater understanding of the appropriate cultural behaviors in the community.

20. *Clinical educator*: Early integration and experiences within the local culture are important before students go into clinical practice. The health environment is not conducive to cultural building and the building of self-esteem – it is not necessarily a safe environment.

Academic programs can also assist these students by developing support systems that help students to question and learn about local cultural practices and language. Courses that teach interpersonal communication, medical interviewing, and counseling skills can be useful mediums for introducing students to the verbal and non-verbal cultural expectations of the health professional–client interchange. Mentoring via a buddy system is another strategy. By linking students of a different culture and/or language background to local students, opportunities to learn more about local customs and social discourse become possible.

21. *Southeast Asian student*: Sometimes I just sit at the side listening to the conversation between the supervisor and [local] student. The way they discuss the treatment program is so mature and clever . . . I just feel like I can't reach that standard now. Maybe it's my knowledge or my poor English from doing so?

22. *Southeast Asian student*: I figured out how to phrase things in a more positive manner. For example, I would usually say, 'Judy, I tried to measure the range of motion of the hip joint but I can't figure it out.' After watching other [local] students, I would now say, I have measured the hip joint using this instrument in this modified position, can you give me some suggestions about a better way to measure? Saying things this way makes you look more clever.

In giving feedback to students from different cultures it may be useful to separate positive and negative feedback. It is also important that the students be asked to paraphrase the feedback so the clinical educator can determine whether the students have understood it in the first place. If the students have not understood the message, the clinical educator will have to re-explain the ideas using different terminology and perhaps even a different approach. Although this may seem tedious, it will demonstrate to the students that the educator understands the challenges the students face in trying to work within a different cultural and language context. It will also save the clinical educator a lot of time in correcting future problems that arise out of students' misunderstanding of feedback.

Clinical educators also have to learn to lose their excess language when speaking to students from different language backgrounds. It is surprising how frequently native speakers of a language use local slang, idioms, and colloquialisms. These language expressions are culturally bound and often outside of the non-native speakers' language repertoire; it is unlikely that they will understand these more colorful aspects of the local language. It is important, therefore, that clinical educators develop their own self-awareness when constructing messages to students who do not speak the host country's language well. Again, getting students to paraphrase back the educator's instructions or feedback is a useful test to see if messages are being misunderstood.

In some cases, it may be necessary to have a specific session with students to review certain words. This is particularly pertinent in the health care professions, which have a lot of jargon. For example, a nursing colleague outlined the difficulty students were having with patients when reference had to be made to the anatomy of the pelvic area. Students often avoided saying specific words or would use inappropriate words. Sitting down with the students and naming the various parts in terms that patients would understand was necessary to ensure effective communication between students and clients.

Perhaps one of the biggest obstacles in cross-cultural supervision is the clinical educator's fear that it will take too much time. Ballard & Clanchy (1991) state that one of the major reasons for staff hesitating to welcome more overseas students is the recognition that these students will invariably take up significantly more of their time. It would appear that this is the case:

23. *Clinical educator*: I find the students [from Southeast Asia] need more time to compensate for their slowness and repetition in comparison to the average [local] student. If they are given this extra time they usually meet the required point by the end of the placement. Knowledge wise they are often better students – it's the cultural and language stuff that needs the extra time.

24. *Clinical educator*: The patients say something and they [the Southeast Asian students] don't pick up on the patient's comment – so they skip it and go on to something else. They may nod approval even though they don't understand what has been said. Because of this, they miss important things. In light of this, I have to be there more often to make sure they process everything.

Because of this additional requirement, academic programs may need to examine their assessment criteria. Without compromising performance standards, how much flexibility is there in the system to compensate for the students' additional time requirement? Unlike academic assignments, which can possibly take into consideration variations in the students' grammar and discourse structure, professional standards are often non-negotiable because of licensing, registration, and patient safety issues. Regardless of the students' cultural and language backgrounds, they still have to meet entry-level standards for their appropriate discipline. The issue of accommodating the language and cultural diversity of students is difficult as well as controversial and probably needs to be examined on a case-by-case basis.

Nevertheless, helping students from diverse cultural and language backgrounds to succeed is not an insurmountable task. Early intervention can minimize many of the issues that have been presented in this chapter. Since many students in health professional programs undertake most of their clinical experience towards the latter half of their studies, there is some time to introduce students to local cultural and language practices:

25. *Clinical educator*: The students [from Southeast Asia] need to be involved both conversationally and culturally. They are very closed. They don't interact outside. If they did so they would improve their understanding and quickness [of English] so that by the time they reach 4th year their communication patterns would be more automatic.

SUMMARY

The challenge of cross-cultural supervision by clinical educators will increase as world populations move freely about the planet. In the rehabilitation profession, it is not uncommon for students to travel abroad as part of their development. Students may also be sponsored by national or international agencies to study overseas in order to enhance the breadth of their clinical skill. As a result, clinical educators need to develop their cross-cultural supervisory skills because of the likelihood of being required to teach a student from a different language or cultural background during the course of one's career.

The challenge for the clinical educator in a cross-cultural clinical supervision situation is to try to incorporate some of the information in this chapter into daily practice. It is difficult to provide a checklist of instructions because of the myriad of cultures and languages that interface in today's world. Even within specific cultural and language groupings, diversity will exist. Two students from the same cultural background may differ substantially because of their experiences in the host country. Thus, the specific challenge for the cross-cultural supervisor is to determine whether you are faced with a cross-cultural dilemma or a student who truly does not have the requisite skills and knowledge to effectively perform as a health professional.

REFERENCES

Ballard B, Clanchy J 1991 Teaching students from overseas. Longman Chesire, Melbourne, pp. 1–26

Bisong J 1995 Language and choice and cultural imperialism: a Nigerian perspective. English Language Training Journal 49: 122–132

Hall S 1992 Developing anti-discriminatory teaching practices in a primary school. Discrimination in government policies and practices S.80, Report No. 9, Equal Opportunity Commission, Perth, Western Australia, p. 21

Kember D, Gow L 1990 Cultural specificity of approaches to study. British Journal of Educational Psychology 60: 356–363

Kennedy K 1995 Developing a curriculum guarantee for overseas students. Higher Education Research and Development 14: 35–46

Ladyshewsky R 1995 Clinical teaching. Higher Education and Research Development Society of Australasia, Australian Capital Territory, pp. 35–38

Millwater J, Yarrow A 1992 Supervision of international practicums. In: Yarrow A (ed) Teaching role of supervision in the practicum: cross faculty perspectives. Queensland University of Technology Publications and Printery, Brisbane, Australia

Mullins G, Hancock L 1991 Educating overseas students at the University of Adelaide: how do we rate? Lumen 20: 3–4

Mullins G, Quintrell N, Hancock L 1995 The experiences of international and local students at three Australian universities. Higher Education Research and Development 14: 201–231

Samuelowicz K 1987 Learning problems of overseas students. Higher Education Research and Development 6: 121–133

Scollon R, Wong-Scollon S 1995 Intercultural communication. Blackwell, Oxford, UK

Shih F 1988 Asian-American students on college campuses. Education Digest 52: 59–62

Waller D 1993 Teaching marketing to Asian students: are they missing the message? Journal of Marketing Education 15: 47–55

Yee A 1989 Cross-cultural perspectives on higher education in East Asia: psychological effects upon Asian students. Journal of Multilingual and Multicultural Development 10: 213–232

Zhang Y 1995 Asian students in the United States: lessons that can be learned. Singapore Journal of Education 15: 14–20

The practice of rehabilitation in cross-cultural and international environments: case examples

Section 3, The Practice of Rehabilitation in Cross-Cultural and International Environments: case examples, offers a glimpse of disability and/or rehabilitation in a variety of cultures throughout the world. Because this book introduces students and practitioners to the world of cross-cultural and international rehabilitation, and because little published material on this topic is easily accessible to the average rehabilitation practitioner, these authors describe an array of experiences from a range of viewpoints. The authors are from a variety of professional backgrounds and personal experiences, and their chapters are a mix of ethnographic case reports and personal narratives. There is an attempt to describe a culture – the culture of disability and/or the culture of rehabilitation, as well as the culture of a particular geographic location or ethnic group. These chapters add to the body of knowledge defining the social construction of disability in varying contexts, that is, how the meanings and identities of people with disabilities (PWD) are constructed by the events and social processes they experience in their lives.

These selective illustrations of practice, representing 'anthropology in action', point to the need to understand how each culture specifically addresses PWD and how each situation must be addressed within its own unique cultural context. The chapters in Section 3 do not necessarily offer 'best practice' rehabilitation models but rather a range of practice realities. The examples, often involving community based rehabilitation (CBR) programs, demonstrate how adaptations can be made to meet the local environmental realities. The authors generally take an advocacy position, as is the case with applied medical anthropology, attempting to support and promote changes that would benefit PWD.

As noted in Chapter 1, it is expected that the reader will usefully generalize information learned about one specific geographic location or population group and apply it to another context if it is appropriate. For example, although not originally intended, many chapters in Sections 3 and 4 focus on a pediatric population. The reality is that much of the physical rehabilitation effort in many of the countries cited does involve children with disabilities (CWD) and there are few, if any, programs specifically for older adults. Certainly, the salient themes can be applied to any population group with a disability. We can all learn from the experience of others.

Chapters 15–18 describe specific examples of attempts to incorporate CBR programs into communities where there is little or no rehabilitation for PWD. Despite the proliferation of CBR models throughout the world, it is very difficult to access detailed information on these efforts. It rarely exists in written form, and when it does, it is not published in mainstream professional literature.

The case from Guyana (Ch. 15), by Shoma Stout and Brian O'Toole, describes the evolution of Hopeful Steps, a program that envisions the development of a CBR program as part of a larger model of community development that would become an empowering process for the community. From its inception, Hopeful Steps considered the need to place the problems of PWD in the wider context of their environment. That is, it was recognized that PWD live in extreme poverty and that ignorance, prejudice and superstition limit the cultural belief system of people in the community. At the same time, previous efforts at rehabilitation for PWD were too often inaccessible to people in rural areas, too capital and technology-intensive, too specialized, and too Western in style. Hopeful Steps

regards rehabilitation in its broadest terms. It has become part of the village infrastructure, integrated with education, employment, and other sectors.

The CBR model in Guyana began based on the community identified needs of health, transportation, and education, with particular emphasis on early physical and mental stimulation of CWD. In each village, a CBR team, consisting of a community health worker, a teacher, and a village leader was formed. This structure proved very advantageous and remains useful as later identified broader community needs of health education, literacy, and cultural affirmation were identified by the villagers. Rehabilitation is not a product to be dispensed from the top-down but rather 'a process in which the villagers are intimately involved.' Programs emerged as a response to the local people's needs, rather than a preconceived agenda.

Some of the most significant outcomes associated with Hopeful Steps were the identification of PWD (at first many did not realize their existence), integration of PWD into village life, and changing attitudes toward and help for disabled people by non-disabled villagers. The integration of CBR into the general health and education sectors of the society, as well as the effort to work on grassroots-initiated projects, makes it more likely that the program will be sustainable. Arguably the most significant accomplishment which will enable continued community development has been the nurturing of community participation to empower CBR workers to feel that they can plan for and accomplish their goals.

In Chapter 16, 'Development of community rehabilitation in Nicaragua: training people with disabilities to be trainers', Estelle Schneider and Hector Segovia also emphasize the necessity and process of empowerment of PWD so that they themselves may be a catalyst for the changes in policies and practices relating to disability. The setting for Chapter 16 is Nicaragua during the late 1980s and early 1990s, a period of considerable political turmoil but one also of advancement within the disability rights movement. From the authors' personal points of view, they emphasize the relevance of the historical and political context in which change can take place.

Schneider and Segovia describe CEPRI (the Center for Promotion of Integral Rehabilitation), an organization founded and run by PWD who experienced, first hand, the shortcomings of the health care and rehabilitation system. CEPRI promotes the full integration of PWD into society, with a focus on identifying society's responsibility to change oppressive attitudes toward PWD. This case focuses more on adult PWD, many of whom have spinal cord injuries as a result of armed conflict or sequelae from polio. It suggests that the war-disabled may be in a unique position to promote a change in the public perception of PWD. Thus, the PWD themselves have been empowered to go through a formalized training program (utilizing ideas from the collaborative learning approach described in Ch. 13) to become 'promoters of integral rehabilitation'.

This program's expansion over the last decade demonstrates its success and sustainability. For example, CEPRI has paid special attention to reaching women with disabilities: since this group is often discriminated against to a greater extent based on gender, 'they are much more quickly stigmatized as "sick and incapable"'. The authors expect the collaboration with the physical therapy school in Nicaragua to have positive long-term consequences. Furthermore, along with the models described by Stout and O'Toole (Ch. 15) and Huib Cornielje and Paulo Ferrinho (Ch. 18), as this program solidified it also expanded into more global areas of community development (for example how to develop income generating projects and run small businesses). The development of CEPRI, reinforcing user sensitive guidelines suggested by Neufeldt (Ch. 3), has developed in response to needs that have been identified by the constituents.

Benedicte Ingstad, in Chapter 17, describes the development of CBR in Botswana. It was one of the first CBR programs developed, and is closely allied with the original World Health Organization (WHO) philosophy and structure. Ingstad has participated in a long-standing

research effort in Botswana to look at the lives of PWD (specifically to address her hypothesis that PWD are not hidden or neglected) and to evaluate the results of CBR. The chapter summarizes the main findings of her work with a focus on an analysis of the problems encountered in mobilizing community participation in the CBR project.

Ingstad elucidates many lessons. For example, at the national level, government and non-governmental organizations attempting to serve PWD are working in parallel, without adequate communication or coordination. This leads to duplication of services and the inefficient use of very marginal economic and human resources.

In her analysis of constraints at the local and household level, Ingstad provides several examples that reinforce some of the theoretical concepts introduced in Section 1. For instance, at the household level, there is a conflict between the generally held Western ideas espoused in rehabilitation discourse, such as concern for individual rights as exemplified by the processes of 'integration' and 'normalization', and the more typical ideology linked to collective rights and duties (i.e. a concern for the coping ability of the household unit). Also, reinforcing information given by Groce, Ingstad notes that PWD are not integrated into society because they cannot fulfill the expected adult role for people in Botswana. Another constraint at the household level is the traditional belief system regarding the causes of disability (such as witchcraft, ancestors' anger, 'God's will'), which is not conducive to having members of the community offer their assistive services. Alternatively, the household may be fearful of having outsiders enter the home if they believe a neighbor or kinsman may be the one who has caused the disability through a curse. Ingstad also notes that the cultural inappropriateness of the concept of volunteerism and the environmental realities of considerable poverty are substantial constraints to successful community mobilization.

Ingstad reaffirms that community participation should include more than helping PWD. Ideally, it is a process that gives people greater control over the social, political, economic and environmental factors affecting their lives. This is a process of empowerment. (An additional observation by Ingstad is that the definition of community, a term that is used widely when dealing with the concept of CBR, needs careful thought. That is, what is the appropriate unit that can be reasonably expected to participate in the process of CBR? Is 'community' the village, neighborhood, compound, extended family, etc.?)

In Chapter 18, 'The socio-political context of CBR developments in South Africa', public health professionals Huib Cornielje and Paulo Ferrinho explain the newly emerging policies associated with rehabilitation and the disability rights movement, taking into account the previously prominent system of apartheid and the new, more democratic social system.

Cornielje and Ferrinho contend that existing rehabilitation professionals (largely white) abdicate their responsibilities to the larger society by primarily practicing in private settings in élite or middle-class urban areas. The authors place much of the blame with South African universities which gear training to high-technology academic hospitals, with little mention of alternative, possibly more relevant, strategies. Furthermore, professionals have tended to concern themselves with improved physical performance of the PWD, with little attention to what happens to PWD after they return to their home environment.

As an antidote, the Institute of Urban Primary Health Care (IUPHC) has developed a training program for community rehabilitation facilitators (CRFs). The teaching principles and methodology are similar to the collaborative learning approach described by Sophie Levitt (Ch. 13). The curriculum at IUPHC emphasizes understanding rehabilitation as part of social and community development and the empowerment of CRFs and PWD. The philosophy is comparable to that proposed by Hopeful Steps in Guyana and CEPRI in Nicaragua.

Cornielje and Ferrinho discuss strategies pertinent to developing an appropriate public policy regarding rehabilitation in South Africa. In this case, they recommend that the ultimate responsibility should lie with the national government, but that regions, with flexible, participatory decision-making input from the community, should be allowed to develop their own programs in view of the differing geography, infrastructure, and culture.

Each of the four preceding chapters identifies the shortcomings of the biomedical paradigm whereby only the professionals are expected to be teaching rehabilitation. They suggest that PWD, usually informally educated but living a life of experiences, are generally more capable of teaching others useful information. Chapter 19 describes a model with a somewhat more biomedical focus, although it does recognize the importance of the sociocultural domains. 'Intensive treatment and problem solving to enhance rehabilitation potential in Mexico', by occupational therapists Christine Nelson and Martha Rubi, describes the Centro de Aprendizaje (the Learning Center), a more classic 'model' rehabilitation program that is attempting to provide high level clinical treatment to CWD and continuing education to rehabilitation professionals in a middle-income country.

Mexico is far more developed socioeconomically than are countries such as Bangladesh, Botswana, or Vietnam, yet rehabilitation services have remained a relatively low priority. A considerable disparity between rich and poor leaves many without adequate health or rehabilitative services. Citing the fact that socioeconomic structures in Mexico do not encourage the provision of excellent quality clinical services or the achievement of professional expertise or advancement, these authors have participated in the development of a more Western, biomedical, secondary level facility that does meet an important need.

Although the biomedical model is not emphasized in this book, it is appropriate for certain environments as long as adaptation to the sociocultural context remains paramount. For example, Nelson and Rubi describe sociocultural accommodations that include the idea of treating a CWD comprehensively for 2–3 weeks (providing on-site living arrangements), because a weekly commute is not feasible. Similarly, an emphasis on teaching family members or care-givers more about how to work directly with the CWD responds to the fact that rehabilitative personnel are often not available. Another consideration is how to facilitate independent self-feeding activities, while recognizing that dif-ferent sub-groups may have varying expecta-tions as to when and how independent feeding is appropriate (Mexican children, for example, are spoon fed by their mothers for a more extended period of time than children in the USA).

A description of the Learning Center brings forth questions also discussed by Kay and col-leagues (Ch. 23) and others. For example, should a range of training levels be encouraged to meet the needs of more PWD, or should a country such as Mexico only train professionals at the university, baccalaureate degree level? In Mexico, a range of practitioners use the title 'therapist', although these individuals are not equally trained. The 'therapist' is not necessarily encouraged (or required) to demonstrate com-petence and/or may misrepresent their level of competence to the public. It is also debatable how many, and what kind of resources should be allocated to treating a few PWD, while many in rural areas are left without any resources. Nelson and Rubi believe that the Learning Center is a necessary and appropriate institu-tion to provide important services to PWD and rehabilitation professionals in Mexico.

Chapter 20, by occupational therapist Gale Haradon, 'A cross-cultural immersion in post-communist Romania', is a personal narrative. She describes her volunteer experience as a developmental therapist in a Romanian orphan-age during the 'crisis' after the fall of the Communist dictator Nicolae Ceausescu in 1989 and amid the publicity surrounding the thousands of abandoned children 'found' in orphanages. Although most CWD in the world are not institutionalized, it is presumed that many such children, especially in low-income settings, lack the adequate early stim-ulation that could potentially minimize some of the effects of a child's impairments. This

case example reinforces the idea that dili-gence in this regard is called for.

Haradon's chapter describes an example of a relatively short-term opportunity offered by a non-governmental organization (NGO) to effect change in the lives of CWD. Although not necessary an ideal model, NGO support for short-term projects often meets an urgent need. In sharing her observations of a 'second world' country, Haradon takes into account the historical, political, economic, and socio-cultural circumstances in Romania. Her reflections give an account of some of the everyday personal frustrations and joys she encountered. She also offers a glimpse of how such an experience can lead to further devo-tion to cross-cultural work and research.

Chapters 21 and 22 specifically address two population groups at opposite ends of the globe, along with the impact of their differing cultures on rehabilitation. In 'Cultural envi-ronmental factors in the delivery of rehabilita-tion services to American Indians' (Ch. 21), rehabilitation counselors Catherine Marshall and Sharon Johnson provide a window from which to learn pertinent information about one ethnic group within the USA. Although the American Indian population is small, this sub-group, which further divides into over 500 tribal nations, has the highest reported rate of disability of any ethnic group in the USA. It is typically under- and inappropri-ately served. Marshall and Johnson give sev-eral practical examples that reinforce themes from the theoretical chapters on culture, racism, and poverty, while underscoring the need for cultural competency when working with this sub-group.

Marshall and Johnson identify the need to acknowledge a 'philosophical consistency' among Indian people, yet the necessity of rec-ognizing cultural diversity among various tribal nations. They stress the need to recog-nize PWD as individuals yet members of an ethnic group whose cultural values differ markedly from the dominant society, reinforc-ing the notion of intra-cultural diversity and the concern for negative effects of over-generalization and stereotyping. In keeping with the goal of cultural competency, the authors illustrate the value of learning about the history, values, customs, and culture of the specific tribe with which practitioners have the most contact.

In addressing the strategies for overcoming barriers to rehabilitation of an American Indian, the authors identify three as most important: acknowledgment of a pluralistic society, acknowledgment of the values of a collective society (including the recognition of the importance of family and the possible role of family in rehabilitation outcomes), and support for indigenous self-determination. These themes are also found in many other chapters in this section.

Jo Simister and Ahmed Younis based Chapter 22, 'Culture and its impact on the rehabilitation program: a Palestinian perspective', on both personal experience and a review of the literature. They present some features of the typical Palestinian way of life, including beliefs about health and healing, and they discuss how these features might influence the life or rehabilitation of a PWD. For the Palestinians, as in the case of Nicaragua, political instability has led to an increase in PWD as a result of armed conflict. In both cases, the authors argue that one result is an opportunity to encourage a more positive attitude toward disability within the society. Simister and Younis also discuss some of the inherent limitations of foreign involvement (especially in instances where the expatriate is not culturally sensitive) in the development and implementation of these services. This chapter offers a somewhat different perspective to those of Haradon (Ch. 20) and Nelson and Rubi (Ch. 19), who do see expatriate involvement as a more viable option.

Simister and Younis emphasize the importance of the concept of intra-cultural diversity as well as the need to pay attention to the explanatory models of the people with regard to health and disability. Furthermore, they reiterate the need to understand the nature of a collectively-oriented community, and the need for 'outsiders' to work collaboratively with local planners and PWD.

Within the world of international development many programs offer medical treatment and teaching, but rarely do such programs include any rehabilitation personnel, and more rarely still are they concerned with a formalized attempt to upgrade the skills of clinicians. Typically, individual therapists go into a country as a 'tag on' to a more medically-oriented group, and they function without a plan, goals or objectives. In contrast, the Vietnam Project has been systematically and thoughtfully developed by the Vietnamese Ministry of Health and a non-governmental voluntary organization (Health Volunteers Overseas) in the USA.

Kay, Huong, and Chau (Ch. 23) describe the Vietnam Project, a multidisciplinary effort to improve rehabilitation services in Vietnam in which rehabilitation professionals are the primary organizers and participants in the program. They specifically focus on the physical therapy portion of the project and describe an intervention to upgrade physical therapy in Vietnam through the education of local professionals. The authors note some of the many obstacles to advancing physical therapy in a country such as Vietnam. For example, despite a core group of professionals trained and working within Vietnam, opportunities to update or upgrade information are almost completely lacking. Mentors, continuing education programs, or educational resources such as books and journals are rarely available. To help meet this need, one component of the Vietnam Project offered a series of multi-disciplinary workshops on the medical, surgical, and rehabilitation management of particular diagnoses. The topics were chosen by the Vietnamese. The themes running across all of the workshops – including an emphasis on generalizable assessment and problem-solving skills, the use of the multi-disciplinary team approach, a focus on realistic and appropriate functional goals, and application of skills and knowledge to a range of environments from a central or provincial hospital to a community based project – are all essential, generic skills required of any competent rehabilitation professional. Ideas presented by Levitt on a collaborative learning approach (Ch. 13) and by Brice and Campbell (Ch. 8), and Ladyshewsky (Ch. 14) on the challenges of cross-cultural communication underlie this chapter.

Chapter 23 also identifies a generic concern regarding the education of professionals and their employment once they are trained. Extensive attention has been paid to expanding and updating the current physical therapy training curriculum and improving teacher effectiveness. Once trained, it is not unusual in the Third World, where there is a tremendous shortage of professionals to begin with, to find that there are no governmental or privately supported employment opportunities. Thus, part of the Vietnam Project has been a concurrent effort to get the government to effectively utilize existing therapists rather than just training new ones. (After the chapter was written, the project added the specific training of clinical educators. That is, training on-site clinicians to serve as educators and role models for students and new graduates. Historically, and typically where rehabilitation services have not yet been fully developed, this aspect has been grossly lacking.)

A related issue is how to meet the needs of a profession as it develops (in this case physical therapy), while keeping the best interests of the population as a whole in mind. There is potential conflict between increasing professional capabilities and status, especially for practitioners in urban areas or hospitals, while also working to foster the development of community level workers who can serve more rural and isolated areas. Should schools offer a training certificate to community workers after 6 months or 1–2 years? Should credentialed therapists receive a 3-year diploma or a 4-year baccalaureate degree education? What does the decision mean with regard to the marketability of therapists in a different country? Within their own country? In essence, the question becomes, how, with

limited resources, to convince the government to support all of the efforts suggested, not one at the expense of the other. These concerns are prevalent in many less developed nations struggling to advance the field of rehabilitation. In Vietnam, Kay and her colleagues have been involved in addressing these concerns through direct negotiations with the Vietnamese government. They expect the Vietnam Project eventually to lead to the formation of a national association for physical therapists and participation in the World Confederation of Physical Therapy.

The next two chapters, by furnishing more detailed illustrations of appropriate assistive technology, supplement Chapter 11 by Zollars and Ruppelt. 'Appropriate prosthetics and orthotics in less developed countries' (Ch. 24), by physical therapist Lawrence Golin, addresses the challenge of transferring appropriate rehabilitation technology to a less developed country. Golin specifically describes the establishment of a self-sustaining artificial limb and brace shop in Bangladesh.

Golin notes the difficulty of convincing Bengali people with an amputation of the viability of buying and wearing a prosthesis. No wonder, he explains, for a Western-style prosthetic foot is completely inappropriate for the South Asian culture; it is not suitable for wet, rural areas nor can a wearer squat to socialize, eat, toilet, or work in the fields using the traditional Western foot. Equally frustrating has been the laborious process by which a more culturally compatible design has been invented, fabricated, and mass produced. The development in India of the Jaipur foot and the use of an aluminium prosthetic shank is part of the answer. Now, how to mass produce such a prosthesis in Bangladesh?

The Jaipur Foot Artificial Limb Center in Bangladesh has opened, but the necessity of importing foot pieces from India continues and the cost still remains insurmountable for many. The ongoing effort to produce a polyurethane version of the Jaipur foot is a reminder that the process of development and indigenization is lengthy. Based on 30 years of work in Bangladesh, Golin suggests certain principles. For example, he suggests that national workers (prosthetists or others) be trained within their own culture, using cost-effective material, and not go to a more developed nation where the conditions are entirely different and irrelevant.

Harry Finkenflügel, in Chapter 25, 'Paper technology and community based rehabilitation: cultural adaptation in Zimbabwe', gives a concrete, culture-specific example of the use of a simple technology that reinforces the principles outlined earlier by Zollars and Ruppelt (Ch. 11). He provides a practical, technical guide to making a specific form of adaptive technology. Although there is a manual (see resource list, p. 136) describing paper technology in detail, this material is included in *Cross-cultural Rehabilitation* because many therapists, trained to use highly sophisticated and expensive technology, do not know that such alternatives exist. When working in any resource stressed environment, whether in the developed or less developed nations, one needs to consider alternative options.

Paper technology has become a part of CBR programs in Zimbabwe. It is a good example of how to develop resources for rehabilitation that are inexpensive, socially acceptable and readily available, one of the philosophical tenets of CBR. Paper technology is used both to make aids and appliances for PWD as well as to fabricate works of art or functional household items to be sold as an income-generating activity. An advantage to using this technique is the ability to involve family members, and sometimes PWD themselves, in production. Because rehabilitation is most commonly the purview of mothers, it is noteworthy that the fathers of CWD have become involved in the paper technology training workshops in a way deemed culturally acceptable.

In sum, Section 3 addresses very specific sub-cultures with regard to their beliefs and behaviors in response to the presence of PWD. There are a variety of rehabilitation models and viewpoints represented for consideration, but no single model is deemed appropriate in all circumstances. Each chapter draws upon the theoretical material found in Sections 1 and 2 and contributes to an understanding of the social construction of disability and rehabilitation throughout the world. Rehabilitation practitioners can use this knowledge in their quest for cultural competence.

15

Community based rehabilitation with indigenous peoples: a case description from Guyana

Shoma Stout
Brian O'Toole

INTRODUCTION

While services for persons with disabilities (PWDs) have been well established for generations in areas close to the capital of Guyana, the challenge of caring for people with special needs in the vast interior areas of the country had largely been ignored within the health sector until recently. In most villages, PWDs were hidden away or shunned because the indigenous folklore attributes disability to possession by evil spirits. Nevertheless, a survey carried out by the Guyana community based rehabilitation (CBR) program in 1994 found that the prevalence of people identified as disabled was roughly comparable with other areas of the country – 0.76% in the Rupununi, compared with 1.5% nation-wide (Hopeful Steps 1994a).

VISION OF DEVELOPMENT

Hopeful Steps, the Guyana CBR program, envisions development as an organic, empowering process for the community. In contrast, previous rehabilitation efforts were accessible only to the privileged few in urban areas, and were often too capital- and technology-intensive, too specialized, too isolating from normal life, and too Western in origin, practice, and prejudice.

Hopeful Steps recognizes the need to perceive the problems of PWDs in the wider context of poverty, malnutrition, ignorance, prejudice, and superstition. All these interrelated factors affect the quality of life of PWDs. In the Rupununi, therefore, disability issues were presented as part of an integrated model of development. This focus was adopted in response to listening to the needs identified by the people of the region rather than adopting a preconceived agenda.

In CBR, a person from the community learns how to design individual, simplified rehabilitation programs for PWDs and how to train parents or family members to administer these programs. The goal is to demystify the rehabilitation process and give responsibility back to the individual, family, and community. The basic premise of CBR is that the greatest resource in developing countries for helping disabled persons lead fulfilled and productive lives is a well-advised and supported family. The goal is for rehabilitation to be perceived as part of community development as the community seeks to improve itself. In such a process, rehabilitation becomes one element of a broader community integration effort. CBR moves from regarding rehabilitation as a product to be dispensed to offering rehabilitation as a process in which the villagers are intimately involved.

As Hopeful Steps evolved in the Rupununi the program became even more oriented toward an empowering process that transcends 'rehabilitation' in the strict sense. A program staff member, when asked to identify the major need of Rupununi people, replied that it was: 'the realization that their destiny is in their own hands . . . that they don't need to wait to be told the direction in which they should be going. They need to realize that they have the capacity to go where their paths to development should take them' (Stout 1996).

Hopeful Steps is committed to a process that helps people recognize that they can set their own development agendas. Asked to articulate the vision the CBR program has for the people, a staff member replied: 'that villagers are better equipped to make their own decisions, villages can decide for themselves what they want. I hope that CBR can stimulate the people to start thinking for themselves. We hope that they will be more proud of their own culture' (Stout 1996).

These responses illustrate the attempt made by Hopeful Steps to place considerable importance on developing an empowering process that affirms culture and puts control of the process of development back into the hands of the community. In doing so, it addresses rehabilitation in the context of wider community issues, through integration with existing infrastructure and through education of parents and community members, rather than through a top-down delivery system.

GUYANA: BACKGROUND INFORMATION

Guyana, located on the Atlantic shoulder of South America, is bordered by Surinam on the west, Venezuela to the east, and Brazil to the south. It is a land of 83 000 square miles with an estimated population of 800 000 and therefore has a very low population density. This number is declining due to a falling birth rate and a high rate of emigration. Life expectancy at birth dropped from 70 years in 1985 to 64.2 years in 1992, although the infant mortality rate is improving, falling from 49 per 1000 live births in 1987 to 42.2 per 1000 in 1992 (EIU 1994).

Guyana achieved its political independence from Britain in 1966 and declared itself a co-operative republic along socialist lines in 1970. The economy, based primarily on sugar, gold, rice, and bauxite, is very vulnerable to fluctuations in world trade.

The Rupununi region

The Rupununi region covers 33 000 square miles in the south-western part of Guyana. About 17 000 people live in the region, concentrated in 42 villages. 80% of the population of Rupununi is classified as Amerindian. These Amerindians represent 24% of the indigenous people within Guyana.

The Rupununi is the second poorest region in Guyana and has been growing increasingly impoverished. Its main industries are farming and cattle ranching. Rainforest covers half of the land; the rest is savannah. Because the economy is subsistent and agricultural rather than industrial, cash is limited. The problem is heightened by the lack of transportation, which increases the cost of basic goods. The presence of a flourishing economy in neighboring Brazil has led to a large degree of emigration, further depleting the economic and human resources of the region.

Rupununi is underdeveloped in structural, capital, and human resources and transportation is scarce and haphazard. Although the health sector provides radio communication in the five major villages of the region, it is very difficult for the people to access basic curative and preventive health services. When there is a health emergency, the patient must travel to the nearest health center by foot, bicycle, or bullock cart, a trip that might take 10 hours to complete.

The crude mortality rate is reported at 2.94% and infant mortality at 35 per 1000 live births (Guela 1994), and there appears to be significant underreporting of both mortality and morbidity statistics. Malaria, diarrheal disease, acute respiratory infection, accidents, dental caries, worms, arthritis, and conjunctivitis are the predominant health problems. Rupununi is the only region in Guyana where leishmaniasis, tuberculosis, and conjunctivitis present as significant health problems (Ministry of Health 1994). The overall immunization rate hovers around 25% for children under 5 years. Nutritional status measured by weight is quite good, but the primary staple is cassava, which provides a predominantly carbohydrate diet. Greens are lacking in the indigenous diet. Nutrition becomes particularly poor during the rainy season, when access to markets is cut off. The Rupununi has the highest incidence of low-birthweight births in the country, with 41.8% of infants born weighing less than 2500 g.

Education in the region, though buttressed by a core of extremely dedicated teachers, is compromised both by the lack of availability in some areas of basic resources (books, papers, etc.) and by a lack of certified teachers; this leads to a system of 'trickle-down' education provided by untrained teachers who have not passed the certification test.

HISTORY OF THE GUYANA CBR PROGRAM

The idea for the Hopeful Steps CBR program was conceived in 1986 when an educational psychologist, Brian O'Toole, and a physiotherapist, Geraldine Maison-Halls, began formulating a simplified model of rehabilitation that could deliver services to rural areas of Guyana, where the vast majority of the country's disabled people live. In 1986, with a small grant from the Canadian International Development Agency, they established two pilot projects in two coastal regions of Guyana, one using nursery school teachers as community rehabilitators and another using community volunteers. Independent evaluations of these two projects showed significant improvement in children's scores on standardized tests. The children were perceived to be happier, better behaved, more mobile, and more motivated. Parents felt more supported and more confident (O'Toole 1989). One of the most interesting outgrowths of the project, particularly among the volunteers, was the involvement of the larger community in the rehabilitation process, shifting some of the responsibility from the individual with a disability to the community at large.

Hopeful Steps has since expanded throughout three major coastal regions of Guyana. In each of these areas, it focuses on empowering communities and community members to care for their PWDs and to value them as a resource, while also encouraging them to discover or reveal their special talents to their communities. When the program expanded to the Rupununi, which became the fourth site in Guyana, the focus shifted dramatically in response to priorities identified by people in this region.

DEVELOPMENT OF THE RUPUNUNI CBR PROGRAM

Hopeful Steps began expanding into the Rupununi in 1992, despite concerns about the applicability of such a specialized program in an area where basic subsistence needs governed people's lives. Dr O'Toole, the director of the program, initially visited the region in early 1992 and was invited to address a conference of Rupununi head teachers, who were attending a Ministry of Education conference. The head teachers' response was lukewarm, since they felt that there were no PWDs in the Rupununi.

Dr O'Toole next made six 1-week visits to about 20 of the 42 villages to get a sense of community needs. In contrast to the head teachers, the villagers responded warmly and enthusiastically; the Rupununi region had been isolated for so long that very few groups visited and those who did rarely travelled to the outlying villages. People seemed to appreciate the effort that Hopeful Steps made to go into the Amerindian communities.

The people of the Rupununi identified health, transportation, and education as their most important needs. From this discussion, early physical and mental stimulation of children emerged as an area within the scope of the CBR program that would be of considerable interest to both teachers and health workers.

Early goals

At this stage, the goals for Hopeful Steps were quite modest. The plan was simply to organize a 1-week workshop for the key health workers and teachers each year. The first workshop was held in October 1992, conducted in association with the Ministry of Health. Open to all the community health workers in the region, it focused on identifying children with disabilities, early stimulation, and simple rehabilitation methods.

The workshop participants were so enthusiastic that Dr O'Toole asked the international funders of the CBR program (Amici di Raoul Follereau (AIFO) from Italy) to develop a broader and expanded vision for the Rupununi. An integral part of that vision was presenting workshops in various locations throughout the region. The funders agreed and a CBR 'team' of three people was created in each village. The teams were composed of the community health worker, a teacher, and a village leader. Hopeful Steps is fortunate to have a funder, AIFO, that

allowed such an evolutionary approach; as one staff member put it: 'the CBR project has a funding agency of whom nothing more could be asked ... they have contributed greatly to the project' (Stout 1996).

The workshops

The initial plan had envisaged a 1-week workshop in the regional capital for 30 health workers per year. The expanded vision entailed organizing five sub-regional workshops each year for 3 years in collaboration with the Institute of Distance and Continuing Education of the University of Guyana. Each workshop would be attended by the CBR team members from the villages in the sub-region (about 20–25 people). Many people made great sacrifices to attend the workshops. On three occasions, teams travelled by foot and canoe for 13 days and nights to reach the workshop.

The formation of such teams served a number of valuable functions. Partnerships between the existing education and health sectors within the village were formalized. The inclusion of a villager allowed more general issues concerning the village to be brought to the leadership of the village. These three people began to serve as representatives of the program at the village level, increasing people's awareness of the program. Moreover, the CBR team members began to develop a sense of ownership and identity with the program. Finally, the selection of a team of people rather than an individual from each village both eased the burden of work on the volunteers and made the team a part of the accepted, regular system of village committees, thereby integrating it into the existing administrative infrastructure of the village. As a committee, most CBR teams received time during monthly village meetings to report to the public and raise awareness of the program. All of these factors increased the program's name recognition, identification, and acceptance by the mass of villagers very quickly.

Once the CBR teams were established, the 3-year training program began in each of the sub-districts. Hopeful Steps attempted to respond to the community identified needs of health, literacy and basic education as their major priorities, while at the same time offering training in meeting the needs of PWDs.

The first series of sub-district workshops, held in January and February 1993, focused on different ways to stimulate children through play and ways to make stimulating toys out of locally available and inexpensive materials. For example, participants learned how to make puppets and use them both in play and as tools in educating their fellow villagers through skits and role plays.

A second series of workshops was held in March, April and May 1993 in each of the sub-districts. These workshops focused on normal and delayed child development with special reference to the applicability of the material to children with disabilities. This raised awareness of the needs of disabled people in the area. During the second series of workshops, participants also had the opportunity to have their village participate in an art competition on disability. Hundreds of children submitted entries.

Focusing on disability

The last workshop in the second series proved to be historic. At their own behest, one of the CBR teams brought seven people with disabilities to the conference; the entire workshop began exploring what could be done to help these people. This open acknowledgment that there are PWDs within the Rupununi, along with the way in which the CBR teams seemed prepared and even excited about their work, gave the program the confidence it needed to address the issue more directly in other sub-regions.

This new focus was identified and consulted upon by the CBR teams during a region-wide conference in September 1993 in Lethem. During this conference, the participants assessed their accomplishments and made new plans for the future. These plans reflected an increasing emphasis on addressing the needs of PWDs.

The third CBR workshop series, which began in December 1993, reflected this new focus on disability. The workshops dealt with screening, early identification of disabilities, toy making, and simple physiotherapy. A video series called 'A New Tomorrow', highlighting disability needs specific to the Rupununi and filmed in the region itself, was produced and shown. The script was developed in consultation with the CBR teams at the workshops. A book containing stories about PWDs was written and translated into the two major indigenous languages. Plans were made to carry out a survey to identify PWDs throughout the Rupununi. PWDs who had previously been 'hidden away' were now identified as being part of the community.

The CBR teams began to work actively to promote the integration of PWDs into every aspect of village life. Health workers began encouraging mothers to bring their children with disabilities to the clinic. The teachers in the CBR teams became more responsive to children with special needs, and about 20 school-age children who had previously been kept at home began attending school. One CBR team made sure that every disabled person in its community always attended village events and meetings. The CBR teams began to make simple rehabilitation tools and shared simple ideas with PWDs and their families to improve their functioning to the highest extent possible.

Changing attitudes

These acts of integration broke down age-old barriers and profoundly affected the attitudes of villagers in the Rupununi about disabled people. Stout (1996) carried out over 100 in-depth interviews of persons involved in Hopeful Steps in the Rupununi as PWDs, family and community members. She identified changing attitudes toward and help for disabled people as a major impact of the CBR program. Of those interviewed, 35% felt that disabled people were better adapted and less shy, and 27% identified the integration of disabled people into village life as the main strength of the program.

Up to this point, the CBR teams had largely been responding to suggestions given by the director of the program. The CBR teams now began to formulate their own village-level plans to integrate disabled people into their communities. Thus teams began to 'own' the process and see themselves as actors rather than simply recipients. In the words of one CBR team member: 'Until recently we felt that CBR was something outside. This was evident by the way in which we constantly asked our 'parent body' for assistance in the form of aids, wheelchairs, etc. However, more recently, we have begun to realize that WE in fact are the CBR program' (Pierre Hopeful Steps 1994b, p. 3).

Broadening the focus

Hopeful Steps did not abandon its commitment to address broader development priorities in the region as it took advantage of the newfound focus on disability. While the third series of workshops were held in December 1993, three other major areas of focus developed in response to needs expressed by villagers or needs perceived by the program in the areas of health education, literacy, and cultural affirmation. There were very few other development agencies operating in the region. Hopeful Steps therefore decided to try and respond to as broad a range of needs as possible. The feeling was that if Hopeful Steps focused solely on disability issues it would be dismissed as irrelevant by the majority of people in the region who faced urgent challenges in the areas of health and basic education. The hope was that if CBR responded in some ways to the broader needs of the region, the villagers themselves would see the needs of PWDs as one of the challenges that they needed to address in bringing about change. Hopeful Steps therefore invested time and resources in the areas of health education, promotion of literacy, and cultural affirmation in addition to training in disability issues in an attempt at promoting an integrated model of development.

Health education

The focus on health education developed as a collaboration with the Bahá'í Community

Health Partnership (BCHP). A 50-minute video called 'Facts for Life', depicting the key health messages in the UNICEF document of the same name, was filmed in the Rupununi. Using portable equipment, the video was shown in villages throughout the region. Training manuals for teachers and health workers and brochures on basic health messages were produced. A series of 'Facts for Life' festivals were held in every sub-district and at the regional level in 1994. Hundreds of poems, songs, skits, stories, and drawings were produced. UNICEF funded the publication of a book featuring the winning entries.

The combination of video, teaching manuals, and art competition proved to be extremely effective in both communicating health messages to the general public and in empowering health workers to teach these messages themselves. Health education was identified as a major impact of the CBR program by 35% of respondents in the Stout (1996) study. This focus on health education helped to identify new cases of disability at early stages and prevented the development of secondary complications in existing cases.

Literacy

The teachers of the region requested help in the promotion of literacy. A 3-day workshop was held in each of the five sub-regional workshops each year from 1994 to 1996. All the teachers of the region therefore attended three workshops. Hopeful Steps developed a 'Steps to Reading' package of 15 books, including workbooks, teachers' manuals, and story books. This package took the teacher step by step through the process of promoting literacy.

Cultural affirmation

The final area that reflected the broadening of the CBR program's initiatives in the Rupununi lay in cultural affirmation. This was done by producing eight video films documenting the development of children within the context of the region. Indigenous music was recorded on audio cassette and produced for widespread local and international distribution. Use of locally available materials, particularly those utilizing cultural craft forms, was encouraged in the early stimulation program. Cultural shows and art competitions encouraged people to translate program themes into their own culture and environment. A book of stories around CBR themes was written and translated into the local languages, Macushi and Wapishana. All of these steps showed respect for the culture of the Rupununi people and helped to make the program and process culturally relevant.

Hopeful Steps' concern about preserving the culture of Rupununi people transcended the mere desire to convey its messages in a culturally sensitive way. The program invested a great deal of time and energy in preserving and affirming the culture of the Rupununi people for its own sake. The focus on these elements within the program attempts to show respect to the integrity and value of the Rupununi people's culture. This is badly needed.

DEVELOPMENT OF INFRASTRUCTURE

The development of human infrastructure and resources constituted a critical component of the CBR program. In the beginning there was simply a national director and the village-level CBR teams. In February 1994 the program was able to attract two Voluntary Service Overseas workers (VSOs). These VSOs were recently replaced by a special educator from Trinidad.

Initially, village visits were made through a partnership with the Bahá'í Community Health Partnership (BCHP), which already provided a mobile health service throughout the region. The purchase of a Land Rover, in 1994, which was used to travel to the various villages, facilitated this process. The formation of what essentially became a mobile resource unit added another element to the CBR infrastructure. It also made the program and its resources far more accessible to the people and helped the program to understand the community better.

As the program grew in scope and the participants gained more power to define their own development agenda, a parallel system of planning, organization, and administration developed that focused on initiatives that arose from the grassroots level. This system, which had its early roots in the village CBR teams, achieved its fruition in October 1995. That date symbolically marked the simultaneous graduation of CBR team members from the university training program and concomitant election of sub-district and regional level CBR committees, elected from the CBR teams. Each team can fully function to carry out its own projects independent of the support of program staff. In essence, the development of this parallel infrastructure reflects a critical transfer of responsibility for the development process in the Rupununi into the hands of the community.

This transfer of responsibility is not just theoretical; it is a functional reality. Between October 1995 and March 1996, for example, the regional CBR committee oversaw the construction, staffing, and supplying of a school in an extremely isolated village that did not have any way of providing education for its children. Now, 66 children are attending school for the first time in their lives. The most important aspect of this achievement lay in the fact that they were able to do this completely on their own.

It is clear, from the breadth, effectiveness, and level of independence of projects which are going on at village, sub-district, and national levels, that sustainability has been achieved in the CBR program in the Rupununi. People know how to identify a need, make plans to meet the need, and carry out the plans in an effective, empowering and unified way.

Several aspects of the CBR program infrastructure deserve special mention. First, this infrastructure does not duplicate existing governmental or non-governmental infrastructure. Second, it brings into partnership existing elements of the government infrastructure that would be interested in a project related to CBR. All CBR workshops in the Rupununi are carried out in partnership with the ministries of health and education at both national and regional levels. These national ministries periodically review the program's plans, excuse teachers and health workers from their posts to participate in workshops, and sometimes co-sponsor workshops with the two programs.

Because CBR participants are drawn from existing health and education infrastructure and because regional and national authorities were carefully consulted during the planning process, CBR has become integrated into existing village, regional, and national systems of organization. The CBR team in each village is part of the village system of committees. At monthly meetings of head teachers throughout the region, CBR work is discussed as a standard part of the agenda. Reports of ongoing activities are included in sub-district, regional, and national reports in health and education. The new health plan for Guyana, which identifies the goals and objectives within this sector from 1994 to 2000, articulates CBR as the centerpiece of rehabilitation care in Guyana: 'A program objective will be to increase access to rehabilitative care by introducing Community Based Rehabilitation as the main strategy for delivering rehabilitative services at the primary care level' (Ministry of Health 1994, p. 120). This inclusion of CBR in the health and education systems adds greatly to the acceptance and sustainability of the CBR program at the political level.

HUMAN RESOURCE DEVELOPMENT

A major focus of the CBR program has been the development of human resources. This development has taken place in two forms: the training of people to carry out the program's goals and objectives and the training of people to take over the process of development. This occurred at the grassroots community level with the development of the CBR teams in each of the villages.

In 1995, the CBR program developed a 'Trainer of Trainers' approach by providing a course to raise up a cadre of workers who could introduce the program to neighboring regions of Guyana. This training took the form of a 1-week workshop in the capital for members of the CBR team who had displayed the aptitude for further training. The workshops focused on literacy, health education, and disability identification, awareness, and management. These resource persons from the Rupununi have now run a series of CBR workshops in three new interior Amerindian areas of the country.

These trainers feel deeply invested in the CBR program and identify highly with it. In Stout's research sample, 46% of the people that they are teaching feel proud or happy to have someone from their own district teaching them and 71% feel positively in general about their leadership (Stout 1996).

Hopeful Steps has been able to develop human resources effectively by combining educational workshops with practical projects to apply, develop, and gain confidence in their new skills. As the program evolved and people became more and more confident, the program was able to support participants in developing and carrying out their own projects. The development of managerial and leadership skills of the original CBR teams and the further training of some of the most motivated CBR workers to support the goals of the CBR program significantly adds to the sustainability of the program.

Each CBR team was also asked to conduct their own workshops in their own villages. These workshops focused on child development, early stimulation and toy making. The process of organizing a workshop was one that taught the team members fundamental organizational and management skills necessary to continue the CBR program in its current form.

The CBR team members learned essential skills and knowledge necessary to run the program at the grassroots level. Training in how to conduct the initial survey to identify PWDs helped the teams assess the basic needs in the area of disability in their village. In 1995, a participatory evaluation of the project was conducted by two researchers from Holland (de Roos & Van Elk 1996). The researchers trained CBR team members from within the region to gather data and develop skills in the area of evaluation. These skills add to CBR team members' sense of empowerment and ownership in the program. These efforts improve the prospect of sustainability by both increasing identification with the program and increasing the community base of skills necessary to run the program.

The promotion of human resources has been developed through a combination of centrally initiated workshops and grassroots-initiated projects. Beginning in 1995, the CBR program strengthened its partnership with the Bahá'í Community Health Partnership (BCHP) by beginning to hold jointly-sponsored workshops for local health board (LHB) members and CBR team members. The BCHP tries to empower and educate people to prepare them to take over the development process and assist in addressing the needs of PWDs. Through small group discussions, role plays, and stories, the participants are urged to recognize their own inherent value or nobility, and explore their capacity to be of service to their communities. During the workshop, participants learn skills relevant to their position as facilitators of the development process, such as conflict resolution and consultation. By the end of each workshop, participants begin to develop a vision for their communities and create a plan for that vision to come to fruition. This process also makes participants conscious of their role and responsibility as leaders of their village and enables them to articulate a vision of their future to development agencies. To the extent that it accomplishes this goal, it adds greatly to the process of sustainability of both the LHB and the CBR teams.

As a result of the workshops, the CBR teams became involved in a number of projects such as the formation of nursery schools, the construction of health posts, the improvement of water and sanitation, the building of wells, and the formation of a cooperative to sew mosquito nets. These projects required CBR team members to consult and gain the participation of both fellow villagers and funding agencies in the region.

PROMOTION OF CBR TEAMS

Hopeful Steps has succeeded in developing a sense of community and identity among the CBR team members. The fact that the volunteers were enrolled in a 3-year university training course in CBR served to reinforce this sense of distinctiveness and identification as CBR workers. The program used a number of other touches to help participants share a sense of community: they created a CBR T-shirt for the Rupununi, developed a CBR theme song, and a Rupununi section to the CBR program newsletter. A whole culture grew around participation in the CBR program that added greatly to a feeling of community and identification with the program.

The act of meeting together with other participants throughout the Rupununi during workshops and during annual regional and national CBR conferences gave CBR team members a feeling of being part of a greater whole that did not exist before. The importance of coming together is highlighted by one team member: 'I think one of the strengths of the CBR program is that it has brought the wider Rupununi together at these seminars, we always came together. We've learned that we are as good as anybody; people in the Rupununi are as good as anybody, anywhere else in the world. People never appreciated or understood it before' (Stout 1996).

This sense of discovery, empowerment, and excitement permeates the manner in which active participants talk about the program. There is a strong sense of identification in the way that people talk not about 'they' but 'we' when referring to the program (Stout 1996). This intangible but real identification with and ownership of the program translates to participants being willing to go to great lengths to make it come alive in their villages. Given that these people do not get paid for their time, the level of effort invested into the program is considerable.

CONCLUSION

Hopeful Steps has attempted to develop a management style that would allow the lofty concepts of 'community participation' and 'empowerment' to be nurtured. There was no predetermined script for the project and many of the most creative features of the program emerged from the participants over the course of time. This process has resulted in the Hopeful Steps program in which a modest beginning in the area of early stimulation has resulted in a wider integrated development program involving many persons.

Hopeful Steps worked in a very poor and isolated region of the country. Initially the leaders of the community denied that there were in fact PWDs in the region. Hopeful Steps responded by providing training in a number of areas identified as priorities within the region. Only after the trust and the confidence of the community leaders was won did it become realistic to introduce training programs to help PWDs within the community. The result of this integrated model of development has been that PWDs are now perceived as one of the largest groups in need of assistance within the community and they are able to receive this assistance within the constraints of the realities of the environment in which they live.

REFERENCES

de Roos T, Van Elk V 1996 Participatory evaluation of Guyana CBR program. University of Amsterdam, Amsterdam
Economist Intelligence Unit 1994 Country profile: Guyana. EIU, London
Guela N 1994 Base line health data of the Rupununi district in Guyana. University of Berkeley, California
Hopeful Steps 1994a Survey of persons with disabilities in three regions of Guyana. Guyana CBR Program (mimeo), Guyana

Hopeful Steps 1994b Interview. Hopeful Steps CBR Newsletter 10 (June): 3
Ministry of Health 1994 Health statistics on Guyana. Ministry of Health, Guyana
O'Toole B 1989 Evaluation of Guyana CBR Program. PhD thesis, University of London
Stout S 1996 Sustainability of CBR and BCHP programs in Guyana. Master's thesis, Department of Medicine, University of Berkeley, California

16

Development of community rehabilitation in Nicaragua: training people with disabilities to be trainers

Estelle Schneider
Hector Segovia

INTRODUCTION

The purpose of this chapter is to highlight a unique and humanistic model of teaching developed in Nicaragua, in which people with disabilities (PWDs) are active participants rather than passive recipients of knowledge and services. The model is part of a broader vision that seeks to restore personal dignity to PWDs who have been disempowered by social and political inequality, injustice, violence, and deeply ingrained cultural stereotypes. Much work has been done in Nicaragua toward constructive change in attitudes, policies, and practices in the social, educational, professional, and governmental spheres relating to disability. The disability rights movement has played an outstanding role as a catalyst for these changes. This chapter provides a window through which to view these developments and learn from the experiences of Nicaraguan people who have much to teach about disability, social change, and dignity.

I [Estelle Schneider] lived in Nicaragua from 1988 to the end of 1993, and spent those years immersed in working as a physical therapist both inside and outside of the health care system. I was part of a groundswell of international support for the Sandinista revolution and the social transformations that were taking place. It was a profound experience in many respects, but the aspect most relevant to this chapter is the re-examination of the role of a health care professional, and a recognition of the shortcomings of the medical expert paradigm which is one of the fundamental underpinnings of professional preparation.

The settings that I worked in took me from the central offices of the Ministry of Health in the capital, Managua, to a rural outpatient clinic to which patients would travel up to 3 hours for treatment, as well as to people's modest dwellings in the more remote areas of the country, accessible only by foot, mule, or horseback. With the assistance of local government agencies and the organization of PWDs, I helped initiate a home-visiting program for the war-disabled. I studied Nicaraguan traditional medicine in order to learn the uses, preparation and scientific properties of commonly used plant remedies, including those used for spinal cord injury complications such as pressure sores and kidney infections. I was privileged to be able to participate to a small degree in the reconciliation process whereby people who became disabled fighting on different sides of the conflict saw their disability as a way to overcome differences, and at the same time work collaboratively to transform society's attitudes toward them.

After almost a year of working in a rural outpatient setting, I was invited to join the staff of the Center for the Promotion of Integral Rehabilitation (CEPRI), based in Managua. CEPRI is an organization, founded by PWDs, whose philosophy, programs and activities are the subject of this chapter. Hector Segovia, a founder and executive director of CEPRI, is the co-author of the chapter. Hector Segovia was also one of the founders of the Organization of Revolutionary Disabled (ORD) in 1980. He became paraplegic in March 1979 as a result of being ambushed by the National Guard, Somoza's military force, while driving to his home in eastern Managua. Hospitalized for several months in what was euphemistically called a specialized rehabilitation hospital, the main thing he learned was how little health professionals knew about spinal cord injury. His response to his own personal tragedy and the overwhelming medical ignorance he encountered was to become a fighter for the human rights of PWDs.

NICARAGUA IN A NUTSHELL

Nicaragua is a small Central American country bordered on the north by Honduras and on the south by Costa Rica. It covers 51 000 square miles (about the size of Iowa, USA). With a population of about 4 million people, it is the least densely populated country in Central America. The terrain is lush and varied, with rugged mountains, towering volcanoes, rainforest, steamy lowlands, tranquil beaches, rivers, pine forests, and many lakes. Climatic conditions can be volatile, and natural disasters such as earthquakes, volcanic explosions, tidal waves, tropical storms, and hurricanes as well as droughts play a major role in Nicaraguan history and everyday life.

Nicaragua's economy is primarily agrarian, with coffee, cotton, beef, and sugar the principal exports, followed by secondary exports of bananas, tobacco and sesame. Approximately 70% of the country's export earnings are generated by agricultural production (Barry 1991). Industries on the eastern or Caribbean coast include gold mining, shellfish production, and lumber.

In spite of its rich natural and human resources, Nicaragua is a poor country. Key economic indicators are generally characteristic of low-income dependent countries. Income is approximately $730 per capita, unemployment in 1992 exceeded 54%, and infant mortality is estimated at 67 per 1000 live births (World Bank 1992). Dependency refers to a situation in which the economy of a weak country is oriented toward external factors and the government is controlled by national and/or international élites that benefit from this economic relationship (Walker 1986). Many of Nicaragua's problems are rooted in this economic and social phenomenon.

The population on the Pacific side of the country is mestizo (of mixed European and Indian ancestry), but the indigenous legacy remains through aspects of the language and the culture. The Caribbean coast is home to the Miskito, Sumu and Rama Indian peoples, as well as the Afro-Nicaraguans, Garifunas and the English-speaking Creoles.

HISTORICAL BACKGROUND

In order to understand the development of community rehabilitation and the role played by PWDs in Nicaragua, one must examine the historical context. Nicaragua's history is indelibly intertwined with the history of conquest, colonization, military intervention and foreign occupation by countries such as Spain, England, and the USA. Colonialism ended in the 19th century with formal independence from Spain in 1821, but for much of that century society was dominated by ongoing internal conflicts among the élite classes and the interference of new foreign powers. Nicaragua began the 20th century facing sharp conflicts among these groups, which were frequently suppressed by US military intervention during the following 2 decades. However, US Marines were not able to defeat the nationalist and peasant-based movement led by Augusto Cesar Sandino (from whom the Sandinistas took their name and legacy), and the USA withdrew its troops. Before leaving, they helped train and install a new force called the National Guard whose control they handed over to Anastasio Somoza Garcia (Walker 1986).

From 1936 to 1979, the country was ruled by the Somoza family dictatorship, during which time the family amassed enormous personal fortunes by controlling most of the country's exports and industry. At the same time, the vast majority of Nicaraguans lived in abject poverty. Illiteracy among the rural population was about 90%, the leading cause of death was intestinal parasites, childhood malnutrition was endemic, and the life expectancy was the lowest in Central America (Garfield & Taboada 1986). The National Guard carried out brutal repression against any attempt at dissent or reform. In 1979, a popular revolution led by the Sandinista National Liberation Front (FSLN) overthrew the dictatorship. With the country in chaos and up to 50 000 dead, the new government immediately began to address and reverse the problems of illiteracy, infant mortality, and land distribution, among others.

The new health care system was based on the conviction that health care is a basic human right guaranteed to every citizen. The public health sector was streamlined into a national unified health system under the Ministry of Health. The number of primary health care facilities was tripled, the social security hospital system was collapsed into the government system, private medicine was restricted, and user fees were reduced (Garfield 1993). The budget allocation for health, a scarce 3% under Somoza, was gradually increased to 14% by 1986 (Henson 1990).

A cornerstone of Nicaragua's initiatives to improve the nation's health was the strategy of promoting the direct participation of the population in health and education efforts. Illiteracy was reduced from 50% to 13% in 5 months by a National Literacy Campaign in which half the country literally taught the other half how to read (Walker 1986). In 1981–2 80 000 volunteers, known as 'brigadistas', received training in basic health and hygiene as well as how to administer vaccinations (Henson 1990, Scholl 1985). In coordination with popular organizations and the Ministry of Health, they carried out national public health education campaigns, vaccination drives, and malaria control programs that reached the most isolated areas of the country. Polio was eradicated, while malaria and infant diarrhea were substantially reduced. Infant mortality was reduced by 50% from 121/1000 to 60/1000 live births (Norsworthy & Barry 1990). By 1983, Nicaragua had received recognition, both from the World Health Organization and from the United Nations Children's Fund, for its innovative primary care programs and public health accomplishments (Norsworthy & Barry 1990, Walker 1986). Even life expectancy, where improvements are generally seen over a longer period, increased from 52 years before 1979 to 59 years by 1985 (Garfield and Taboada 1986)

In the early 1980s, the US government initiated a series of measures to destabilize the Sandinista government. These included diplomatic pressure, economic embargo, and support for the formation of a counter-revolutionary army known as the 'Contra', whose objective was the overthrow by force of the new government by 1983 (Robinson & Norsworthy 1987). When this rapid overthrow failed to materialize, the strategy was changed to low-intensity warfare, which focused less on conventional military engagement and instead relied on eroding popular support for the Sandinistas. Infrastructure targets such as health care centers, schools, social service centers, oil storage tanks, and grain silos were mined, bombed and attacked by the Contras (Garfield 1989, Garfield & Williams 1992). Civilians in rural areas who worked in health, education, and development projects, as well as religious workers and agricultural cooperative members were targeted by the Contras (Brody 1985). As Muecke (1992) observed, in working with refugee populations displaced by political conflict and affected by state terror: 'Violence against health care personnel and sites is a political strategy to instill fear in the populace, penetrate everyday life with oppression, and deprive people of recourse when ill and wounded'.

In 1990, the government of the Sandinistas lost the parliamentary elections, and power was peacefully transferred to the new government headed by Violeta Chamorro. This was the first democratic transfer of political power in Nicaragua's history. It was hoped that a new government with close ties to the USA would bring some relief from the economic pressures and an end to the war. It was a vote in anticipation of peace and economic prosperity.

Since 1990, however, the anticipated peace and prosperity have proved elusive. The post-1990 economic restructuring policy required by international finance institutions has resulted in a shift from the Sandinista model of mixed ownership (state, private, and cooperative) to a model favoring privatization of public and state-run institutions. The health system is in the process of becoming desocialized and has been severely affected by decreased government funding, layoffs, and buyouts of public health sector jobs (Garfield 1993, FETSALUD 1994). Particularly hard-hitting for PWDs was the closing of two out of three vocational

rehabilitation training centers in Managua (SOLIDEZ 1995).

Official figures place the unemployment rate at 25%, while independent organizations report 1994 unemployment levels at 60% of the economically active population (Barricada Internacional 1995). Unemployment levels for PWDs are far higher. SOLIDEZ, an organization of PWDs whose focus is vocational training and work integration, conducted an investigation of the status of 700 women with disabilities on the Pacific coast. The rate of illiteracy was found to be 43% and the rate of unemployment was reported at 83% (SOLIDEZ 1991). On the Caribbean coast, a similar study of 800 women with disabilities revealed a 32% illiteracy rate and an unemployment level of 81% (SOLIDEZ 1993). PWDs are further disadvantaged in this economic climate.

CHANGING VIEWS OF DISABILITY

During the period from 1979 to 1990 there were profound changes in how PWDs saw themselves, and how they were seen by others and by society. Under the Somoza regime, medical rehabilitation as a concept did not exist. After the polio epidemic of 1959, the government responded with some rehabilitation services, but no structure was created to guarantee ongoing assistance for PWDs. Those with financial resources in need of rehabilitation sought services in other countries.

The dominant social and cultural view was that the disabled were deserving of pity or were considered as sub-human and ignored. Prevailing attitudes ranged from overprotection, to pity, to hiding and even beating PWDs. Disability was seen as punishment for an offense committed in this or a previous life (see Ch. 4). In the case of children born with disabilities, the father would often claim that his partner had been unfaithful, since his ego could not bear the thought of having an 'imperfect' child. There was no context to challenge these beliefs, much less replace them with more positive constructs. In general there was a bleak panorama for PWDs.

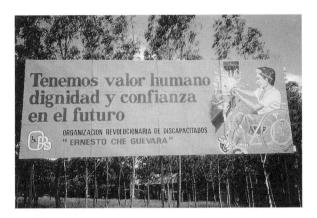

Fig. 16.1   ORD billboard in Managua – 'We have human worth, dignity and confidence in the future'.

The stage was set for change in the wake of the 1979 triumph of the Sandinista revolution. Tremendous energy was generated by people who were able to speak in their own voices, be heard, and advocate and organize themselves for the first time in their lives. This included the war-disabled, who did not want to become either invisible or be seen as a burden to the new government. Their fervor for changing society was carried over into the arena of struggling for full rights as citizens with disabilities (Fig. 16.1). During the 1980s, following the lead of the ORD which was founded in 1980, many organizations of PWDs emerged. These included associations of blind people, deaf people, and parents of children with disabilities. Wheelchair building and repair workshops run by PWDs, sewing collectives, and projects addressing mental health and disability issues also developed, as well as income-generating projects. In the words of a disabled activist, 'The revolution provided the opportune space for us to organize, and to transform the attitudes and prejudices of society' (CEPAD 1990). This was a new reality for Nicaragua, and prompted a change in public image and perception of PWDs, particularly the war-disabled (Bruun 1990).

Although scarce government resources and the need politically and psychologically to support the war-disabled meant that preferential treatment was accorded them in health care, education, housing and other social services, there seemed to be a positive spillover in attitudes toward PWDs in general. An attempt was made to redefine all PWDs as full members of society. This concept was deepened by the influence of visiting US disability rights activists who advocated the ideal of equal rights for disabled people – to participate in society, live independently, and bear the same responsibilities as other citizens.

Nonetheless, the situation facing PWDs was daunting. The number of people severely disabled in the war overwhelmed the infrastructure of the health care system. The one national rehabilitation center in Managua often had a 2-month waiting list for rehabilitation after acute hospitalization for people with diagnoses such as amputations and spinal cord and head injuries. A shortage of adequately trained medical and rehabilitation personnel complicated the picture further, and treatment often focused on providing basic medical care and not on long-term rehabilitation. The delay prior to admission for rehabilitation often meant that people had already developed severe complications, ranging from contractures to decubitus ulcers to kidney and bladder infections, as well as depression and other emotional and psychological problems that created obstacles to social reintegration. Sexuality was a total taboo, and both men and women with disabilities suffered severe consequences in their personal lives as a result. The vocational training services that were available were limited to those traditionally acceptable for the disabled, such as sewing, tailoring, manual skills, and small appliance repair. Employment was hard to come by.

RESPONSE OF PEOPLE WITH DISABILITIES

In the midst of this situation, a small group of people with spinal cord injuries who had been active in the larger organization of PWDs, began to question the appropriateness of the health care system. They raised concerns about the training and quality of health care personnel, the lack of adequate medical supplies (such as leg bags and catheters), the absence of adequate nutrition, the lack of emphasis on self-care (such as bowel and bladder retraining), the minimal psychosocial support services available, and the shortage of wheelchairs and of training in their use and maintenance for people who did have them. They challenged the concept that only the war-disabled were worthy of respect and demanded that society change its handicapping attitudes toward all PWDs.

This committed group of activists went on to form an organization called CEPRI. It was founded in 1986 by five people with disabilities, all of whom had spinal cord injuries of different etiologies – three of them were civilians who became spinal cord injured as a result of the war, and two had sequelae of polio. The three men and two women were from different geographical areas and backgrounds.

The distinguishing characteristic of CEPRI's philosophy is its focus on identifying society's responsibility to change oppressive attitudes toward PWDs. Its principal objective is to promote the full integration of PWDs into the economic, social and political life of the country. In the words of one of CEPRI's founders, Orlando Perez, a person with quadriplegia since 1975:

Rehabilitation is more than just learning how to move your legs and arms or getting on a bicycle and doing exercises. It's the combination of medical, psychological and social changes necessary for the disabled individual to be fully reintegrated into society, with all of his or her rights as a citizen. In order for we disabled people to be fully integrated into society, it's obviously necessary to rehabilitate society as well. (CEPAD 1990)

This need to 'rehabilitate' society is reflected in CEPRI's other objectives. CEPRI works to promote appropriate measures by governmental and non-governmental organizations and agencies that will guarantee adequate assistance, services and training for PWDs, thus assuring them the tools to achieve full integration into the society. CEPRI also advocates for improvement in the level and quality of training for professional and technical rehabilitation and medical personnel who are then more able to provide information necessary for physical, mental, and spiritual rehabilitation to PWDs and their family members.

Hector Segovia initially underscored the importance of the attitudes toward disability that are reflected in language and semantics. 'One of our earliest accomplishments was a campaign to demystify the use of the word *minusvalido* (of less value) and replace it with *discapacitado* (person with a disability), which is less stigmatizing.' 'A physical deficiency converts to a disability because one loses the aptitude to carry out a certain activity owing to lack of adequate conditions. It's the society that actually forms "minusvalidos".' In CEPRI seminars a group dynamic, called 'what words are used to identify people who are disabled', yielded long, seemingly endless lists of descriptive terms like *deschincacados* (literally, 'spineless'), as well as other pejoratives. This set the stage for a discussion on the importance of changing the attitudes of disrespect and self-deprecation behind the terminology so that words used for PWDs would reflect different values.

FROM PHILOSOPHY TO ACTION

In the years between 1988 and 1991, when CEPRI was developing its programs, circumstances were far from optimal. Nicaragua was experiencing post-war trauma in all respects – politically, economically, and socially. There were constant fluctuations in the currency with major financial instability as a result, a shortage of material resources, and transportation problems. There was distrust between people who may have had different allegiances during the years of conflict, which created ongoing polarization and episodes of violence, especially in regions of the country most affected by the war. There were many PWDs in these regions and also great obstacles in reaching them. At times activities were postponed or canceled because of armed clashes, or lack of safe conditions on roads. Funding agencies and international organizations expressed concern about whether programs could be carried out under these conditions, creating much financial uncertainty for CEPRI. In this context, the accomplishments and achievements are yet more remarkable.

During this period, CEPRI's programs concentrated on the twin objectives of affecting change in societal attitudes toward disability, as well as education and training of PWDs and their family members. Activities were designed to inform the public about the physical and social barriers preventing disabled people from active integration and to suggest ways to eliminate these barriers. CEPRI met and established relationships with organizations that provided support for activities. These included the Ministry of Health, Ministry of Social Welfare, the Commission to Support the Combatants, the Interministerial Commission on Rehabilitation, and community organizations as well as organizations of PWDs. Meetings were also held with rehabilitation specialists from Nicaragua and other countries and other individuals (both disabled and without a disability) involved in rehabilitation.

Consultations with the above-named groups led to the presentation of two 3-day seminars entitled 'Constructive attitudes toward disabled people in social transformation'. The topics discussed were concepts of disability and the philosophy of integral rehabilitation, self-care for people with spinal cord injuries, how to handle depression, sexuality and disability,

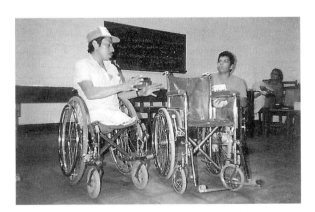

Fig. 16.2 Juan Gonzalez of the Foundation for Independent Mobility, giving a class on basic wheelchair maintenance and repair during a CEPRI seminar.

basic maintenance of mobility devices (Fig. 16.2) and accessibility. Participants included health professionals, representatives of government and non-government agencies, and PWDs and their family members. Instructors included rehabilitation as well as other professionals, and PWDs. It is in keeping with the spirit of CEPRI to work collaboratively with all who share its principles. Laypeople and professionals, whether formally or informally trained, disabled and non-disabled, all work together with equal opportunity. Everyone's experience, whether professional, empirical, or practical, is respected.

Another seminar, called 'People in a barrier-free environment for integral rehabilitation', was held for participants concerned with accessibility issues and the shared goal of seeking possible solutions. A seminar called 'The reality of disabled people in Nicaragua' was held with the objective of increasing the awareness of high-level government officials about the problems faced by PWDs. And finally, a seminar was held with physical therapy students on sexuality and disability, emotional adjustment to disability, and the self-help movement of people with disabilities in Nicaragua, topics which had never been addressed previously in any professional or technical health training curriculum. These courses were taught by CEPRI leaders and were the springboard from which a broader collaboration with the physical therapy school was to develop in later years.

Other unique activities in this period included a photography contest entitled 'The disabled in Nicaragua'. Its objective was to motivate photographers to take into account the problems people face with societal integration, and to reflect this awareness in their work. Over a dozen photographers participated to create an exhibit that was held in a major Managua gallery and received extensive publicity.

A library of documents, videos and other resources was established to be of assistance to associations of disabled people, institutions that have rehabilitation programs, government agencies and officials, and PWDs and their family members. This project grew from the need to produce educational and resource materials on different aspects of disability that are reflective of the Nicaraguan reality. This too became the springboard for a larger, more ambitious project to develop in later years – an extensive library and documentation center on disability and rehabilitation issues, in Spanish and English.

Given the consequences of spinal cord injury, which are grave if untreated and can be fatal, and the experience of CEPRI founders in living this reality themselves, CEPRI decided to focus on spinal cord injury in the educational seminars. CEPRI's education and training team (Equipo de capacatacion') had the responsibility to prepare, coordinate and teach the seminars. Initially this team consisted of CEPRI founders and several rehabilitation health care professionals – a psychologist who was team coordinator, a nurse, and me [Estelle Schneider], as a physical therapist. The seminar was called 'Integral rehabilitation and self-care for people with spinal cord injuries' and included the following topics:

- basic concepts and philosophy of integral rehabilitation
- what is a spinal cord injury? (including spinal anatomy, spinal shock, defining the level of injury and complete and incomplete lesions, and potential complications of spinal cord injury)
- skin care and prevention of pressure sores
- self-care of the urinary system (including different types of catheterization)
- bowel and bladder education
- emotional adjustment to disability
- sexuality and spinal cord injury
- prevention of contractures
- autonomic dysreflexia
- medical complications
- use of plants and natural medicine for complications of spinal cord injury.

A major part of 1991 was spent in writing, translating and collectively producing what became CEPRI's major educational and teaching resource, *A Manual of Self-Care after a Spinal Cord Injury* (CEPRI 1991). A second manual, a revision of a similar manual done by two occupa-

tional therapists from the USA, called *A Manual of Sexuality after Spinal Cord Injury*, was produced (CEPRI 1993). While it provided information about sexuality, its main purpose was to promote communication between a couple that included a spinal-cord injured member, and it was used for participatory group activity in the seminars. Two additional publications include a comic book version of the self-care manual, and an edition of the spinal cord self-care manual by and for women.

DEVELOPMENT OF THE CONCEPT OF TRAINING PROMOTERS

During a period of evaluation and reflection of programs and objectives in 1991, several issues of concern were discussed. Chief among them was the sense that although the seminars were reaching a number of PWDs, it would take close to forever with this particular methodology to reach all the people in need. A smaller pilot program of home visits to people with severe disabilities drew the same criticism. The home visits by CEPRI's team would evaluate and assess people's situations and make recommendations for appropriate measures and interventions and work with family members (Fig. 16.3). While productive in certain aspects, they were labor- and time-intensive. It was concluded that the most likely way to increase the number of

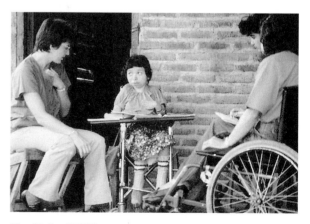

Fig. 16.3 CEPRI team pays a home visit to 13-year-old Ana Mercedes, Matagalpa (author Estelle Schneider is seated on left).

people that could be reached in different parts of the country was to change to the methodology of the 'multiplier' concept. Along parallel lines, the CEPRI team had observed that the response of the participants to being taught by PWDs was very positive. Seeing people similar to themselves as role models seemed to have as strong an effect on people as learning about the actual material itself. This was also in keeping with CEPRI's philosophy to continually empower PWDs in all levels of practice. It was therefore decided to formalize a training program for PWDs to become 'promoters of integral rehabilitation,' so that they could function as teachers, leaders, and peer advocates.

By early 1992, funding was secured from a US aid agency, a curriculum was developed based on the topics taught in the seminars, and a selection process, based on interviewing interested candidates who had been participants in previous seminars, were all in place. In addition, the project provided funding for a Nicaraguan physical therapist who became my partner and counterpart. Four people with spinal cord injuries, two men and two women, were selected to receive the training, and CEPRI's team was about to double! (Fig. 16.4)

After 4 months of training, the promoters began to assume teaching responsibilities in CEPRI's seminars and workshops. Beginning with one or two themes, they gradually

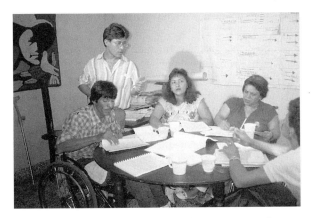

Fig. 16.4 Carlos Lopez, physical therapist, with the first four promoters, from left to right: Claudio Castro, Janeth Rosales, Lilian Anador, Pedro Joaquin Guerrero.

assumed teaching more topics during the six seminars carried out throughout 1992. Team meetings and evaluation sessions after the seminars, as well as feedback from seminar participants, provided constructive criticism to all team members regarding teaching weaknesses and strengths.

Evaluation of the projects performed in 1992 was overwhelmingly positive, yet there was a sense that there were regions of the country and numbers of people that were still not being reached, and the role of the rehabilitation promoter continued to evolve and expand. Based on feedback from PWDs in more isolated areas, the team believed that the promoter should be able to respond to broader social concerns. There were suggestions to provide training in how to prepare project proposals, develop appropriate income-generating projects, conduct feasibility studies and run small businesses among others. The concept of integral rehabilitation was expanding even further according to the needs and interests of the people it represented.

EXPANSION OF THE PROMOTER CONCEPT

After a period of consultation with PWDs and rehabilitation organizations, a very ambitious project called 'Promoting the integral health of the spinal-cord injured' was designed, and funding was secured as a follow-up project to the previous one. The role, function and training of the promoters was expanded, as well as the geographic scope of the regions covered. The goal was to train 30 new promoters from five different regions of the country over a period of 18 months and to select a coordinator who would have the responsibility of coordinating between CEPRI and the rest of the promoters in the region. CEPRI team members traveled to different parts of the country to explain the objectives of the project and set up the local selection process. The promoters and coordinators received small monthly subsidies, but were essentially community volunteers (Fig. 16.5). The promoter, in addition to having teaching

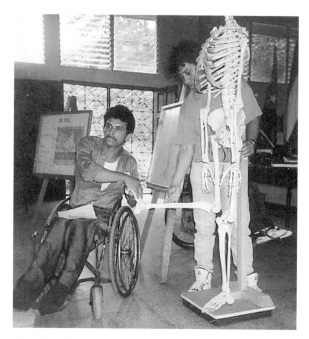

Fig. 16.5 Pedro Joaquin Guerrero, rehabilitation promoter, teaching a class on range of motion and prevention of contractures, Juigalpa.

responsibilities, was to be a community volunteer trained to serve as an advocate for PWDs and provide support, referrals, and information to those in need. The coordinator, in turn, was responsible for coordinating and supervising the base work of the promoters in their respective communities, and to provide information to CEPRI that could be used to generate future projects to meet the needs of the constituents. Other responsibilities included attending supervisory meetings with CEPRI's technical team, developing projects that would generate income for PWDs in the communities, and carrying out a local census to identify people with spinal cord injuries. In order to prepare the promoters for their new functions, the following topics were added to their training:

- concepts and methodology of popular education
- interpersonal skills and leadership training
- human rights and disability
- community based rehabilitation
- national and international organizations of people with disability

- alcoholism, drug addiction and disability
- preparation of project proposals for income-generating projects.

Instructors for these topics were solicited from agencies such as the Nicaraguan Commission on Human Rights, the National Training Institute for Small Business, the mental health team of a regional health clinic, and the rehabilitation program of the Ministry of Health. This once again served the function of expanding and strengthening CEPRI's institutional ties. The training was carried out in four seminars, each a week long, over a 7-month period and 25 promoters (13 women and 12 men) graduated from the training. They included 15 people with spinal cord injuries, 6 people with other disabilities, and 4 people without disabilities. At the conclusion of the final seminar, an overall evaluation of the four seminars was conducted to evaluate organization, logistic support, content and methodology, and group participation

Once again, the accomplishments of this program must be seen in the context of the Nicaraguan reality. The first seminar of this sequence took place in September 1993, with 40 participants expected from around the country. The first day was 2 days after an 18-hour tropical storm had devastated the country, leaving 30 000 people homeless. It also coincided with the first day of a national transportation strike that within 24 hours paralyzed transport throughout the country and blocked access to Managua where the seminar was being held. Fortunately, the planning called for participants to travel and arrive on what turned out to be the day after the tropical storm and before the national transport strike. The majority arrived safely and spent a calm week in the seminar while the rest of the country was battered by the strike and the aftermath of the storm.

WHERE ARE THE WOMEN?

All throughout the seminars held in the late 1980s and early 1990s, the participants included very few women with spinal cord injury or any disability. When a meeting of women with disabilities was held in 1989, the women expressed a need for support to face the double and sometimes triple discrimination based on gender, disability and class. Women stated that often they were either overprotected or hidden away by their families, and in very few cases were they encouraged to pursue education and training, or even socializing.

Lesbia Solorzano, a Managua physician who became paraplegic and deaf in 1985 as a result of a procedure known as *raquidea*, an epidural anesthetic technique used in cesarean births that has left many women disabled (Shrader 1996), shares the sentiments of the women expressed in their support group in 1989. Currently the coordinator of CEPRI's women's program, she states that women with disabilities, compared to their male counterparts, 'are much more quickly stigmatized as "sick and incapable" '. She says they are more likely to be abandoned by their spouses and families, and have greater difficulty finding sex partners and building healthy relationships. Additional problems include job discrimination: 'When we look for a job, we face an employer who always thinks of the woman as a secretary or receptionist who greets the public. The employer doesn't want someone in a wheelchair, or who uses crutches, because it's somehow not aesthetic. He doesn't think about our capability to do a particular job, he just goes by our physical appearance.' She declares that women with disabilities want to work, but social prejudices often prevent that. Women are thus left as a burden to their families and the society around them.

At a seminar in 1990 for spinal cord injured people and health workers, the scope of the problem became more apparent. A female participant was noted to have a wheelchair without footrests, and she was beginning to develop bilateral plantarflexion contractures. In general, the wheelchair was not in good condition and was not adequate for her needs. Two CEPRI team members spoke with her to try to address these issues. Reticent at first, she eventually revealed a startling story. In the first place she informed us that the wheelchair was a loan and

that she didn't have her own chair. This one had somehow been obtained by a supportive family member in order for her to attend the seminar. She became disabled the year before after giving birth by cesarean section and being administered the epidural known as 'la raquidea'. Since that time her husband rejected her and kept her in the back room of the house while he became involved with another woman – 'una mujer buena' (a non-disabled woman) whom he installed in their house as his new partner. Sympathetic family members brought her food, and she had never been out of the house during that year. Under these circumstances, it was very brave of her to attend the seminar and disclose her story, a first step in her transformation to gain dignity and self-respect.

This situation highlights the multiple and overlapping issues facing women with disabilities – powerlessness and abuse within their primary relationships, economic dependence, lack of self-esteem, and lack of opportunities for advancement and independence. Although the initial concern was the development of plantarflexion contractures, the mobilization required to change her situation touched on deeper and more profound issues. The problem of physical, sexual, and psychological abuse and violence toward women with disabilities has not been an easy concern to address. When CEPRI became aware that one of its own disabled male associates was physically and psychologically abusing his disabled female partner, CEPRI offered support to the woman so she could make necessary changes and also confronted the male partner so that he could begin to understand that such behavior was unacceptable and damaging to him as well.

Further analysis and discussion of these issues led CEPRI to initiate a 'Program of attention to women with disabilities'. The first step was finding the women with disabilities, which turned out to be no easy task. Local community organizations were consulted to identify women with disabilities on a neighborhood level, and at times the search was literally house-to-house. A suspicion that there were many women with disabilities who rarely left the house, either for lack of mobility devices or lack of something to do, was confirmed. For example, in a small town, a group of women who had participated in a CEPRI seminar through their church carried out an assignment to find, identify and become familiar with PWDs in their community. They identified a woman who used a wheelchair, lived alone with her husband, and never left the house, which was inaccessible. The local church women's committee got together, and eight women spent a day building a ramp into the woman's house. The woman reports that her life changed dramatically simply because she can now get in and out of the house by herself.

CEPRI developed a format for small workshops for women with disabilities that started out with the theme of building self-esteem. A gender-based approach was taken to question the subordinate position of women in society and the further subordination of disabled women, and to provide alternatives for change in relationships between men and women. The workshops are a source of information for the women on sexuality and reproductive health, violence and abuse, human rights, self-care, equal access to property and credit, formulating income-producing projects, and a host of other issues (Fig. 16.6). The participants in these workshops went on to form small local groups

that developed their own activities in nine towns around the country. What began as an occasional support group has grown to a fully-fledged autonomous program that has helped spawn smaller networks of women with disabilities throughout the country, as well as at least two new organizations. Women with disabilities have gone from being hidden at home to becoming active players in the social and political movements in Nicaragua and have participated in such international forums as the International Interdisciplinary Congress of Women, the Disabled Peoples International Conference in Vancouver in 1992, the United Nations Conference on Human Rights in Vienna in 1993, and the United Nations Fourth World Conference on Women in 1995 in Beijing.

INTEGRAL REHABILITATION AND PHYSICAL THERAPY STUDENTS

Under the Somoza regime, rehabilitation services were practically nonexistent. Physical therapists were trained informally on the job with no didactic preparation. In response to the polio epidemic in 1959 there was some improvement in services, with approximately 25 physical rehabilitation workers with minimal formal training and two physiatrists providing services. The number of people in the field remained virtually unchanged until 1979 (Koren 1987).

The physical therapy school in Nicaragua is located at the Polytechnic Health Institute of the National Autonomous University in Managua. The school was established in 1979, and provides a 3-year curriculum which was developed by reviewing physical therapy programs in Mexico, Cuba, and Argentina. Students come from all over the country and during the period 1979–90, tuition, housing, and transportation costs were subsidized. About 25–30 students graduate yearly. Students receive 1500 hours of theory and 1500 hours of practical training, during which they are supervised by the faculty in conjunction with supervisors from the hospitals. Since there is only one national rehabilitation

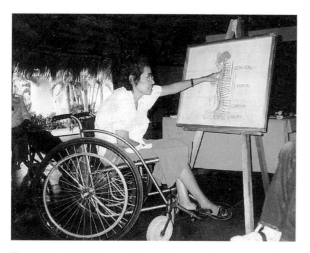

Fig. 16.6 Socorro, a participant in a seminar on sexuality and women with disabilities, learning about spinal cord function and injury.

hospital, and physical therapy services are not uniformly available at all hospitals, it is difficult to guarantee a variety of clinical experiences to all students. Nonetheless, the formation of this school is a major accomplishment and has provided a steady stream of nationally trained physical therapists. Academic teaching is hampered by a chronic shortage of books and equipment – it is not uncommon for a group of 10–15 students to share one photocopy of a manual muscle testing book.

The curriculum on spinal cord injury did not include any preparation for the students on psychosocial issues or on sexuality and disability and was also limited in training on self-care. These deficiencies were in turn perceived by spinal cord injured patients, who felt that the physical therapists were not adequately prepared to teach them what they needed to know to avoid serious complications such as infected pressure sores, contractures, kidney infections, and depression.

CEPRI stepped into the breach in 1989 by offering a seminar with physical therapy students to address issues of sexuality and disability and to introduce the students to the disability rights movement. It was evaluated very positively by all concerned. As a result, a more ambitious collaboration with the physical therapy school was initiated the following year. A once a week class called 'Promoting the integral health of the spinal cord injured' was introduced and has since become a part of the curriculum. It is planned, coordinated and taught by CEPRI's team of PWDs and health professionals, and focuses on psychosocial issues related to disability in general and spinal cord injury in particular. Students are encouraged to view a person who is disabled in a broader social context, rather than just in a limited medical environment. To that end, the seminar starts out with a round-table discussion to familiarize students with representatives from organizations of PWDs. The goal is for students to become aware of issues facing people in the broader community and society once their hospital based rehabilitation is completed. This course is unique in that PWDs and their per-

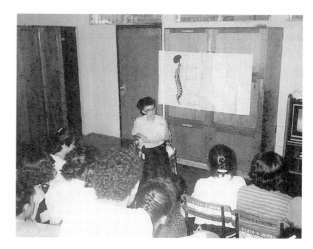

Fig. 16.7 Lesbia Solorzano of CEPRI teaching physical therapy students in Managua.

spectives are the central focus of the presentation, and in that they are orienting the students to their responsibilities to their future patients (Fig. 16.7).

REFLECTIONS

Toward a new model for professional collaboration

The model of community-based rehabilitation carried out and developed in practice by CEPRI is constantly evolving and is based on the needs that are identified by the constituents themselves. Once the needs and objectives are identified, resources and support are solicited from appropriate governmental, non-governmental, or community organizations and agencies. The planning, execution and evaluation are led by PWDs, who by virtue of this are the central players and active subjects of the process. This is in direct contrast to other models where plans for community rehabilitation are developed on a more central level by professionals who are not as familiar with local conditions and cultural influences (Woelk 1992). Without input from PWDs, they become transformed into objects rather than subjects of the rehabilitation process (Werner 1995).

There have been many positive outcomes of

CEPRI's model of community-based rehabilitation. Physical therapy students and health professionals subjectively report a change in awareness of the reality of PWDs, which translates into compassion and respect for them. PWDs express feeling more purposeful and able to fulfill their potential as a result of improved self-esteem. They also report an improvement in their self-care routines such as skin care, range-of-motion, and wheelchair maintenance. Family conflicts caused by negative attitudes are sometimes resolved as new understandings emerge, or as the disabled family member achieves a greater degree of independence. In addition, traditional gender roles are challenged as women with disabilities who were previously economically dependent on male partners and socially inactive become wage earners and public figures such as teachers, speakers, and consultants. These were not easy or smooth transitions but they are deep-rooted and reflect the personal ramifications of developing and practicing new social roles.

Furthermore, this model challenges the predominant model of professionalism with its assumptions that professionals teach and everybody else learns from them. Conditions in Nicaragua are such that many people are educated informally and through their life circumstances, rather than in a school or university setting. The methodology of popular education used by CEPRI is based on the principle that one's life experience is a source of knowledge to be built upon and shared. This model eliminates barriers between professional and non-professional, while at the same time it effectively acknowledges and uses all available resources. It also equalizes the teaching and learning processes. It is humanistic in that it promotes self-esteem and empowerment of PWDs and respects all people's knowledge and experience.

Toward a social model of disability

CEPRI's philosophy is an example of the social model of disability that emphasizes the removal of barriers, both physical and attitudinal, on an individual and societal level (Coleridge 1993). It is a necessary departure from the medical expert paradigm, which emphasizes providing a 'cure', or a 'return to normalcy' for the PWD. An implicit dependency is created by the medical model since it is based on the premise that professionals have solutions, regardless of whether or not they are acceptable to PWDs. In addition, medical expertism does not acknowledge the skills, abilities and creativities exhibited by PWDs internationally who have developed innovative and accessible rehabilitation technologies and systems in such areas as orthopedics (Myers 1987), prosthetics (Staats 1993), community rehabilitation training and education (Loveday 1990, CEPRI 1991, 1993, 1995a, 1995b), early childhood intervention (Butler 1993), and wheelchair design and repair (Hotchkiss 1985).

Developing countries are continuing to contribute their own culturally appropriate and practical solutions to problems facing PWDs using designs, materials, techniques and programs that are based on scientific principles, are locally produced, and are low cost and therefore accessible (Butler 1993). Faced with this development, professionals will of necessity have to change focus and consider a shift to a model of interdependence. Rather than promote hierarchy and dependency, interdependence stresses partnership (Condeluci 1991) and collaboration. Nobody is arguing for fewer professionals. What is at issue is the definition of the professional's role and the underlying attitude toward PWDs, who would much prefer that professionals collaborate with them in all respects ranging from formulating rehabilitation policy to determining treatment plans. This is a challenging approach that enhances professional input rather than detracting from it as some may fear. Rather than 'patient management', this approach emphasizes the professional as being a resource so that a greater goal can be accomplished, and it promotes the idea of popular participation rather than professional dominance in health education and practice (Stone 1992). Acting as a resource may require not only a higher degree of skill but a set of different attitudes and training (Coleridge 1993). According to Finkelstein, the nature of the helper/helped relationship needs to be questioned:

Professionals acting as a resource to be used by others need special education and training so that they are able to promote control by disabled people. . . . To do this, professional workers will need new communication skills, new professional codes of practice, new ethics, new rules of confidentiality and new concepts of clinical responsibility. In all this the professional rehabilitation worker needs to learn how to listen to clients, while at the same time helping the client to identify the central rehabilitation issue. . . . The need is for new relationships to develop between helpers and those they help. (Finkelstein 1981)

War-time and scarcity rehabilitation technology

Lack of medical supplies and medicines provoked ingenious responses from many quarters. Most sobering was the use of a Coke bottle and straw as a substitute for a leg bag and catheter on the part of a man who is paraplegic. CEPRI encountered another man who is paraplegic who rarely left his house owing to the lack of a functional wheelchair and lack of urinary supplies. Faced with this situation, he had a hole cut in his mattress and bedboard, placed a bucket underneath, and took care of his elimination needs in this way. When examined, he was found to have puzzling scratches on his genital organs, abdomen, and buttocks. Unbeknownst to him, a cat playing under the bed had inflicted these potentially dangerous wounds. The reality and consequences of these conditions are almost unfathomable. Less potentially deadly was the use of old brassiere straps as a substitute for velcro to secure condoms for intermittent catheterization. These are the desperate prerogatives of the poorest of the poor, and reveal far more than words or statistics regarding the reality of PWDs. Rather than cultural differences, they reflect differences in economic development and access to needed resources.

On a more positive note, the shortage of medicines during the 1980s was one of the catalysts for a policy to discover, systematize and pro-mote the use of natural medicine and plants for the treatment and cure of certain health problems. The use of medicinal plants is rooted in centuries of Nicaraguan culture. In a strategy designed to rescue and document the popular practices of the *curandero(a)s* (healers), *parteras* (midwives), and *sobaduras* (bone setters), brigades of high school students and teachers went to the countryside and interviewed traditional practitioners on the use and preparation of the most common herbal and plant remedies. The founding in 1985 of the National Center of Popular and Traditional Medicine in Esteli created an institution whose mission is to continue the promotion, research, training and cultivation of medicinal plants and remedies. During CEPRI's seminars, several participants mentioned using plant based remedies for healing pressure sores, using the liquid from papaya, and treating urinary infections with a tea made from *cola de caballo* (horsetail). Curious to learn more about this, CEPRI members signed up for a 10-day course given by the center that taught the use, preparation, and botanic and scientific properties of 43 of the most commonly used plants, as well the health and healing paradigms of the indigenous cultures. The information was then integrated into CEPRI's seminars and included in its educational materials. This is a clear example of the use and promotion of national resources and culture, and a departure from the practice of dependency and domination.

In closing, the teaching methodology, disability model, and redefinition of the professional role discussed in this chapter, permit participants to strive for ways all of us, whether disabled or not, can live lives of greater value and compatibility with each other. It maximizes and humanizes the quality of rehabilitation practice, and emphasizes mutual respect. The very positive outcome in Nicaragua justifies exploration of its application in educational and community settings in industrialized nations. It proves beyond a doubt that countries of the south have a great deal to teach countries of the north.

REFERENCES

Barricada Internacional 1995 Nicaraguan economy: a numbers game (January): 21–24

Barry T 1991 Central America inside out. Interhemispheric Educational Resource Center, Albuquerque

Brody R 1985 Contra terror in Nicaragua: report of a fact finding mission, September 1984–January 1985. South End Press, Boston

Bruun F J 1990 Hero, beggar, or sports star: negotiating the identity of the disabled person in Nicaragua. In: Ingstad B, Whyte S R (eds) Disability and culture. University of California Press, Berkeley, pp. 196–209

Butler C 1993 Effective solutions in rehabilitation: learning from each other. In: Woods D Developing awareness of disability in the world: looking at issues relevant to disability in Asia, the Pacific, and Africa through the eyes of U.S. Fellows. International Exchange of Experts and Information in Rehabilitation, University of New Hampshire, Durham, pp. 16–17

CEPAD 1990 CEPAD report. CEPAD, Managua, Nicaragua

CEPRI 1991 Manual de auto-cuido despues de una lesion medular. CEPRI, Managua, Nicaragua

CEPRI 1993 Manual de sexualidad despues de unia lesion medular. CEPRI, Managua, Nicaragua

CEPRI 1995a Nosotras . . . despues de una lesion medular. CEPRI, Managua, Nicaragua

CEPRI 1995b Hablemos del auto-ciudo de las personas con lesiones medulares. CEPRI, Managua, Nicaragua

Coleridge P 1993 Disability, liberation, and development. Oxfam Publications, Oxford

Condeluci A 1991 Interdependence: the route to community. Paul M Deutsch, Orlando

FETSALUD 1994 Las reformas en los servicios de salud a partir de 1990 [Report of the Confederation of Health Workers]. FETSALUD, Managua, Nicaragua

Finkelstein V 1981 Disability and the helper/helped relationship: an historical overview. In: Brechin Handicap in a social world. Hodder and Stoughton, London

Garfield R 1989 War related changes in health and health services in Nicaragua. Social Science and Medicine (28): 669–676

Garfield R 1993 Desocializing health care in a developing country. Journal of the American Medical Association 270(8): 989–993

Garfield R, Williams G 1992 Health care in Nicaragua: primary care under changing regimes. Oxford University Press, New York

Garfield R M, Taboada E 1986 Health services reforms in revolutionary Nicaragua. In Rosset P, Vandermeer (eds) Nicaragua: unfinished revolution. Grove Press, New York

Henson D 1990 Ten years of revolutionary accomplishments in EPOCA Update, Spring 1990

Hotchkiss R 1985 Independence through mobility, Whirlwind Wheelchair International, San Francisco

Koren T 1987 Regaining autonomy: rehabilitation in Nicaragua. Links 4(2): 4 [New York]

Loveday M 1990 Community-based rehabilitation workers: a South African training manual. SACLA Health Project, Cape Town, South Africa

Muecke M 1992 New paradigms for refugee health problems. Social Science and Medicine 35: 515–523

Myers A 1987 Studying health during war. Links 4(3): 14–15 [New York]

Norsworthy K, Barry T 1990 Nicaragua: a country guide. Interhemispheric Education Resource Center, Albuquerque

Robinson W I, Norsworthy K 1987 David and Goliath the US war against Nicaragua. Monthly Review Press, New York

Scholl E A 1985 An assessment of community health workers in Nicaragua. Social Science and Medicine 20: 207–214

Shrader E 1996 disability and reproductive rights: complications after regional anaesthesia in Nicaragua. Reproductive Health Matters. 7 May pp. 135–143

SOLIDEZ 1991 La mujer discapcitada en Nicaragua un informe. SOLIDEZ, Managua, Nicaragua

SOLIDEZ 1993 La situacion de la mujer discapacitada en la costa Atlantica: un diagnostico. SOLIDEZ, Managua, Nicaragua

SOLIDEZ 1995 Information Bulletin. SOLIDEZ, Managua, Nicaragua

Staats T 1993 A cross-cultural model for appropriate technology prosthetics. In: Woods D Developing awareness of disability in the world: looking at issues relevant to disability in Asia, the Pacific, and Africa through the eyes of U.S. Fellows. International Exchange of Experts and Information in Rehabilitation, University of New Hampshire, Durham, pp. 9–10

Stone L 1992 Cultural influences in community participation in health. Social Science and Medicine 35: 409–417

UNICEF 1991 Effects of armed conflict on women and children: relief and rehabilitation in war situations. 10: 2–3

Walker T W 1986 Nicaragua, the land of Sandino. Westview Press, Boulder

Werner D 1995 Disabled people as leaders in meeting their needs. Newsletter from the Sierra Madre No. 32, Palo Alto, California

Woelk G B 1992 Cultural and structural influences in community health programs. Social Science and Medicine 35: 419–424

World Bank 1992 World development report. Oxford University Press, New York

17

Problems with community mobilization and participation in CBR: a case from Botswana

Benedicte Ingstad

BOTSWANA – THE BEGINNING OF CBR

Botswana, a landlocked country on the southern tip of Africa, is in many ways a remarkable country. It has had a multi-party democracy since its independence in 1966 and has not been seriously troubled by internal or external conflicts. Its most unique characteristic is, however, a rapid economic development. From being one of the poorest countries in the world Botswana has now changed its status to upper middle-income country largely because of the mining and export of diamonds. However, the development has largely taken place in the urban areas. The majority of the population in the rural areas is still very poor.

Botswana has one of the longest histories of community based rehabilitation (CBR). Its national development plan for 1973–8 stated that so far insufficient attention had been paid to the problems of people with disabilities (PWD). Following this, it was recommended that the government seek assistance in the preparation of a program for detection, care, training and rehabilitation of disabled people. This, of course, did not happen in a vacuum. Botswana was already ahead of most other countries in the developing world in establishing a primary health care (PHC) system with the aim of reaching the whole population with healthcare facilities within a reasonable walking distance (15 km). Thus, the idea of community based services for disabled people fell well in line with the PHC ideology.

In 1977 a consultancy was carried out by Dr Einar Helander, who was later to become head of the World Health Organization (WHO) rehabilitation department and one of the co-authors of the first CBR manual (Helander et al 1983). This exercise contributed significantly to the development of the WHO CBR program (personal communication from Dr E. Helander), and Botswana became one of nine pilot countries chosen for field-testing (WHO 1982). This chapter will analyze the problems encountered in mobilizing the community for participating in CBR in Botswana.

A special service unit (SSU) was established in 1976 under the Ministry of Health and given the responsibility for matters concerning PWD and their rehabilitation. The unit has from its beginning been led by a commissioner and assisted by two senior welfare officers, one for the northern and one for the southern part of the country. Social welfare officers (SWO) with special responsibility for PWD are placed in the district health teams attached to each district council. The SWOs are responsible for instructing the family welfare educators (FWE) assigned to each clinic and health post in the training of and care for disabled people. The FWE is the Botswana equivalent to the village health workers found in many developing countries as part of the PHC system. They are chosen by the village and given a 3-month training course in basic health skills. Their task is mainly of a preventive and case-finding nature and they are expected to use a large part of their time doing home visits.

The main task assigned to the SSU was to develop a CBR program according to the WHO guidelines. The beginning of this effort was initiated in 1981, the same year as the International Year of Disabled Persons, with a national workshop for key personnel expected to be involved in CBR. The program was intended to be launched simultaneously in all districts and to cover all PWD. The actual number of PWD to be considered was not known at the time although a few local attempts at screening had been made. A population census carried out in 1991 found a disability rate in the population that now counts 2.2% in a population of 1.3 million (Stats Brief 1991).

In late 1981, Botswana Red Cross (BRC) started another CBR program as part of its ongoing program for PHC (Armitage 1982, Ingstad & Melsom 1985). The project had the same objectives as the national one, to give help to as many PWD as possible in their home communities. The target was set to reach 10 000 by the year 1985, based on the expectation that all Red Cross volunteers who were already trained in first aid would be active trainers for PWD in their home communities. After a 3-month trial period, followed by an assessment, the program was intended to expand all over the country.

Thus, by the end of 1981, CBR in Botswana had come to be organized as two pyramidal structures. The structure headed by the commissioner for the handicapped ranked above the second, which was implemented by BRC, since the commissioner is formally the head of all activities for disabled persons in the country. This ranking should have been reflected at all levels, with the BRC field officers referring to the SWOs and the BRC volunteers referring to the FWEs. In reality there was very little communication between the two structures.

A FOLLOW-UP PROJECT

In 1984, I was asked by the WHO rehabilitation department and the Norwegian Red Cross Society (NRC), which was sponsoring the BRC program, to do a follow-up study of 100 PWD who had been helped by CBR for at least 1 year. With support from the Norwegian Agency for Development Cooperation (NORAD), this was later extended to a research project with a 2-year (1984–5) follow-up of the CBR program in one health district (Kweneng). Being a social anthropologist by training and also the mother of a multi-handicapped teenage son, I was particularly interested in finding out how PWD and their families experienced their life situations in general and their encounters with CBR in particular. I also wanted to look into what I have elsewhere called 'The myth of the hidden disabled' (Ingstad 1997) in order to ascertain the truth of the often-stated comment that parents in developing countries tended to hide and neglect family members with disabilities. My hypothesis was that when looked into further, and understood in the sociocultural context of family life, the issue of hiding or neglect would not be a prominent one.

Method

To some extent, a study of PWD in their local communities becomes a choice between getting to know closely one community with a relatively small number of households with disabled family members, or trying to reach a larger number of people who live scattered over a larger area. I tried to compromise by using a combination of methods. I carried out participant observation, close follow-up of a few households with family members with disabilities, combined with informal interviews of other key informants in the village of Molepolole in which I lived with my family for 2 years. I also used a variety of other methods such as semi-structured interviews, focus group discussions, and time-use studies in getting to know PWD and their families from the whole of Kweneng district. Since Kweneng is one of the largest districts in Botswana, stretching from the border of the capital Gaborone a considerable distance into the Kalahari Desert, this involved extensive traveling.

Frequent follow-up visits (1987, 1989, 1990, 1991, 1995 and 1996), sometimes twice a year, have given me the opportunity to continue my contact with some of the PWD and their families as well as see the developments in the CBR program and rehabilitation in Botswana in general.

Sample

Semi-structured interviews with PWD and/or their carepersons formed the basis for the follow-up of the CBR program. The 95 households interviewed included a total of 100 family members with disabilities. The households were interviewed twice, with 1 year between each

interview. The first interview concentrated on the life situation of the PWD and her family from the onset of the impairment and up until the time of our meeting. Those interviews also touched upon experiences with CBR and other rehabilitation efforts. The second interview concentrated mainly on experiences with CBR in the year gone by as well as whatever important changes might have taken place in the situation of the PWD and the family members.

Out of the total sample of PWDs, 44 were males and 56 were females, which corresponds fairly closely to the over-representation of females in the total population of Botswana shown in the 1981 census. Those below the age of 15 made up 47% of the sample, which is exactly the same as in the census (Brunborg 1987). A total of 45% of the sample had multiple impairments. Physical impairment alone was a problem for 31%, while 51% were mentally affected. Epileptic seizures were a problem for 14%, while 19% were sensory impaired in one way or another.

The sample was obtained in close cooperation with the officers in charge of both the CBR programs in the district (SSU and BRC) as well as with the FWEs, and is believed to be very close to the total number of PWD in the district that had been in contact with CBR at the time, although poor registration and record keeping made it impossible to determine the exact number.

Main findings

The main findings from the study are briefly summarized below:

1. There was hardly any use of the CBR manual in spite of several training courses for FWEs. This was partly explained by the delay in its translation into Setswana. But even in 1985, when the translated version was available, only two families with a fairly high level of education had been able to utilize it.

2. There were also problems with referrals to higher levels of special services. At the first interview in 1984, as many as 52 needs for referrals were identified. One year later, only 15 of

these had been followed up. One of the main reasons for this was transport problems. Another important reason was lack of capacity at centers of referral.

3. Follow-up of families was not sufficient. During the study year, only 38 households with disabled members had been visited regularly by local supervisors or CBR field officers, 47 of the households had been seen a few times, and 12 households had not been seen at all.

4. A total of 42% of the disabled people in the sample had experienced no improvement in their condition or general life situation in the time between the two interviews, 39% had experienced some improvement, 12% had experienced much improvement, while for 7% the situation had actually worsened.

5. There was almost a complete lack of participation in CBR by the local communities. Only in two villages in the district had any significant community activities taken place to support PWD.

6. Families were generally found to be taking care of their disabled members as well as possible within their means of subsistence.

A more detailed discussion of these findings can be found elsewhere (Ingstad 1997).

PROBLEMS IN COMMUNITY PARTICIPATION AND MOBILIZATION

The problems in community participation and mobilization in Botswana can be analyzed at three different levels: the national level; the local or community level; and the household or individual level. These are of course closely interrelated.

National level

Coordination and cooperation

As mentioned above, CBR in Botswana was introduced through two pyramidal structures with their administrative and planning activities located in the Ministry of Health and Botswana Red Cross headquarters respectively. Consequently, both programs very soon took on the character of being top-down. There was

very little cooperation between them at any level, which complicated matters even more. Sometimes the field officers from SSU and BRC were not aware that they were helping the same PWD until they happened to meet in her yard. The client on the other hand, was not likely to offer the information, thinking that what help she could not get from one officer she might get from the other.

The introduction of CBR to a community would often take place in the form of a workshop in which administrative officers from the headquarters would come for a day or two to demonstrate physical therapy and use of the CBR manual to the FWEs. The workshops had the triple function of mobilizing volunteers, registering and assessing PWD, and giving the participants basic knowledge of CBR and PHC. Villagers with disabilities and their family members would be brought to attend the workshop. Although they may have been used for demonstration, little or no attempt was made to involve them in a discussion or to ask for their advice or opinion. The effect of this was that CBR was defined as something *new* to be learned, not something about which PWD and their family members already had a certain amount of valuable expertise. During one such workshop, a CBR administrative officer made a home visit to a family who had a teenage girl with quite a severe case of cerebral palsy. The CBR officer started out with a lengthy speech on how this child should be trained according to the manual. The mother kept very quiet until the end, when she was asked what she herself had done to train her child. Given this opportunity she came up with a lengthy account of her experience in dealing with mobility and toilet training that was much more inventive and suitable than the advice that had been given to her.

Costs

The ideology of 'low cost' was another constraint in making the program community based. The idea of running the CBR program more or less within the existing framework of PHC, which meant minimal additional input of resources, had clearly been one of the motivations of the Botswana government for embarking upon it. Thus, the SWO of the health team had to manage within the general resources allocated to the team, which, for example, meant that she had to share the only two vehicles with other team members. Efforts to go on treks together were not very successful since the needs of various team members rarely coincided. The SWO was stuck in her office for too much of her time, and when able to go on field trips she would try to reach as many PWD as possible and often had to concentrate on those who needed referral to special services in Gaborone. Thus, there was little time to concentrate on community involvement, and CBR soon became an outreach, not a community based program. This problem became even more acute when some years later decentralization of the health services led to the district health teams (DHT) being integrated in the council health services and the DHT vehicles being placed in the pool for the whole council.

For the BRC program, the resource situation was somewhat better in that they were almost fully financed by a foreign donor, the Norwegian Red Cross (for further discussion of this relationship see Ingstad 1995). The BRC field officers had their own vehicles and could plan their field trips when and wherever they liked. In spite of this they also tended to do more outreach than community based activities, with frequent reports back to headquarters in Gaborone. The BRC field officer had the support of an expatriate physical therapist and financial resources to arrange local workshops, as described above, to which SWOs were invited. The fact that BRC, as a non-governmental organization, was the inviter, and the representatives of the government CBR program the invited, also had an impact on how CBR was perceived.

Communications and follow-up

A final problem facing CBR at the national level was the program's aim of reaching the whole country at more or less the same time. With small villages connected by very rough sandy roads within a large country, this soon proved to be impossible with the limited resources available. The field officers were not able to go everywhere or regularly follow up previously visited families. A fairly large turnover in field officers, partly because of dissatisfaction in not being able to do the job for which they were intended properly, added to the problem. New people were employed who had not been to the original CBR training courses, and it took several years before resources were available to conduct follow-up courses.

Local/community level

Poverty

The problems encountered at the national level might have been less serious for CBR had the CBR field officers and FWEs been able to mobilize the communities to support their members with disabilities. There are two important reasons to be considered in understanding why community mobilization was a problem. The first is poverty. CBR was introduced to Botswana in the beginning of what turned out to be one of the worst droughts in history, lasting for 7 years. By 1984–5, most small-scale farmers had lost all their cattle and the crops had failed for several years. With a very high rate of unemployment, especially in the rural areas, there were few possibilities for additional income. A well organized drought relief system was the main factor in keeping Botswana from becoming a famine disaster area during those years.

Faced with this situation, it is not surprising that volunteers for CBR were hard to find, even for the BRC, which had originally counted on utilizing the large number of people all over the country who had been registered as volunteers after finishing their short first-aid course. One woman expressed her views thus: 'My husband would never allow me to work for free when I have five hungry children at home.' It also soon became clear that many of those who initially did volunteer did so in the hope of eventually being employed as FWEs and gave up when this did not happen.

Cultural concerns

Associated with this is the cultural appropriateness of the concept of volunteerism. Foreign planners tend to think of local communities in developing countries as homogeneous societies where people have a strong feeling of collective responsibility. In reality, this is rarely the case. The Tswana tribal society (which makes up around 80% of the population of Botswana) is very hierarchical. Traditionally there is a paramount chief as head of the tribe and local chiefs and sub-chiefs, who are usually his relatives, in each of the villages. The chief could demand services *letsema* (service to the chief) from the villagers but was himself obliged to allocate some of his wealth in return, for instance in the form of meals when the job was done. The villagers could also be ordered to do a certain amount of service *mophato* (service for the common good) for the community. People who went through initiation rituals together as an entrance into adult life would form certain age sets that could be called upon as a group to do such services. These traditional ways are, however, disappearing as the result of the modernization process, and this tendency has no doubt been accelerated by the expectation of handouts through drought relief and voluntary organizations. While participation in *letsema* and *mophato* was conforming to the norms of society, volunteer activities mark out the person as different, a quality that is not regarded highly among the Tswana. Coupled with the lack of material rewards for the family, engagement in such activities is likely to be considered frivolous behavior (Thobega 1980). Thus it seems that the concept of volunteerism built into the WHO's CBR program fits well with the European tradition of charity, but not very well with Tswana culture, especially not in times of hardship.

Similar problems have been encountered in the mobilization of modern institutions like the village development committees (VDC) and village health committees (VHC) consisting of elected members from the community. The extent to which these committees were functioning and able to mobilize in support of PWD varied, most of them paying only lip service to the support of CBR. The drought and need for employment clearly influenced people's willingness to spend their time on voluntary work and meetings. However, in one village the VDC had built a house for a family with five members with various disabilities and in another village a pit latrine for a man confined to a wheelchair. These cases are exceptions, however, and spring from an unusually good working relationship between the particular VHC and the local clinic. The BRC also struggled to keep up the interest of their local branches, except for the few occasions when workshops or visits from the headquarters were arranged. One very dedicated FWE in one village managed to organize a group of parents of children with disabilities. The group had meetings for a while but fell apart when the agricultural season started and people moved away to their 'lands' (agricultural fields) which were sometimes quite far away from the village. Even when rains were scarce people went to the 'lands' in search of wild fruits and berries and to look after their goats. Unfortunately, more formal organizations by PWD in Botswana were at the time either too divided by internal conflicts or too much of a Gaborone phenomenon to have any impact locally.

Education

During the time of fieldwork, a few attempts were made in Kweneng district at integrating children with disabilities in the local schools. Except for two girls with physical handicaps who were 'integrated' already before the concept was formalized or enacted, these attempts failed. To place a child who has a mental or sensory impairment in a class of 50–60 pupils, with teachers who had not been prepared in any way other than being told that disabled children should be integrated, is doomed to failure. Some parents were reluctant to send their children for fear of them either being beaten by the teachers for not keeping up in subjects or being teased by other pupils. Some very poor parents who could afford only to buy uniforms and shoes for a few of their many children would choose to prioritize the able-bodied ones.

Defining terms

A final problem to be mentioned is the lack of reflection over terms and their meanings in the CBR manual, specifically the concept 'community'. The unit that is usually implicated is a village. However, if 'community' means a unit that may act uniformly with some form of common interest, the village in Botswana may not fit the definition very well. Tswana villages are traditionally quite large and today they may number from a few hundred to as many as 30 000 inhabitants. Although there will always be a certain feeling of common belonging, rivalry and suspicions of witchcraft are just as important in determining people's actions. The only unit in which a real joint interest exists is the 'compound', consisting of several small houses, some traditional roundavels made of mud, with thatched roofs, and some more modern housing made of brick with corrugated roofs. A compound is inhabited by members of an extended family. The Tswana recognize agnatic kinship and newly married couples would usually move in with the parents of the bridegroom. In modern days, however, young people often want to establish a household of their own somewhere else. Female headed households are also becoming more and more common (for further discussion of implications of this for dependent household members see Ingstad et al 1992). Such knowledge pinpoints the need to sensitize planners of CBR about what a community really is. Who can be meaningfully mobilized in joint action for PWD, and what are the values, beliefs, options and constraints under which such action takes place? Answers to these questions require thorough studies to be done in an area *before* a CBR program is launched. Unfortunately, this is very rarely done.

Family/individual level

Is it community participation when almost all the responsibility for the training and care for PWD is left to the members of the household where these people live or to the people themselves, if they are able? This may be a matter of opinion, but this author would hardly consider it so. Perhaps, it would be more correct to say household based.

Cultural and ideological differences

Although the individual Tswana is recognized as someone with special needs and desires, this person is first of all seen as part of a larger whole: the family group, the living community of extended kin, and the ancestors through whom they are linked to the universe and its omnipotent god Modimo (a name which is used both for the traditional Tswana deity and the Christian God). Thus when referring to the sorrow of realizing that a child has a serious disability, a parent in Botswana would not say (as a Norwegian might), 'I am sorry because he cannot play football, get an education, have a career, etc. . . .', but rather, 'I am sorry because he cannot contribute to the family, support me when I am old, marry and have children, etc. . . .'. This distinction is important because it refers to the difference in an ideology linked to collective rights and duties in contrast to one of individual rights, reflected in the ideas of 'integration' and 'normalization' in rehabilitation discourse (Ingstad 1995). Thus, when asked about their needs, the disabled people themselves and their family members will most often ask for help that will promote the coping ability of the household unit as a whole. Similarly, what help is offered will be accessed in view of the life and values of the household units before it is eventually accepted. For example, a young woman, sent by the family from Gaborone to a remote village in order to care for a nearly blind mother-in-law, flatly refused to comply with the CBR instructions in mobility training. She claimed that having the old lady walking around in the village by herself would mark her as an inadequate daughter-in-law.

The CBR manual is based on the biomedical model in which the body consists of separated parts to be trained to regain their full or improved functioning. This is also reflected in the way CBR is practiced. In the Tswana culture, however, illness and impairment are seen in a much wider context, as part of a general misfortune in which close relatives, other members of the community, as well as ancestors or Modimo himself may have a role to play. It may be believed that illness and impairment are caused by witchcraft, break of sexual taboo by oneself or one's parents, ancestor's anger, or 'God's will'. 'Natural reasons' or 'just happened' are also used as explanations when none of the previous causes can be confirmed. In cases of permanent impairment people tend to resort to the more 'traditional' explanations, believing that ancestral punishment, witchcraft or break of taboo may be cured if the right rituals are performed in time, otherwise not.

The implications of this for CBR are twofold. First, there is no clear understanding of improvement as such. Since impairment caused by witchcraft is believed to be completely cured if one finds a 'strong' enough traditional healer, the values of the minor improvements that can be seen in the individual quality-of-life perspective are rarely fully appreciated. This is particularly so when there is limited usefulness for the household. This does not mean that the value of improvement is not understood and appreciated once it is pointed out, but it becomes an important task of the CBR workers to do so and to understand the viewpoint of the family without being prejudiced. A severely physically disabled child may be 'hidden' inside the house and thus easily become severely understimulated simply because this is the coolest place in the hot summer months and the family is busy with other tasks outside, not because they are ashamed or want him out of the way.

Second, traditional explanations have implications for community participation and involvement of people outside the household in care for the PWD. If witchcraft is suspected as an explanation for the disability, one cannot be certain who has caused this misfortune. Witches are usually sought among kinsmen or neighbors who for some reason might be envious or wish to cause harm to the household. Therefore, it is not surprising that there is a certain reluctance to have local people come in and do exercises or initiate other forms of CBR activities. To receive help from a CBR officer coming from outside

the community seems like a safer, more attractive alternative, especially since people tend to perceive CBR as something new and not as something in which they may use their own creativity and already gained expertise.

LESSONS TO BE LEARNED

There are several lessons to be learned from the Botswana CBR experience. First, the program that was started was too ambitious. Although the population at the time was less than 1 million, the area to be covered is more than 581 000 square km and the resources put into this (field officers, training and vehicles) was far from being sufficient. This was particularly consequential in that it was one of the very first CBR programs in the world, intended to be a model for other countries, and there was no previous experience to build upon. A similar program in Zimbabwe, launched by the Zimbabwean Red Cross in 1982, started out in one district. After being evaluated and considered a success (Modise et al 1984) it moved on to another district, leaving its first activities to be taken over by the government. Eventually the Zimbabwe Red Cross joined with the government in expanding the CBR program to the rest of the country. This overlapping model has the obvious advantage of concentrating resources (material, manpower, knowledge and training) in order to get the most effect out of them and to be able to learn from experiences.

The second lesson has to do with the relationship between the service of the government and that of non-governmental organizations (NGO) in CBR. Clearly, the unfortunate overlap between two programs that was seen in Botswana in the initial years of CBR should be avoided. It may easily lead to competition and represents a waste of resources. Another issue is the coordination of rehabilitation activities between various NGOs and such as these, giving special education to particular groups (school for the blind, the deaf, etc.) and that of a government rehabilitation program. Such coordination is often lacking in a developing country where each NGO may be building a 'white elephant' with no guarantee of sustainability once the foreign donor withdraws its support.

A third lesson has to do with the costs involved in launching and running a CBR program. Although undoubtedly cheaper than the more specialized rehabilitation services, a well functioning CBR program needs continuous input in the form of training of field staff, transport, and options for referral to more specialized services. This will easily make it more expensive than WHO's initial calculations (Helander 1984, 1993). It is important to make the calculations realistic, otherwise a government will easily lose interest once the real requirements for economic involvement become obvious.

Finally, it is necessary to emphasize the importance of a knowledge of local conditions, and of people's values and traditions. Without such knowledge there is the risk of constructing CBR programs that are felt to be of little relevance to the people concerned. A CBR program, in order to avoid a top-down approach, should start with identifying the needs of PWD and their family members looked at from their own point of view. Then it should find ways to promote better coping with life in general and overcoming the burdens of impairment in particular. It will often be more fruitful to focus on the household (care unit) than on the subfunctioning of a limb, sense, or mental competence.

Community participation should include more than helping the individuals and households to help themselves. A process whereby people gain greater control over the social, political, economic, and environmental factors affecting their lives should be promoted. According to Morley (1983, p. 323) such participation usually amounts to the government coercing the people into mobilizing their own resources to subsidize government-planned and -operated programs in which the people have little to say. This problem is exactly what has been seen in Botswana as well as several other countries in which the CBR program has been implemented according to the WHO model (Kalyanpur 1995). What is needed is to accumulate cross-national and cross-cultural knowledge so that each new CBR project may learn from the experience of others.

EPILOGUE

More than 10 years have gone by since the data on which this chapter is based were gathered. It is interesting to take a brief look at some of the developments that have taken place in CBR in Botswana since then. During the years following 1984–5, there was a continuous decline in both the government's and the BRC'S CBR programs, and their cooperation did not improve. The government-run program was faced with a rapid turnover in SWOs, and eventually there were a large number of vacancies. The reason was said to be a combination of job dissatisfaction and low salary level. Soon, hardly any of those that had initially been trained to do CBR remained. Facing a near collapse of the program and seeing a need for more expertise, a foreign donor funded several positions for expatriate physical therapists to work alongside the SWOs in some districts. The physical therapists tend to be more in charge than the SWOs. This situation still prevails, and it has clearly elevated the quality of help given to some PWD, albeit keeping much of its outreach character. However, the sustainability of the program after the donor withdraws technical assistance is questionable, since there are very few trained physical therapists in Botswana. Although a few multi-purpose rehabilitation workers have been trained in Zimbabwe, there are not enough to fill all SWO posts and some of them have already gone on to other types of jobs.

The BRC program, following a critical evaluation in 1985, was reorganized to concentrate on two smaller areas, one in the south and one in the north. The one in the south soon ended while the one in the north continued quite successfully for some years, partly because of the assistance of an expatriate physical therapist. When the donor period ended, however, the whole BRC CBR program was terminated.

The gap in service caused by the decline of the two CBR programs was eventually filled by various NGOs and foreign donors. Two rehabilitation centers were built, one in the northern part of the country and one near Gaborone (see Ingstad 1995 for a more detailed discussion of this period). Although practicing CBR to some extent in nearby districts, the policy of these centers is mainly to bring in people for assessment and a limited time of training, following them up in the community when possible. Although the quality of these services is relatively good, there is clearly a limit to how many PWD can be helped in this way. For a while, it appeared as if the center in the south would take over the government responsibility of training FWEs for CBR. Lately, however, this seems to have changed.

Following the first report and recommendations from my 1984–5 project, a consultancy was initiated to draft a national plan for rehabilitation. The resulting document (Omphile et al 1987) included quite detailed recommendations for government responsibility for special educa-

tion and services as well as training of CBR workers at various levels. It also gave recommendations for coordination of government and NGO activities. Following a workshop in which the plan was discussed by all parties involved, the process of revision and acceptance through the various ministries was begun. This turned out to be no easy road, and it took 9 years before the plan was finally accepted (Ministry of Health 1996). The second document is much less detailed and more vague in its formulations than the original draft, but contains several statements about the government's policy toward PWD that may prove valuable as a foundation for rehabilitation work in the future.

This new policy document coincides with a revival of the Botswana Council for the Disabled, a national umbrella organization embracing all NGO and government activities in rehabilitation. Thus, in 1997 the picture of rehabilitation in Botswana and hopefully also for CBR is characterized by a new optimism.

REFERENCES

Armitage J D 1982 League of Red Cross Societies development of Red Cross rehabilitation services: report to the executive committee Botswana Red Cross Society. Botswana Red Cross Society, Gaborone, Botswana

Brunborg H 1987 The population of Botwana. In: Hasse R, Zeil-Fahlsbusch E (eds) Botswana – Entwcklung am Rande der Apartheid. Arbeiten aus dem Institut für Afrika-Kunde, 61. Institut für Afrika-Kunde, Hamburg

Helander E, Hendis P, Nelson G 1983 Training in the community for people with disabilities. WHO, Geneva

Helander E 1984 Rehabilitation for all: a guide to the management of community-based rehabilitation, vol 1: Policymaking and planning. RHB/84.1. Provisional version. WHO, Geneva

Helander E 1993 Prejudice and dignity: an introduction to community-based rehabilitation. UNDP, Interregional programme for Disabled People UN Development Programme, NY

Ingstad B, Bruun F, Sandberg E, Thom S, Care for the elderly: the role of elderly women in the Tswana Society. Journal of Cross-cultural Gerontology 7(4): 379–389

Ingstad B 1995 Public discourses on rehabilitation: from Norway to Botswana. In: Ingstad B, Whyte S Disability and culture. University of California Press, Berkeley, pp. 174–195

Ingstad B 1997 Community-based rehabilitation in Botswana: the myth of the hidden disabled. Studies in African Health

and Medicine, vol. 7. Edwin Mellem Press, Lewiston

Ingstad B, Melsom T 1985 An evaluation of the Botswana Red Cross Society primary health care and community-based rehabilitation programmes. Norwegian Red Cross Society, Gaborone, Botswana

Kalyanpur M 1995 The influences of Western special education on community-based services in India. Disability and Society 11(2): 249–270

Modise T, Ingstad B, Chivuru J 1984 An evaluation of a Red Cross programme for community-based rehabilitation in Zimbabwe. Zimbabwe Red Cross Society, Harare, Zimbabwe

Morley D E 1983 Practising Health for All. Oxford University Press, Oxford

Ministry of Health 1996 National Policy on Care for People with Disabilities, Gabarone, Botswana

Omphile C, Betrancourt B, Mokgadi P, Hoel V, Richter L 1977 Proposals for a national plan for services for disabled people. Ministry of Health/Norwegian Development Cooperation, Gaborone, Botswana

Stats Brief Census 1991: disability in Botswana. Central Statistics Office, No 94/5, Gaborone, Botswana

Thobega M 1980 Which way volunteers? Botswana Red Cross Society, Gaborone, Botswana

WHO 1982 Community based rehabilitation: report from a WHO interregional consultation, Colombo, Sri Lanka, 28 June–3 July. WHO/RHB/IR/82.1, Geneva

18

The sociopolitical context of CBR developments in South Africa

Huib Cornielje
Paulo Ferrinho

INTRODUCTION

In apartheid South Africa, health care delivery and rehabilitation services in particular were primarily geared to the needs of the white minority. The health care system followed a biomedical model not only in the development of its health services but also in the training of its personnel. This medically-oriented paradigm concentrated almost exclusively on university-based training of therapeutic professionals and had a strong Eurocentric focus. As a result, South Africa has not been able to develop a comprehensive national rehabilitation policy, let alone implement such a policy. This does not mean that rehabilitation programs do not exist. Indeed, there is now a strong movement towards the development of regional and national rehabilitation policy. Until recently, however, the country's sociopolitical divisions prevented various participants from joining the ranks. Rehabilitation has yet to be viewed as a serious issue on the political agenda.

Previous difficulties concerning the adoption of a rehabilitation policy in South Africa should be seen in the context of power struggles among the various participants. These are closely related to the political history of apartheid and the swift developments on the political front since the early 1990s. The situation has been affected dramatically as the disability movement moves towards achieving new disability rights and equalization of opportunities. South Africa is finally seriously discussing the development of a rehabilitation policy and the expectation is that the country will be able to design systems and structures for the delivery of effective, appropriate, accessible, affordable and equitable services (Government Gazette 1996).

Health transitions

Every society or social system is inherently predisposed to changes. Social life occurs in the context of two kinds of forces – restraining forces and driving forces – in a quasi-stationary balance. Disturbances in this balance, if followed by changes in the structure of the system, result in social change (Ogburn & Nimkoff 1960, Ferrinho 1971).

When a social system changes it is natural to expect that the health status of a population would reflect this change. After all, the social system is a determinant of health status (Riley 1994). This process is explained by the concept of health transition, which is defined as the change in the health profile of a population associated with socioeconomic development. It involves a shift towards a relatively higher proportion of non-communicable diseases even if the actual mortality rates of these diseases are declining. Concepts associated with the health transition are demographic, epidemiological, and risk transitions.

The demographic transition reflects the influence of evolving patterns of vital statistics (birth and death rates) on population size and distribution (Notenstein 1945). Grounded in the demographic transition is the concept of epidemiological transition (Omran 1971).

Epidemiological transition refers to the changes in patterns of health and disease in relation to social factors. As countries evolve through higher levels of development and social conditions improve there is a transition to increased survival into older ages, with a relatively greater proportion of morbidity, disability, and mortality from non-communicable diseases (Verbrugge 1984).

Risk transition refers to the changing pattern of disease determinants that accompany social development. Such determinants range from traditional environmental exposures (such as bacterial water contamination) to exposure associated with agricultural development, industrialization and urbanization (see Ch. 12).

Health status of South Africa

South Africa is undergoing a demographic transition along the lines of the contemporary delayed model, which is characteristic of many middle-income countries. In these countries, the change in health status has not been accompanied by the expected high rate of decline in mortality and fertility. Significantly, changes in health status are driven by investments in health care and in technology, but high levels of morbidity associated with infectious and parasitic disease persist; the rise of degenerative diseases is apparent; there is an increasingly high proportion of mortality and morbidity associated with lifestyle (such as smoking, alcohol abuse, violence, traffic accidents); and the rising life expectancy of people beyond the age of 50, together with high levels of fertility, becomes a crucial factor in population growth. This demographic transition results in an increased incidence and prevalence of disabling conditions and subsequently influences the ability to provide essential rehabilitation services.

South Africa's sociopolitical history has greatly influenced the development of several community based rehabilitation (CBR) pilot programs. Similarly, it set the scene for specific training for CBR personnel, notably the training program at the Institute of Urban Primary Health Care (IUPHC) in Alexandra, a slum north of Johannesburg.

This chapter examines sociopolitical influences on the development of CBR in South Africa. It uses the experiences of the CBR training program at the IUPHC to illustrate some of the most relevant issues. Finally, it makes some recommendations regarding the future of CBR in South Africa.

ABOUT PROFESSIONAL PRESERVATION

South African rehabilitation services have basically followed Western models of biomedical intervention. The three physical therapeutic professions (physical therapy, occupational therapy and speech and hearing therapy) have played an active role in this process. As professionals, therapists have restricted their rehabilitation skills primarily to institution based therapeutic intervention, focusing more on alleviating functional inabilities than on integrating the person with a disability (PWD) into society. Their scope has largely been dictated by the high-technology medical establishment which accommodated the needs of the white minority. Therapy has developed into sophisticated and predominantly acute care services responding to the medical demand. Almost all (98%) of all state-subsidized physical therapy services are rendered at – and limited to – secondary and tertiary institutions (Smit 1990). Physical therapy is primarily found in privately owned practice, mainly in middle-class urban areas, and it is both high quality and highly specialized. However, it is unlikely to contribute to any significant improvement in the health and welfare of the majority black population and as such is not a meaningful answer to the marked demographic transition.

The relationship between the number of therapists and the population is more favorable in South Africa than in any other African country (Anti-Apartheid Movement n.d.), yet in spite of the claim made by therapists that they fulfill a key role in the rehabilitation of PWDs, the real needs of PWDs are hardly being recognized, let alone met.

The problem is not that there are not enough therapists to cover the population in need of rehabilitation services. As long as so many newly qualified therapists open private practices serving the privileged élite, these certainly very relevant professionals have failed to act as responsible bodies.

Statistics on professional registration with the South African Medical and Dental Council (SAMDC) reveal, since the early 1980s, a dramatic decline in the number of physical therapists working in the public sector. In 1988, 2784 physiotherapists were registered with the SAMDC, with only 27% working in the public sector ('black', 'coloured', Indian and 'white' institutions). This figure had been significantly higher in 1983 (63%). By 1990 it had declined even further, to 20% (Smit 1990). These figures were confirmed by an official of the Department of National Health and Population Development, who stated that the private sector (in which 80% of physical therapists work), serves approximately 20% of the population, i.e. the wealthy, usually 'white', population (Mostert 1994).

To a large extent, universities are responsible for this situation. This is illustrated very well by the words of a lecturer at the University of the Witwatersrand in Johannesburg: 'With one notable exception, all universities are at present training physiotherapy students in high-technology academic hospitals, and their graduates are most competent to practice their profession in these areas both in South Africa and abroad' (Wallner 1992, p. 2). No mention is made of the role of physical therapists in the rehabilitation of the majority of PWDs, that is, those who live in rural and semi-urban areas. No mention is made of the necessity of informing students of physical therapy and allied health disciplines about alternative, possibly more appropriate, strategies of treating disease, disorders, and disabilities within the specifically African context.

Occupational therapists have, to a certain degree, received more training in the area of integration of PWDs into society. However, among physical therapists, only exceptionally bold and committed people have bypassed the bureaucratic and ideological barriers to become involved in the activities of professional action groups such as the recently disbanded Rural Disability Action Group (RURACT) and the Progressive Primary Health Care network (PPHC).

Probably the most obvious shortcoming of physical therapists has been their failure to acknowledge the individual person who happens to have a disability as an inextricable part of his or her family and community. Arkles (1995) observed this painful shortcoming when visiting a leading Johannesburg hospital for injured mine workers. Noting the excellent medical care provided she asked, 'What happens to these men after being discharged?' The reply from a variety of staff members was, 'We don't know'. This answer implies that the institution based therapist is out of touch with the reality of daily life as it is experienced by individuals with disabilities as soon as the hospitalization ends and clients go home to their shacks in the townships or their huts in the mountains or semi-deserts of South Africa. This leads to situations whereby, for example, people with spinal cord injuries reportedly have been discharged with wheelchairs that are impossible to use in the steep mountains of Lesotho or the barren sandy grounds of Kuruman. This, in turn, means that the efforts of the few dedicated hospital based therapists fade away as soon as the person leaves the hospital.

Contact between therapists and patients at home is usually non-existent. Much competent care and rehabilitation is thus wasted when therapists do not pay attention to the broader needs of PWDs, their families, and the community at large.

Another illustration of the inefficiency of the rehabilitation system during the years of apartheid was the predicament of wheelchair-bound people who needed to visit their hospital regularly for follow-up and check-ups. Their hospital was not always the closest one: health care services were segregated on the basis of race and color. In practice, black paraplegic wheelchair drivers often had to travel long distances to hospitals, passing other 'white' or private hospitals. The PWDs often had to pay their own traveling expenses from meagre disability grants.

Even harder to understand were the hospital authorities and therapists who (silently) accepted, and thus maintained, the *status quo*. If they had voiced their outrage about the waste of funds spent on this inefficiency, the quality of

life for many PWDs and their relatives could have been greatly improved.

Conventional training of rehabilitation professionals in South Africa is the responsibility of the medical faculties of seven public universities. While this training equips professionals to deal primarily with an individual's impairments and loss of function, a number of CBR programs in South Africa focus on the social aspects and consequences of disability. CBR is viewed by PWDs (and increasingly by health planners and rehabilitation professionals) as a more appropriate rehabilitation approach, based on its goal of empowering people and encouraging subsequent social action.

Since it recognizes rehabilitation as an integral part of a broader community development approach, CBR is a sharp contrast to the medically oriented approach of conventional rehabilitation programs (Cornielje & Ferrinho 1993). This community development approach is particularly important to a transitional society where, until recently, there was a marked absence of democracy and where poverty, the most handicapping of all social problems, is a growing obstacle to an improved life situation for rising numbers of PWDs.

The national disability movement, Disabled People South Africa (DPSA), which is the country's leading organization of PWDs, has, time and time again, raised its voice against the ambiguous role of rehabilitation professionals, and even more specifically against the role of the conventional charity/welfare movement in the empowerment of PWDs. Conferences on disability issues often end up with conflict among the participants: defensive professionals on one side, outspoken PWDs on the other.

At the same time an increasing number of professionals (mostly therapists) have joined PWDs in their struggle for emancipation. The Rural Disability Action Group (RURACT), an organization affiliated with DPSA, but now superfluous since other democratic structures are in place, was the catalyzing organization facilitating mutual cooperation between professionals and PWDs. Until it disbanded, therapists and PWDs were able to work together, through

RURACT, toward the promotion of CBR for rural areas. While this mutual action in itself has had a great impact, the ability of interested parties to bridge the gap between these two groups and form a coalition in the struggle for appropriate and equitable services has probably been more important. The increased interest of local South African professionals in CBR is certainly a result of the activities of RURACT.

CBR TRAINING: MORE THAN THE ACQUISITION OF CLINICAL SKILLS

The coinciding emergence of the disability rights and CBR movements in South Africa is a significant development in the Southern African region. More than in any other Southern African country, rehabilitation in South Africa has been promoted as a basic human right of all inhabitants; rich or poor, urban or rural, white or black.

Various CBR models have emerged in several parts (both rural and urban) of the region. One of the models, an urban CBR pilot program, was developed at the Institute of Urban Primary Health Care (IUPHC) in Alexandra.

In 1990, the IUPHC decided to develop a training course to introduce and prepare a new type of rehabilitation personnel, the community rehabilitation facilitator (CRF) as part of the emerging CBR program (Fig. 18.1 and 18.2). The institute developed this program in view of the immense human resource deficit, not only in Alexandra but also in other areas in South Africa. Similar programs, though with a less explicit social action component, have emerged in other parts of the country.

At the IUPHC, CBR training is a 1-year education and instruction program in which empowerment and social integration of PWDs form the underlying philosophies of the training. Students are selected by a panel on the basis of educational background and motivation. The training methodology is based on the ideas of Knowles and Freire (Knowles 1980, Freire 1982). Imperative for this training program, based on humanist and radical views, is

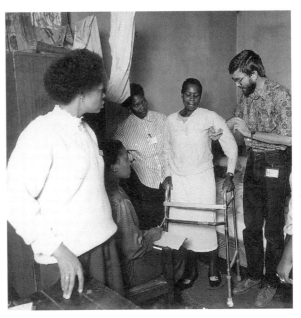

Fig. 18.1 Training community rehabilitation facilitators (CRFs) in Alexandra township, South Africa. Photo courtesy: Mike Goldblatt.

a significant focus on developing human resources (the CRFs in this instance). Such a strong concern with the empowerment of CRFs has been pursued in the conviction that only through their personal empowerment could appropriate CBR programs be initiated and developed (Cornielje & Ferrinho 1995). Besides clinical skills, a very important element of training includes the advancement of knowledge and skills in the area of community development.

The IUPHC training center believes that disability can no longer be seen as a specific anatomical impairment for which there is a rather simple therapeutic solution. Nor can rehabilitation be defined by finding a therapeutic solution outside the community context. As a result of this philosophy, the training places considerable focus on developing students' attitudes towards rehabilitation. This occurs to such an extent that they see rehabilitation as part of social development.

The training methods encourage active participation by the students in the learning process. Various methods are used, such as role play, problem solving exercises, group discussions, and experiential learning. Participatory methods are used optimally to address the transfer of skills in the areas of problem solving and critical thinking (see Ch. 13), both of which are essential for the CRF, who often works independently and therefore needs the flexibility to be able to do new things, to think about local realities and to cope with change in the community.

The first weeks of the course focus on building trust among the participants and enhancing interpersonal skills. Acknowledging the risk of being too abstract and/or theoretical, everyday examples of the difficulties faced by PWDs form the background and framework of the training. This means that both the teaching methods and the course content have to be selected carefully and adapted or re-focused to fit the defined course objectives. For example, the daily struggle by people with a visual disability was made evident when students were blindfolded and asked to construct an animal using Lego blocks while receiving only verbal instructions from their partner. Not only is blindness experienced, but teamwork and problem solving skills are also fostered, not to mention the trust which such an activity forges.

The training topics focus on specific knowledge about community development and relate to the field of sociology. They include such issues as accountability and community analysis, as well as the concepts of power, community involvement and participation, and primary health care. Also covered are the politics of health care, the economics of health care, and the impact of the social, ecological and cultural environment on PWDs.

All of these issues are discussed in global and local contexts. The course developers were of the opinion that a good understanding of local developmental issues would emerge if the students could appreciate the more global developmental issues. This in effect would help them critically to view, for example, their own limited role in national, regional and local power politics, while learning to appreciate the need for collective self-reliance and development.

An element of the training strongly related to

community development is insight into one's own attitudes and those of others. Negative attitudes towards PWDs is one aspect of this. Just as important, cross-cultural communication and management styles form the direct basis of the challenge faced by the course leaders and students. A great deal has been learned about the prejudices even educators have, which are often rooted in Western value systems.

The different disability-aggravating circumstances – such as the prevalence of specific disabilities – that justify different developments of CBR programs receive adequate attention during training. However, in order to accommodate students from a variety of different programs, a curriculum with a certain number of core modules considering the major disabilities plus a number of optional modules has been developed. In addition, the impact of an intervention strategy is considered in both the planning of services and curriculum development. For example, it is debatable whether an intensive module on post-polio paralysis should be included in a CBR training program because this condition often requires more institutional forms of rehabilitation following surgery. However, CRFs need to know when it is appro-

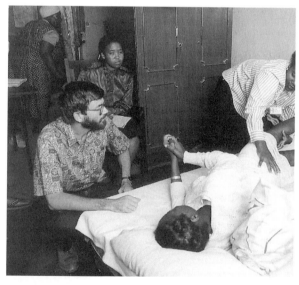

Fig. 18.2 Training CRFs, Alexandra township, South Africa. Photo courtesy: Mike Goldblatt.

priate to refer PWDs to secondary and tertiary facilities.

The course also addresses culturally determined factors (such as the extended family, the role of religion, and attitudes toward time and respect) in community development and health care that influence the management environment in day-to-day relations. In this process of mutual learning, insights are acquired into the dynamics of culture, thus generating a basis for appropriate rehabilitation interventions.

By appealing for solidarity among students, particularly in conflict situations, an attempt is made to reinforce positive attitudes towards communal organization, a typically African cultural strength in the process of community development. Appreciating one's own cultural values is one of the acknowledged cornerstones in empowerment and of much importance in the process of community development. The value of having cross-cultural communication skills and a knowledge of African cultures is too often neglected, while these should form the foundation of any community development program.

One influence on the enhancement of cultural awareness is the sociopolitical context. Considering this issue in a training program like the IUPHC rehabilitation course is of the utmost importance. During apartheid, several students were active in liberation movements. This has influenced some of the ethical issues that have been addressed. For example, some participants have felt that they could never provide services for their political opponents, a topic that has needed careful facilitation. The educators' own Western value system, with a solid belief in medical neutrality, could easily have become an obstacle if the sociopolitical context (family members of the learners were killed) in which these attitudes had developed, had not been acknowledged right from the start.

CBR: PALLIATION OR LIBERATION?

Students from different locations attend the IUPHC training program and, both during and

after training, develop CBR programs in their own communities. Recent evidence shows that CBR programs facilitated by these students can thrive under very different institutional and local circumstances, taking into consideration the specific needs of PWDs in their particular communities (Cornielje et al 1994).

The different CBR programs have succeeded in:

- developing services for and with PWDs in areas where formerly none (or few) existed
- increasing awareness among the community at large and specifically among health personnel about the needs of PWDs
- acknowledging that social rehabilitation is a critical area to be addressed by the CBR movement (Fig. 18.2).

In addition, most programs deploying CRFs have allowed them to take on an empowering role. There is persuasive evidence that support structures determine, to a large degree, the ability of CRFs to fulfill the role for which they prepared at the IUPHC (Fig. 18.3).

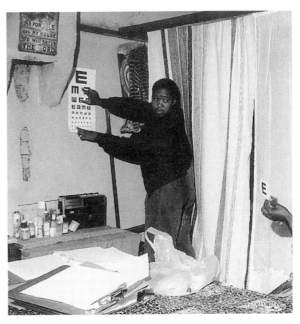

Fig. 18.3 House visit for eye testing. Photo courtesy: Mike Goldblatt.

The main difficulties and problems encountered and reported during the early phase of program development relate to:

- the lack of consensus among policy makers and professional therapists regarding what is to be the accepted CBR paradigm
- the subsequent role of the CRF
- the individual performance of CRFs.

The role as change agent that some CRFs fulfill has resulted in significant progress towards empowering of PWDs. There is a general awareness and acknowledgement among health care managers that the CRFs most important role should be in the area of social rehabilitation, since the needs and demands of PWDs are greatest in this area. However, not all CRFs are allowed by their supervisor to take on such a role. This is partly due to the failure on the part of the training institute to sensitize health care managers to the unconventional roles of CRFs. Consequently, in such programs, a depreciation of the program's impact was noticed. The lack of a common vision at the supervisory and management levels as to what CBR should be appears to correlate with a declining and poor individual performance of the CRF.

On the basis of a recent study (Cornielje et al 1994), it seems appropriate to conclude that in most instances there is a common perception by managers, CRFs and clients about what is feasible within the constraints of existing resources. Individual, home based rehabilitation is very satisfying for clients and CRFs, but has the disadvantage of evolving into individual palliative interventions. There is also the risk of increasing cost. Most rehabilitation efforts should be channeled through disability rights movements, self-help groups, support groups, income generating projects and other projects in the social area of rehabilitation. These projects appear to support appropriate and sustainable interventions for large groups of PWDs, resulting in greater emancipation. A significant proportion of the CRF's time should be spent in supporting the development of these community structures.

TOWARDS A NATIONAL POLICY

You cannot develop by act of parliament. (de Gaay Fortman 1984)

The risk of copying Western systems of rehabilitation persists, particularly in South Africa where excellent forms of rehabilitation have been available for prolonged periods, albeit only to a minority of the country's population. Analysis of the history and experiences of both the IUPHC training program and the actual CBR programs set up by CRFs provides a basis for the further 'maturation' of policy proposals.

Many resources, provided mainly by local and international non-governmental organizations, have been applied in the development of local rehabilitation programs. As a result, several interesting models of rehabilitation have emerged in South Africa in spite of its years of isolation from the rest of the world. The experiences of these, often small-scale, local projects, initiated by individuals with and without disabilities, are worthy of further evaluation and could be used for developing a long overdue rehabilitation policy.

The regional authorities should use these guidelines as a framework to develop systems and structures for the development and delivery of rehabilitation. The interests of PWDs seem best served if the ultimate responsibility for rehabilitation policy and planning is with national government. National policy should therefore, at least, propose firm and binding guidelines that guarantee an appropriate, accessible, affordable, and equitable rehabilitation program. However, regions should be allowed to develop, on the basis of already existing experiences, their own contextualized rehabilitation programs taking into account differing geography, infrastructure, and/or culture. This requires, at least during the implementation process, flexibility and a focus on participatory decision making. Community support should form the basis for policy, planning, and subsequent implementation of rehabilitation programs.

The scaling-up of the small-scale, bottom-up programs requires vision and tact: there is a great risk of losing the essence of these specific programs, that is community participation. Access to rehabilitation for all will result in a rise in the costs of rehabilitation. Therefore, the acceptance of whatever rehabilitation system, whether institutional based or community based, should be viewed in terms of macro-economic efficiency. This in turn will mean that with limited funding available, the South African government would have only one option: to allow, on the basis of minimum but socially acceptable levels, the development of essential regional and local rehabilitation programs.

Those who choose to receive sophisticated high-technology rehabilitation, provided for in private practices and private hospitals, could insure themselves or pay individually. This development could mean that the accusation 'CBR is for the poor' finally would become a reality!

During 1995, DPSA and RURACT were asked to send one delegate each to the Restructuring Development Programme (RDP) of the Government of National Unity. Disability issues seem to have at last been placed on the political agenda. A major breakthrough is the role given to PWDs and concerned professionals: at the highest level of decision making, they will contribute towards rehabilitation for all in South Africa. It is hoped that the conventional participants such as universities will not be ignored completely, but that they will have a role in which they will learn to use their knowledge and skills not only to help those who are wealthy but also for the sake of the thousands of less well-off and poor PWDs in South Africa.

Major efforts towards the advancement of CBR should be placed in the development and support of community based structures. The IUPHC experience shows that the concerns for social change and health transition are best addressed by a community development methodology that guarantees collective problem solving of rehabilitation issues and joint implementation of rehabilitation plans. This can be done by supporting institutions including rehabilitation services and voluntary associations in the community – within a common ecological framework.

This methodology supplies the framework to develop CBR as a social movement. The current social and political changes, following the euphoria of the political transition in 1994, present an opportunity to establish a realistic national policy and provide essential rehabilitation for the majority of PWDs. The various CBR models signify a need for strengthening the community components. This can only be achieved by organizing communities around their felt needs, and by fostering and consolidating democracy as an essential characteristic for the long-term success of CBR.

REFERENCES

Anti-Apartheid Movement (n.d.) Memorandum to the World Confederation of Physical Therapists. Physiotherapy in South Africa: the case for the expulsion of the South African Society of Physiotherapy. Anti-Apartheid Movement, London

Arkles S 1985 Industrial accidents: the social consequences. Dissertation Series No. 7, Development Studies Group/ Critical Health, Johannesburg SA February

Cornielje H, Ferrinho P 1993 Development of a community based rehabilitation programme for a poor urban area in South Africa, part II: programme development. Community Health Association of Southern Africa Journal of Comprehensive Health April 4(2) 56–57

Cornielje H, Ferrinho P 1995 Community development skills: essential component in the training of community rehabilitation facilitators at the Institute of Urban Primary Health Care in South Africa. Community Health Association of Southern Africa Journal of Comprehensive Health 6 (1): 28–32

Cornielje H, Fernandes A, Ferrinho P 1994 An evaluation of the community based rehabilitation training programme of the school for primary health care in Alexandra (South Africa). Internal report, Institute of Urban Primary Health Care, Alexandra, Johannesburg, South Africa

Ferrinho H 1971 The impact of technology on social change in a rural settlement in Mozambique. Arts in Sociology degree dissertation, Department of Sociology, University of Pretoria, South Africa

Freire P 1982 The politics of education: culture, power and liberation. Berger and Garvey, New York

Gaay Fortman de B 1984 You cannot develop by act of parliament: rethinking development from the legal viewpoint. Public lecture, Institute of Social Studies, The Hague, The Netherlands

Government Gazette 1996 Gazette no. 17038, notice 299. March 1996. Pretoria, South Africa

Knowles M S 1980 The modern practice of education, 2nd edn. Follett, Chicago

Mostert K 1994 Report of the World Health Organization rehabilitation management workshop, Mmabane, Swaziland, May 30–June 10 National Department of Health and Population Development, Pretoria, SA

Notenstein F W 1945 Population – the long view. In: Schultz T W (ed) Food for the world. University of Chicago Press, Chicago, pp. 36–57

Ogburn W F, Nimkoff M F 1960 A handbook of sociology. Routledge and Kegan Paul, London

Omran A R 1971 The epidemiological transition: a theory of the epidemiology of populations change. Milbank Memorial Fund Quarterly 49: 509–538

Riley M W 1994 Changing lives and changing social structures; common concerns of social science and public health. American Journal of Public Health 84: 1214–1217

Smit E 1990 Physiotherapy services in Transvaal hospitals. Reach Out Symposium Physiotherapy, Pretoria, University of Pretoria, SA October 4–5

Verbrugge L 1984 Longer life but worsening health? Trends in health and mortality of middle aged and older persons. Milbank Memorial Fund Quarterly 62: 475–519

Wallner P 1992 Physiotherapy in transition – a personal view. Physio Forum No. 1 (Jan): 2–3

19

Intensive treatment and problem solving to enhance rehabilitation potential in Mexico

Christine Nelson
Martha E. Rubi

HEALTH CARE DELIVERY IN THE CONTEXT OF MEXICO

Health care delivery of any kind and the history of rehabilitation must be considered within its surrounding environment. This chapter describes a model rehabilitation center that is unique in Mexico, the Centro de Aprendizaje (Learning Center). This center provides secondary and tertiary high quality care to persons with a disability (PWD) while adapting its programs to fit with the culture of its clients. The center also sponsors continuing education courses for rehabilitation professionals.

Mexico is a country that historically has been so strongly influenced economically and politically by its northern neighbor, the USA, that its name is even the United States of Mexico. The present population is 92 million, with 40 million people at or under the poverty line. Mexico City is the largest city in the world; it surpassed Tokyo several years ago and together with its suburban areas accounts for 22 million people. The minimum wage is approximately $5 (US) per day although few employers in the cities pay only the minimum wage. Mexico has never had a true middle class, even though factories and assembly plants improve the income of those who can adapt to the working conditions. Mexicans have a history of seasonal agricultural orientation, and it has been very difficult for them to adapt to the 'sameness' of factory work. Most factory work requires geographic relocation and often includes substandard housing. Television offers a view of a lifestyle that is inaccessible to most Mexicans.

Approximately 20% of Mexicans live with upper-class standards and tastes. These are the people who have heavy investments in the USA, who travel and buy the goods that are imported principally from the north.

The city of Cuernavaca, the site of the Centro de Aprendizaje, has a population of about 1 million people. Located in the state of Morelos, which adjoins the state of Mexico and Mexico City, it has long served as a recreation area. People still come for weekend visits to escape the air pollution problems of Mexico City.

Public rehabilitation services

Mexicans generally receive health services through specialized hospital systems for workers of various types. These systems have a strong political influence, and their quality varies according to the local forces that determine community government. New leaders are appointed with each new election.

Although many government hospitals and treatment centers employ rehabilitation therapists, therapy services are poorly represented within these systems and are sometimes offered by untrained persons. Typically, large numbers of clients must be helped in a very limited time. Conventional therapies (such as range of motion) and group treatments are often applied. Mothers learn how to help their babies and young children in classes of 10 to 20, depending on how many people come to the centers on that day, with a single therapist who demonstrates the activities with a different child each session. Clients and accompanying family members often spend long hours waiting for their brief period of direct service. Non-profit organizations, such as Asociación Pro Personas con Paralisis Cerebral (similar to United Cerebral Palsy in the USA), also operate programs organized with this group orientation.

Training and education in rehabilitation

Throughout Mexico, therapy has yet to achieve the status it enjoys in the neighboring USA; in many situations the public image of therapists is close to that of a maid. The public also tends to confuse a therapist with a teacher or someone who gives a very general type of massage. Due to poor salaries, it is common to find that therapists, like medical doctors, work in a public facility during the morning and have a private practice in the afternoon. Socioeconomic structures do not encourage the achievement of expertise, nor does society reward professionals who advance or develop special skills.

Physical therapy (PT) and occupational therapy (OT) training programs are traditionally at a technical level with a 3-year program sponsored by the federal government or other large institutions. Schools of therapy are concentrated primarily in Mexico City, and more practicing therapists are in the metropolitan area. A university level program in OT with support from professionals from the USA and the Ibera Americana University in Mexico City is being developed. This program will give a master's degree upon completion and supplement the current 3-year training programs for OTs. There may be some difficulty in recruiting potential therapists who have a basic academic degree in a related area of study, given the continuing option of the shorter, more accessible course. The existing programs in physical therapy are located elsewhere in Mexico City and are still seeking university sponsorship, which may lead to expensive duplication of faculty and facilities. (At one time, therapists had the option of training in both OT and PT, but this is no longer possible.) Speech and language therapists are trained in a program at the University of the Americas, just south of Mexico City.

In an effort to provide more services to a wider population there has been a move in Mexico to train 'therapy technicians' at the high school or secondary school level. Government agencies seek to put in place people who can be of some functional help to families with a disabled member. These training courses run about 6 months and are sponsored by the federal government. However, these superficial courses appear to have resulted in even greater public confusion regarding the services that might be expected from someone with the title of 'therapist.' The graduates of such courses often work with no professional supervision. This is quite easy in Mexico because clients are often treated in the privacy of their own home. There are also many physiatrists and other physicians who prefer to employ their own assistants without formal training. Parents who are unaware of the quality differences in care for their child may be quite comfortable with someone who agrees to come to the house two or three times a week, and this convenience also serves the needs of families who have an adult member who is difficult to move. No laws prevent this type of misrepresentation in Mexico.

It is very difficult to motivate therapists to pursue further learning, although some do complete their curricula with a keen awareness of the incompleteness of their academic preparation and the desire to continue to learn. They save from meager wages and make many sacrifices to attend seminars and courses which unfortunately vary widely in quality.

Therapy associations exist but meet in Mexico City and have little influence on the ongoing educational process. There is no formal licensure of either OTs or PTs and little professional encouragement for continuing education. Recently, the Physical Therapy Association has been revived with a goal of increasing its influence on service quality. The Occupational Therapy Association periodically attempts to organize, but attendance waxes and wanes. Neither the government nor private agencies support the concept of ongoing educational opportunities for therapists in any serious way.

Social orientation for service delivery

Mexican public awareness of PWD has gradually emerged during the last 5 years, as indicated by the occasional talk show that focuses on people who travel in wheelchairs, as well as the more frequent signs that reserve parking for people who are handicapped. Some large stores have provided wheelchairs at the entrance. These are used by people who walk with difficulty, but their presence also provides an important educational message for the public. Since 1986, federal law has mandated that all newly constructed buildings provide access to everyone, regardless of disability. However, respect for the law is inconsistent: architects argue that ramps interfere with the aesthetics of their design, and building owners find ways to avoid the extra expense of accessible construction. Mexico is proud of its history and older established buildings that are renovated to house public facilities, museums, stores, restaurants and schools often remain inaccessible to persons in wheelchairs.

The large crowds in Mexico City further complicate access to public transportation. Rural pueblos (small towns) necessitate walking and the occasional crowded bus with high steps and a driver in a hurry to be on his way. Bus and metro transportation is subsidized by the federal government, and very few *campesinos* who work the fields have access to cars. The compensating factor is that Mexicans are notorious for their willingness to assist anyone with a special problem, and it is not unusual to see two young men hoist a wheelchair with its occupant up five or six steps.

THE CENTRO DE APRENDIZAJE DE CUERNAVACA: A NEW FOCUS IN SERVICE

The Centro de Aprendizaje (Learning Center) of Cuernavaca is a private treatment and education center begun by Mexican psychologist Raquel M. de Benabib, M.S., as a private office in 1974 in response to expressed needs of the community. Benabib had worked previously as a volunteer in the public rehabilitation center in Cuernavaca, after organizing programs in Mexico City for persons with severe visual impairments and teaching at the university.

The original orientation of the center was specific intervention for children with learning problems, with a program of speech, special education, and occupational therapy that supplemented Benabib's background in psychology. By 1976 public demand for services influenced the inclusion of children with birth injuries, speech delays, and other problems that interfere with optimal development. The primary author came to the center in 1977; the center continued its growth and moved to the present facility in 1980. The second author joined the staff in 1990, working with a physical therapist and speech therapist. A major renovation in 1992 modernized the building to provide more efficient teaching facilities for seminars and short courses, as well as to improve architectural access for clients and their families. The staff now consists of an administrative coordinator who doubles as a vision therapist, a clinical coordinator who leads evaluations of all clients, a physical therapist, an occupational therapist, a speech and language therapist, and a secretary.

The center supports advocacy programs and the programs of the newly formed 'human rights' committees that encourage PWD to become integrated into society. With a program that addresses ongoing education for therapists and other professionals while putting equal emphasis on direct and comprehensive treatment of PWD, the center's reputation has grown gradually by word of mouth.

With no outside funding or third-party payments to maintain the center, client and seminar fees must cover its expenses. Nevertheless, the professional staff members, who are better paid than the average Mexican therapist, agree to treat those who cannot pay for up to 15% of their caseload. This independence from outside funding brings with it a freedom to maintain a quality orientation rather than follow the commonly accepted and routine practices.

Patient evaluation and treatment: a problem-solving approach

While the Centro de Aprendizaje is primarily oriented to children, clients have ranged in age from 2 months to 80 years. The awareness that families are coming from rural areas and must accomplish many objectives in a brief period of time created the need for short-term, intensive treatment. The time period is most often 2 or 3 weeks, with one to three individual sessions each day of a 5-day week. Families are housed in small, single-level bungalows one short block from the center. Children who receive this short-term intensive treatment opportunity several times a year seem to have made progress over time comparable to children with similar diagnoses who have received approximately one to two sessions per week throughout the year. This observation is based on children seen in the center and supported by the experience of therapists coming to Cuernavaca.

In Mexico, as in other Latin American countries, therapy is not available in many rural areas. To offer assessments without time to recommend a program and change the effect of the presenting problem on the client leads only to frustration for everyone. It has been found that a 2–3 week stay permits some daily treatment; on this basis, intervention recommendations are made to the family. The center is oriented to an interdisciplinary model and intervention efforts are closely coordinated to work toward the agreed upon goals. The center stresses the problem-solving approach of neurodevelopmental (Bobath) treatment (NDT), with the addition of manual therapies, such as soft tissue mobilization, myotherapy, and other preparatory treatments. The client is helped to change physically and behaviorally while planning is done for the family needs when they return home.

In addition to local clients with neurologically based diagnoses who come for evaluations or treatment, families come from outside the city and from other countries for consultation and direct intervention to make the maximum change possible in the time available with the client. Orthotic support, visual function, communication skills, and family needs are taken into account by the staff.

The staff help clients find a local therapist or appropriate local program when possible and provides the family with videotapes and written reports to bring home. Some people return to a local therapist who has trained at the center. Others have no local therapist or for some reason have not been able to obtain pertinent services due to local politics, inadequately prepared professionals, or other reasons.

Each visit presents the staff with the rehabilitation challenge of finding helpful positions and activities for home, after working intensively with direct handling to bring the child forward to a new level of function. Many children have lacked specific analysis of their postural problem, have never had visual dysfunctions considered, or need orthotics to facilitate controlled movement. Parents have an opportunity to focus on the special needs of their child and often come to understand more completely the child's personality during this time in a new setting. Parents or principal caregivers learn infant massage, special feeding techniques, and assisted dressing or other modifications of daily care that are appropriate for their family member at the time.

Another group of clients comes for a period of direct hands-on treatment in order to determine whether a suggested surgery or other treatment is advisable or to assist the child to an optimal level of physical function for a planned medical intervention. In addition to the staff working at the center, an orthotist and an orthopedic surgeon have local offices and are available for consultations. A pediatrician is also available for consultation, primarily for children who might have some illness during their time in Cuernavaca. Neurological consultation is available in Mexico City in the event that a child needs more definitive diagnosis or tertiary-level testing and care.

Limits on the treatment sequence of a particular child or client have an interesting psychological effect on the therapy staff; everyone is more focused on specific objectives. It is essential to listen carefully to the goals and motivations of the family and to evaluate the child's potential to reach the functional goals with appropriate intervention. Families are encouraged to bring photos of home seating and typical activities so staff can understand better the challenges faced in home care. Changes in positioning extend to OT, PT, and speech therapy sessions, as well as vision therapy.

While formal psychological testing is not done at the center, the staff are alert to the possibility that a child understands more than he can communicate as the therapy sessions begin. All professional staff meet for half an hour each morning to discuss the current treatments and responses or to determine whether an electronic communicator or other augmentative communication should be introduced. Electronic communicators have offered a new and valuable resource for families who speak languages other than English. Families are encouraged to observe all treatment sessions and to participate fully in the program of the child. In most cases, the family will need to carry out many or most of the home handling recommendations.

Functional vision problems are a primary interference in school performance, so the Centro de Aprendizaje sponsors five consultations each year that are shared by three experienced behavioral optometrists. The child is observed carefully during the evaluation for correspondence between visual responses and conversation or hand activity or moving through space. The doctor checks basic visual skills of fixation, pursuits, saccades (the rapid, involuntary eye movements that are used to examine written material) and binocular focusing skills. Home vision therapy is planned in many cases, and lenses are prescribed by the optometrist as needed. Children with strabismus or other conditions that need close follow-up are scheduled to return for therapy with the optometrist. Visual dysfunction often explains why a child on a walker is unable to keep the eyes forward and manage changes in space or why an infant walks well along a support but is unable to completely let go of that contact. Competent function of the visual system relaxes the physical body and becomes an integral part of physical treatment for movement control, particularly for children with neuromotor dysfunction.

Setting priorities during evaluation

Two or three staff members attend the initial evaluation of the client, whether a family is arriving for the first time or for a return visit. For example, they observe the client's postural and movement control in different positions and challenge, with physical assistance given as necessary, balance and righting reactions. Dissociation of the arms and hands for functional independence is evaluated in keeping with the age of the individual. The ability to shift the weight forward over the feet to move from sitting to standing is fundamental for client independence, even when the person may be limited to walking with the assistance of an adult. Infants and small children are observed closely for their responses during feeding, dressing and daily care.

Observations of this type are the basis for consequent decisions about the most efficient way to help the person improve his control of posture and movement. The therapist explains to the family and the client why the missing components of control are important and how they might be achieved.

The age of the child and the wishes of the family determine the priorities set. In Latin American upper classes, a full-time person is often available to care for the child at home. For such families, the therapist needs to establish a working relationship with the caregiver, in addition to confirming the parent's authority to assure that the program will become a part of the child's life. This dual caregiver assignment can be very complex, and even more so when the child has special needs. Sometimes, conflict arises between the mother and the nanny regarding care so the therapist must be alert to signs of these differences of opinion and find a way to work positively with both maternal figures in the child's life.

Practical self-care skills are checked by interview and then confirmed when necessary by direct observation. Dressing skills for children with neuromotor dysfunction can become an important activity for sensory and postural organization even when the culture does not

dictate the need for early independence. If at all feasible, the child sits in a straddle position on a bench, with the assisting adult seated behind. Clothing is laid out systematically in front of the child so that choices and sequences can be followed by the child regardless of his level of independence. For some children, the reaching, pushing, or other selected activities receive more emphasis to correspond with individual treatment objectives.

Independence in self-feeding for the young child is not a strong objective for many families in Latin America, because children without impediments are often helped with spoon feeding until they are 5 or 6 years old. However, preparing the movement patterns and postural control necessary for self-feeding as part of the direct treatment gives the young child a feeling of accomplishment and competence within the family environment. An early start also improves the child's physical control. For example, the shoulder activation that permits lifting of the spoon is a useful preparation for writing or other hand activities and fosters dissociation of the shoulders. Because use of the baby bottle is often prolonged for Mexican children, it may represent a challenge to the therapist to introduce cup drinking to a family with deeply ingrained cultural attitudes about this. However, some infants with neuromotor dysfunction are more successful at cup drinking than they have been with the bottle, so this reassures parents.

Feeding programs must take into account cultural, religious, and medical beliefs of the family and the child. The process of taking in food is perhaps the most intensive cultural behavior that is encountered. A high percentage of children with neuromotor dysfunction have food allergies that directly affect brain function, or the family may have diet restrictions that they wish to respect for the child with a developmental problem. In Mexico, babies often get sweets very early, and parents have difficulty in understanding the need to restrict sugar. Respect for these individual preferences assists the bonding process between the family and the professional staff.

In Mexico, and in Latin American countries generally, the extended family still exists and is an important resource for families with a member who has a disability. A wheelchair or other permanent assistive device that represents a major investment often is paid by voluntary contributions from the extended family. In some cases one part of the family has a better socio-economic status than another and will volunteer to provide resources for treatment services. This is particularly important because an insignificant number of persons have any health insurance, which is extremely expensive in Mexico.

To walk independently is a primary goal of most families for a member with a physical disability. In Third World countries this becomes a practical issue because of the difficulties in moving around in a wheelchair or the lack of a wheelchair of any type. Family members often help a child or adult to practice walking daily even when therapy in a rehabilitative setting is not available. The ever-present concern for 'what will happen when we're not here' is very real when residential facilities and group homes are essentially non-existent. Most newer styles of equipment for independent mobility are imported to Mexico (and to Central America) from the USA but lightweight designs and balance that permits easier use of wheelchairs and walkers tend to be missing in locally produced items. The cost of the imported equipment is a limiting factor for many families, so chairs and other equipment are often the worse for wear, even with reasonable care, and are seldom fitted to the owner.

The extended family also represents a source of information and recommendations for intervention. As such it may become a stronger influence than the staff of the rehabilitation setting. It can be very difficult for a young couple with an infant or small child in therapy to feel secure in the choices of how to proceed with rehabilitative intervention. As a secondary problem, this cultural characteristic makes the family vulnerable to highly advertised programs of intervention that tend to be repetitive, costly and essentially the same for every child. Such programs often originate in the USA. They can serve to deplete financial resources so that families have difficulty paying for local care after they have become disillusioned with the imported program's failure to deliver on advertised promises.

Systematic preparation for function

An effective rehabilitative program begins with the need to move around the environment and control the body. Each individual will have particular goals that are important. As an example of the problem-solving approach, the development of hand coordination must consider the accompanying postural adaptations that position the body.

Hand use represents an area that does not always receive the attention it merits when the individual has a moderate to severe neuromotor limitation. There may be an assumption that change will not be possible or the family may feel that standing and walking are of paramount importance. In fact, the individual confined to a wheelchair, and possibly unable to get into the community because of architectural barriers, has even greater need for hand use merely to achieve some independence within the home. If at all possible handwriting should be pursued to the level of signing one's name and perhaps noting a telephone number. This is not to minimize the possibilities that computers and electronic devices can offer, but the keyboard is not consistently available and few Latin Americans have routine access to these marvels. The ability to dial a telephone or push the sequence of numbers on a number pad can offer some level of independence.

Hand-use objectives during treatment are primarily functional. There are a very limited number of sheltered work situations available to the Mexican person with multiple disabilities. However, some individuals may work as computer programmers, secretaries, or at other jobs that do not necessarily require extensive movement from one position to another. Personal independence, hand use, and communication are fundamental to holding down such jobs.

Professional development

To improve the clinical preparation of therapists, the Centro de Aprendizaje began to bring skilled American professionals to Mexico, providing translation so that motivated Mexican therapists could improve their level of function and their self-image. Over the past 20 years therapists from Guatemala, El Salvador, Columbia, and later Argentina, Chile, Bolivia, Puerto Rico, and Venezuela have joined the classes that give them access to more current information in their own language.

The seminar program and the certificate course in NDT (Bobath) at the center have been the most clinically-oriented educational opportunities for therapists working with children and adults who have neuromotor complications. A certificate is issued from the US based Neuro-developmental Treatment Association, Inc., on the basis of the standard curriculum for this 2 month course taught by an established 'coordinator-instructor.' This pediatric course was first offered in Mexico in 1978. A 3-week NDT certificate course, 'Treatment of Adult Hemiplegia and Head Trauma', has been offered since 1984. This course is also given in Cordoba, Argentina, with translation by the administrative coordinator of Centro de Aprendizaje.

MODELING TO IMPROVE QUALITY OF REHABILITATION

What is the purpose of such attention to detail in a country that has so many overwhelming needs for the larger population? The establishment of a model center in the midst of the Mexican environment has not been easy, but it has served to show what can be done. Some therapists and medical professionals trained in Latin America have changed their concept of their role in the rehabilitation effort. Mechanized programs of intervention in government-sponsored centers have been modified slightly and increasing numbers of therapists have opened private offices. The public is learning that its support of education for rehabilitation personnel affects the quality of service they will receive. Mexican professionals have better skills and are beginning to have confidence in their own abilities. They no longer feel that they always have to wait passively for another country to bring them information.

The education of therapists and special educators and the availability of informative seminars for consumers of health care help those who are interested obtain the desired information. Providers of care become better known to the general public. In this information age, some of the citizens of Third World countries are also turning to the Internet to obtain information on syndromes and other health-related topics. This inevitably creates greater gaps between social classes, but it does make current information available to those with computer access.

There continue to be marked differences in rehabilitation service availability between cities and rural areas. Therapy service in smaller towns generally depends on the training of a person whose family lives in the area or the marriage of a therapist to a local person. Due to the importance of the family constellation, therapists often work near where their parents live. Families who cannot travel to services must depend on local centers that are staffed by the government or by volunteer agencies. Hospital services are available to government workers and workers who have health benefits paid by their employers. Rehabilitation centers are funded with donations but seldom have trained staff that stay over time due to extremely low salaries.

Quality services need to be built from the ground up. Public education must create the need for better qualified professionals delivering consistently effective rehabilitation services. Families need help in assisting their members with disabilities to a better quality of life. With time, public education, and the sharing of professional information and experience, all levels of service can begin to improve simultaneously. This will provide a stronger base for all programs of rehabilitation so that the concept of improving independent function in spite of some neuromotor dysfunction becomes ingrained in the culture.

20

A cross-cultural immersion in post-Communist Romania

Gale Haradon

INTRODUCTION

December 1989 marked the end of the era of Nicolae Ceausescu, the Communist dictator who dominated life in Romania during the Iron Curtain years. Following a revolt, in December 1989, Nicolae and his wife, Elena, were executed. With these events, Romania was plunged into a wider exposure in the world news than had been the case for decades. Most Westerners, like myself, had even less knowledge about Romania than about other countries in the closed Communist Eastern Bloc, owing to the lack of news coverage. More media attention followed when reports such as the *New York Times Magazine* (Romania's Lost Children, a photo essay by James Nachtwey, pp. 28–33) (June 24, 1990) and *20/20*'s television program (October 5 1990 ABC Television network) flashed disturbing images of institutionalized children. These sensational stories on international television and in the press depicted overcrowded orphanages filled with thousands of abandoned babies and children.

The events that occurred in a relatively unknown country thousands of miles from my home in the USA entered my life in the summer of 1990 through a short local newspaper article. A story in the *Denver Post* (June 22, p. 1E, 1990) featured a photograph of a forlorn 2-year-old child and was accompanied by a plea for developmental specialists to go to Romania to work with the orphans. The sponsoring organization, World Vision, was joining the international response of non-governmental organizations

(NGOs) to provide humanitarian relief to the abandoned and institutionalized children in Romania. World Vision is a Christian relief and development organization with programs of emergency relief, international health and water development in 94 countries. This chapter will share the unusual journey and events that occurred when the author, a seasoned occupational therapy clinician and educator, decided to respond to this plea for help. The journey goes into a country that had just reawakened to the outside world. Changes were occurring so rapidly that in 1990 computers were not even allowed into the country, yet only 2 years later, private computer stores operated in competition with each other. Personal emotions and enhanced cultural awareness will be shared throughout this chapter as the rehabilitation life of post-Communist Romania is explored through one set of clinical eyes.

The beginning of the journey

The abandonment of thousands of Romanian babies and children to orphanages did not happen suddenly, but was the gradual result of policies of the deposed dictator. To increase the government workforce in Romania, Ceausescu planned to increase the population by prohibiting family planning and birth control. Romanian State Decree No. 770, issued in 1966, declared abortion illegal for any woman under 45 years of age who had not yet had four children (Bridges for Children in Romania 1995). The burden of the policies fell most heavily on women with limited resources. The economic policies also imposed by Ceausescu caused many parents to abandon thousands of children to the care of orphanages (News from Helsinki Watch 1990, published by Human Rights Watch, NY).

Scant travel advisory information on country conditions was available at the time of my departure for Romania on October 6 1990, since I was the first clinical person employed by World Vision for this mission. The *20/20* film depicting the appalling conditions of children, aired in the USA on the eve of my departure,

gave a very alarming glimpse of the country that I was about to enter. As I boarded the plane and left my family for 3 months, I felt that I was traveling to an unknown fate. Upon arrival in Romania, the sight of uniformed soldiers carrying weapons on the airport runway confirmed that I had arrived in an unfamiliar part of the world. The ability to be extremely flexible was necessary throughout my stay. The first week in the country was spent getting oriented to the city of Bucharest, getting to know the World Vision staff and the orphanages, and in beginning to learn the language. To facilitate language acquisition, I was provided with individual tutoring by a Romanian couple. My graduation test was to communicate some basic phrases to my tutors' 6-year-old-son who already knew five languages.

THE COUNTRY, CULTURE, AND LANGUAGE

Romania is a country approximately the size of the state of Colorado or Oregon (USA), with a population of 23 million. It is beautiful, with easy access to the Carpathian mountains and the Black Sea. Romanian, a Romance language, sounds similar to Spanish and Italian. Castles, where people of title once lived, dot the countryside, and traces of the grandeur of previous years were clearly visible amid the evidence of years of neglect (Fig. 20.1). Romania had once been a well-developed country of culture and education and Romanians developed an early awareness of art, music, ballet and poetry. Even pre-school children could recite long poems of their best-known lyric poet, Mihail Eminescu.

My earliest impressions of the country were of the prevalence of long bread and food lines and the absence of merchandise in the department stores. Even major department stores in Bucharest did not have escalators that worked and very few goods were on display. At this particular time, toilet paper was in demand and word of its appearance would circulate from mouth to mouth, prompting workers to leave their jobs to be able to go to the particular store that had just received the special shipment of

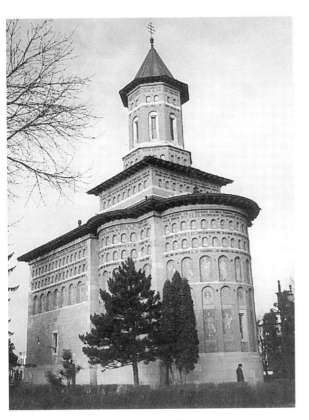

Fig. 20.1   This monastery is a reminder of the former grandeur of Romania.

this needed item. Families who had grandparents who did not work outside of the home were considered fortunate because they could spend long hours waiting in the food or milk lines. Some of the lines themselves observed formal conventions whereby a milk container placed in the line by an earlier individual maintained that position in lieu of the actual person. Despite the material inconveniences in 1990, I felt safe walking alone in Romanian cities.

Gracious demonstrations were easy to become accustomed to, such as the kissing of a woman's hand following an introduction and being the first to board an airplane while the men stepped to the side. Most Romanians ate their meals at home and despite food shortages insisted on serving delicious meals to their international visitors. Women worked hard preparing food, which was the center of social gatherings for friends and family. The pattern of

eating, drinking, and talking for many hours was one of the most prevalent and pleasant of the Romanian customs that I was privileged to observe and join. The charm, hospitality, warmth, and graciousness of the Romanians toward me was extraordinary.

Surprises and startling events continued to occur, partly because of my limited knowledge of the language. On one occasion during my second week in Romania, I was invited to attend a pediatric conference that included speakers from neighboring Moldova, which was still, in 1990, a part of the Soviet Union. As I was entering the lecture hall, my Romanian translator asked that I speak slowly to enable her to translate my English more easily. I assured her that I was not a speaker at the conference so that she need not worry about translating for me. As I was being led to the speakers' table, she assured me that indeed I was scheduled to be a speaker. As I surveyed the room of 150 pediatric delegates and the television cameras, I sought for appropriate words with which to address this audience. Ultimately, I reasoned that my purpose in speaking to the delegation must primarily be a courtesy invitation since I was an international visitor from the USA. I was then able to convey some words of appreciation for being included in the meeting and to tell them of the purpose of my visit to Romania.

A sobering experience that I encountered during this pediatric conference involved meeting a visiting professor from the Soviet Union. During a banquet the night before the conference, we enjoyed a convivial, spirited discussion about pediatric health problems in our respective countries. We shared information and left each other in a very friendly mood. The next day this same professor did not look at me or display any awareness that he had met me the previous night. This behavior contrasted with everyone else I had met, who would greet me with smiles and nods of recognition. I later learned that this medical professor had been warned against continuing further discussions with me by his traveling companion and was threatened with severe negative consequences

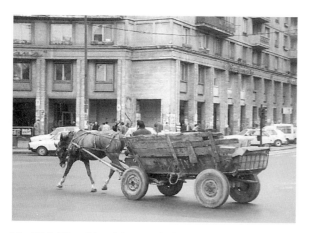

Fig. 20.2 The old and the new in Bucharest, 1992.

should he continue to talk to me. The realization that a mere discussion with me about professional matters could have dire consequences for a man of his distinction made me aware that free speech, which I had taken for granted as an American, is truly a privilege and not available to all people.

My strongest impression of Romania was that of continual contradictions and contrasts. Contrasts were prevalent in the colorful, handmade dresses of many Gypsy (Roma) minorities, sheepskin coats and hats of villagers and the western dress of the majority of the Romanians. Other contrasts involved the transportation on the city streets, which consisted of automobiles and electric trolley cars, alongside horse-drawn wooden wagons (Fig. 20.2). Interacting with Romanian families left me with the especially vivid contrast between the way that children were treated in the community and the way in which they were treated in the institutions. Romanian families in the community appeared to be generally devoted to their children and were strong advocates for their education. Education stressed memory of information with great emphasis on math, science and languages. During the Communist era, emphasis was not placed on psychology, social work, nursing and allied health professions (personal communication, 1991).

Awareness that established attitudes and relationships do not instantly change following a political revolution became clear during my first stay in Romania which occurred only 10 months after the Communist era had ended. As a health worker, it was essential to be impartial and not to become involved with the political situation. Unlike the Romanians, I had no prior knowledge of any roles that individuals had occupied under the Communist regime so that I was easily able to enter into unbiased relationships with everyone I met.

THE ORPHANAGES

The orphanages where I worked, taught and consulted were part of an organized system of institutions. Babies were delivered at state run maternity hospitals and mothers who chose not to take the newborns home would typically abandon them at this stage with the knowledge that they would be cared for by the orphanages. Since the orphanages were run like hospitals with physicians and nurses, many families rationalized that they were making the best decision for their children by leaving them where they would receive good care. Many parents believed that they would return for their children when they enjoyed better economic circumstances. The orphanages for babies of 3 months to 3 years, called *leagans* (cradles), were operated under the auspices of the Romanian Ministry of Health. Children were arranged by age within each orphanage and were moved to different groups and buildings as they grew older. In the north-east Romanian city of Iasi, there were five *leagans*.

When children reached pre-school age, they typically would be assessed by an evaluation team who would determine where they would next proceed. If judged to be normal, children moved to a pre-school orphanage directed by the Ministry of Education. There the education facilities were similar to boarding schools, where children lived in dormitories and received their education in classroom settings. As children advanced to adolescence, they would be supervised by the Ministry of Labor where they could perform jobs and continue to live in group home settings, sometimes in remote villages and small towns. If children were assessed to be mildly or moderately mentally retarded at the time of the pre-school evaluation, they would be sent to special orphanages that offered rudimentary vocational and educational activities. If children were found to have other disabilities such as cerebral palsy, Down Syndrome, or congenital anomalies, they could be sent to institutions called *camin spitals* (community hospitals). These homes, generally located in small towns, were custodial in nature, not providing educational or recreational programs. One such institution that I visited was very barren of toys or stimulation. Later, with the influx of NGOs, portions of institutions or entire facilities were adopted by various groups. Donated clothes, toys, equipment, personnel, consultants, and sometimes funds for partial or total facility renovations were provided. It was not unusual during these times to see groups of volunteers painting walls or murals and pounding nails to build or repair playgrounds. The programs in the schools for community children with a disability, in contrast to the *camin spitals*, provided an array of vocational and recreational programs. Such curricula included cosmetology, hairdressing, cooking and pastry and rug making. The teachers at one such school that I visited were interested in learning about wheelchair sports for their students.

The Romanian Orphan Social Educational Services (ROSES) project, envisioned and directed by an American developmental pediatrician, Dr Barbara Bascom (first for World Vision and later for the Brooke Foundation), called for staffing orphanage sites with two expatriate health professionals to provide direct care and in-service training (World Vision 1990). The ROSES project was designed to deliver exemplary services to children and the developmentally disabled and to foster professional health training (Brooke Foundation 1993). Expatriate occupational therapists, physical therapists, psychologists, educators or speech therapists could be employed for these positions. The two professionals at each site were intended to complement each other. My job

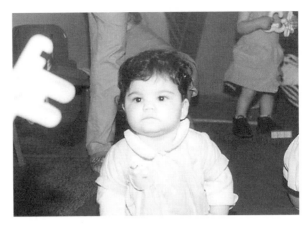

Fig. 20.3 Developmentally delayed baby.

description as an occupational therapist specified providing diagnostic services and direct treatment to developmentally disabled and delayed orphan children, who could have a wide spectrum of disorders. My role was also to participate in teaching Romanian allied health professional counterparts, medical students, and community para-professional aides. In order to establish a base for determining the efficacy of intervention programs, I also organized and participated in data collection and analysis for studies (World Vision 1990). One of the major projects developed involved examining the progression of growth and development of failure-to-thrive children in the orphanages (Fig. 20.3).

Ordinarily expatriates lived in apartments that were rented by the World Vision organization. Since I came alone and was the first clinician to arrive, I was invited to live in a large house near the Medical University in Iasi with Barbara Bascom and her spouse, Dr James Bascom. Barbara Bascom was the project director for the ROSES program, and James Bascom was the director of the medical education redevelopment program (MERP), which worked with medical schools to introduce computers for their libraries and assist with updating sources of medical information. An American educator, Thelma Roach, was the expatriate assigned to the orphanage in Iasi with me. She worked with the ambulatory orphans to engage them in educational tasks. The 250 pre-school-aged children in the orphanage had heretofore received minimal educational or developmental stimulation. In the absence of organized activities and lack of toys, the children were expected to nap for hours in the afternoon and find their own diversions. Under these sterile conditions, any adult stranger who walked into a day room was literally mobbed by a room of children with outstretched arms, demanding to be picked up and held. Shortly after my arrival, several Romanian educators were newly employed to work with the children and to implement programs. The desperate need to be held by strangers diminished when opportunities for interaction with adults increased.

The variety of environmental stimuli is diminished in an institutional environment (Provence & Lipton 1962, Spitz 1945). Infants raised in institutions with insufficient staff and sterile environments are known to be exposed to prolonged deprivation of maternal care and sensory stimulation (Provence & Lipton 1962). The early study by Spitz (1945) also recognized the development of psychiatric disturbances and asocial behavior of children who were institutionalized. Our experience with institutionalized children corroborated the progressive developmental deficits that occur with longevity in an institution.

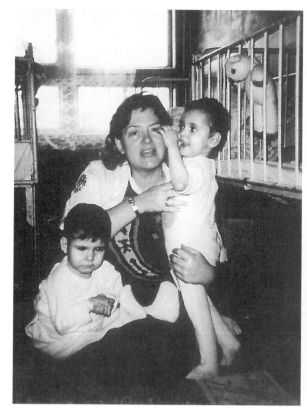

Fig. 20.4a Gabriela (right), aged 3, weighs 9 kilos, has no vocalizations, and crawls and pulls to stand. Reproduced with kind permission of Jan Grosshans.

THE PROGRAM

The two directives given to me prior to my departure for Romania were to establish relationships with the Romanian staff and to choose a caseload. Selecting a caseload proved to be a difficult decision. The large numbers of needy children and the scarcity of providers necessitated prioritizing services. Most of the pre-school-aged children in the orphanage would probably have been in some type of special program because of lack of age-appropriate stimulation if they had been in a North American school. Many of the pre-school children spread throughout various rooms lacked muscle tone and were not sitting or walking (Figs 20.4a, 20.4b). Their ambulatory dorm-mates would sometimes climb into the cribs of these children

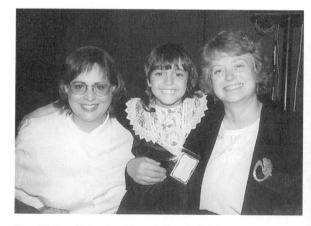

Fig. 20.4b Following intervention, Gabriela grew and developed. She was adopted, age 7, in the USA. Today she attends public school and is a happy child. Shown, age 8, with her mother (left) and Gale Haradon (right). Reproduced with kind permission of Jan Grosshans.

and hit them. Upon questioning, I learned that most of these nonambulatory children carried a diagnosis of dystrophia or 'failure to thrive', a condition that affects growth and development (Drotar 1985). I decided that this population would serve as my target group for intervention and that if progress could be shown with this regressed population, then it might serve as a dramatic demonstration of the effects of developmental intervention.

Compounded by my lack of understanding fluent Romanian, I found that I felt continuously surprised and uncertain about what daily events I would encounter. A few days after talking about my plans for targeting the dystrophic population, I walked into the orphanage to find a flurry of activity with crying children being carried by personnel to various rooms. When I inquired, I was informed that the children were being changed to two separate rooms as I had suggested on previous occasions and the very best aides were being assigned to them. Although considerable discussion had undoubtedly taken place among the orphanage staff to gain the orphanage director's approval for these changes, these activities surprised me when they happened since they were not usually communicated to me beforehand. Therefore, I assumed that suggestions I made which were not implemented had been rejected and was continually amazed when suddenly they were adopted. With this flurry of activity, a collaborative intervention began for the benefit of the dystrophic children.

The two rooms where the children with dystrophia were moved each housed 25 children. Each room contained iron cribs juxtaposed to each other with a table, bench, and large group playpen in the room. In 1990, few toys or play equipment were present in the day rooms and the children were rarely taken outside to the playground. Diapers were not used, resulting in soiled clothes and beds that required continuous changes. My description of diaper pins horrified the Romanians who demonstrated concern for the possibility that the children could be injured by the pins. The activities of feeding and bathing were carried on in the dorm rooms

although according to Day (1982), the amount of play and stimulation provided by feeding, holding and carrying in a home was substantially more than children received in an institution. Since most of the children were unable to walk, much of the day was spent in their cribs. Developmental assessments determined that these children were functioning far below their chronological age and were substantially smaller than the other children in the orphanage population.

For these 'failure to thrive' children, the effects of institutionalization that I observed involved abnormal posturing of the arms while lying supine, perpetual rocking motions, delayed development (especially affecting speech and language acquisition), sensory deprivation, and varied reactions to interpersonal contact ranging from clinging behaviors to withdrawal and aggression. The nondystrophic children, who were able to progress more easily through the orphanage system, were closer to their chronological age for development. Thus they were able to ambulate, climb, and talk despite minimal environmental stimulation. The resiliency of human life and the genetic imperative toward growth was one of the amazing lessons learned from working in an institutional setting where deprivation was the norm.

Experience in assessing developmental status taught me that standardized developmental tests more involved than a screening test were too time-consuming and difficult to administer to the orphan children who were not accustomed to interacting with adults. I first began to remove individual children from the crowded dorm room to a separate room for assessment and intervention. I quickly realized that these children were terrified to be away from their beds and from their rooms. Sometimes they spent an unresponsive hour where they would not touch or interact with any objects or persons. This observation was consistent with the classic study of 75 infants raised in orphanage settings by Provence & Lipton (1962), in which they described the crib as the primary boundary for the infants' activities during the first year. The duration of inactivity and fear reactions from separation from their familiar environment diminished dramatically when I evaluated and interacted with the children in their rooms. Even with the security of their rooms, some of the more severely involved children would scream when touched or picked up, and scoot under their cribs on the floor with bodies turned away in order to avoid interaction. A common behavior that became known as the 'orphan salute' consisted of children shielding their faces and eyes with their arms to avoid visual contact.

The orphans with dystrophia were delayed both in their physical growth and in their development. Tactile, vestibular, visual, auditory, and proprioceptive input was diminished because of the small number of adults available to interact with them. Adequate sensory processing allows infants and children to make adaptive responses to sensory experiences (Ayres 1972). Two sensory systems that are of primary importance in the development of sensory integration are the tactile and vestibular systems because the sense of touch and the vestibular apparatus develop early in infancy (DeGangi & Greenspan 1989). Developmental theorists agree on the importance of the foundation of the early sensory motor period for development and believe that the lack of opportunity to experience a variety of normal stimuli affects the course of normal growth and development (Drotar 1985).

Aylward (1990) suggests that the quality of the mother's interaction with the infant, in addition to opportunities for stimulation and health care, are included under environmental risks contributing to developmental delays. Thus, therapy was targeted both at altering the environment in which the orphans spent their time and at stimulating their development and sensory systems. Play equipment that provided rocking and swinging actions was moved into the rooms. Romanian medical students were recruited as volunteers to spend time with selected children. The first indication of change among the children with dystrophia was that they showed a significant weight gain following intervention. They continued to gain weight incrementally and to advance in their gross and

fine motor abilities. Initially only one of the 3-year-old children with dystrophia could walk unassisted, but within 6 months, a majority of the intervention group were taking their first steps. Language was severely delayed for these children but language skills also began to develop slowly.

The Romanian staff had also been victims of the Communist system as much as were their small charges. Education for the orphanage staff was provided by visiting health professionals. The program aimed at empowering them. Prejudicial attitudes toward abandoned children and limited job choices affected the behavior of other staff toward the children. Nevertheless, faced with one aide to care for 27 children, limited heat, water, food and electricity, many Romanian orphanage staff had still continued to advocate for their charges during the Communist era (personal communication 1991). When support, encouragement, and additional resources became available from international organizations, many of the staff attitudes and behaviors changed in a positive direction (Fig. 20.5).

Nonjudgmental attitudes toward the Romanian staff were essential for developing positive relationships. The Romanians seemed delighted to work with representatives from other countries when given consideration of courtesy and equality. When progress was demonstrated by these children, the Romanian staff became

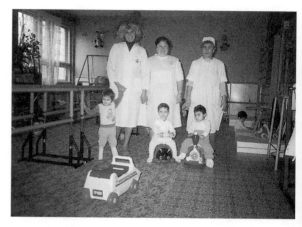

Fig. 20.5 Therapy staff and children, Iasi, Romania.

excited and determined to help more of the orphans achieve new abilities.

One of the more perplexing cultural differences arose regarding discontinuing the use of a particular institutional garment to clothe the children with dystrophia. Even after the donations of suitable alternative clothing, and continual education about the problems that the garments caused, the use of the one piece footed cotton garments which restricted full range of motion of weak extremities continued. Other cultural differences involved our desire to have the nonambulatory infants and children placed on the floor in order to develop appropriate muscle strength and mobility. Strong cultural attitudes about the negative effects of air currents prevented transition to the floor for activities. Cultural concerns about the children getting cold on the floor needed to be appreciated.

I was fortunate to work with three talented Romanian health professionals, psychologist Melanie Ciuperca, kinetotherapist Alice Visan (Fig. 20.6), and logopedist Carmen Frunzetti. Because of staff shortages, their professional assessments of the children's abilities were not being used to implement intervention programs. New staffing models were introduced to facilitate greater application of diagnostic information to develop treatment programs. International organizations sent specialists to teach various theories and treatments. Those

organizations that valued and directed their programs in collaboration with the Romanians had better results than those groups that disregarded their status as guests of Romania. Clinical work in Romania was not primarily developing new programs as much as aiding with the redevelopment of previous ones or adding new methods and techniques that had evolved during the closed Communist years. Although medicine is socialized and available without charge to all people, many patients seek to ensure competency and special consideration by giving gifts and funds to the doctors. Clinic patients would wait for their appointments holding favors, from simple flowers, cheese and wines to more elaborate presents, according to their means.

CONSULTATION

When I left Romania after my initial 3 months in 1990, an Australian occupational therapist, Carolyn McTurk, replaced me to continue working with the same children at the orphanage. After my return home, I found myself preoccupied with the Romanian orphans and was determined to continue to address their overwhelming needs and to retain contact with the Romanian health professionals. I developed a consultant relationship with World Vision to orient new health professionals to the culture, logistics and country of Romania. I also served as liaison and coordinator of allied health professional resources.

Barbara Bascom's visionary plan was to have involvement from Western health professional organizations to support redevelopment efforts for children in Romania. As a consultant to World Vision, I helped implement this plan by working with the American Occupational Therapy Association (AOTA), American Physical Therapy Association (APTA) and the American Speech-Hearing Association (ASHA) to choose representatives to travel to Romania for a needs assessment of the children, and to explore ways to develop rehabilitation professional organizations and partnerships. The

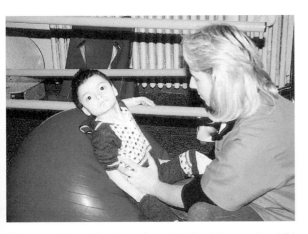

Fig. 20.6 Romanian kinetotherapist Alice Visan and a child in the orphanage.

information gathered from Satoru Izutsu (AOTA), Noel Matkin (ASHA) and Jane Sweeney (APTA) contributed to the understanding of the development and focus of these professions in Romania from the spring of 1991.

Occupational therapy (OT) was not an established profession in Romania although I was shown references about this profession for the treatment of mentally ill persons in old texts for psychiatrists. The existing professions most closely related to OT were psychologists, educators, ergotherapists and kinetotherapists. In my experience, psychologists were responsible for the assessment of all the children and the supervision of the educators. Romanian psychologists were graduates of university curricula, although in 1977, all psychology courses and training programs were discontinued by the government until after the December 1989 revolution (personal communication 1991). The educators in the orphanage had typically graduated from a special 5-year high school and worked with the children on traditional educational skills. Ergotherapists were also university graduates who appeared to work in psychiatric institutions where they operated sheltered workshops for adult patients and were under the department of ergonomy in the Ministry of Labor. *Physioterapie* and *Kinetoterapie* were the professions in Romania that were most similar to the profession of physical therapy in the USA. Dr Sweeney found that professional education courses for these professions had not been conducted since 1981. The physiotherapists had 12 years of education followed by 3 years of school where they received technical training. While the first 2 years of the professional training were spent in medical education, the third year consisted of applying physical modalities such as heat, cold, ultraviolet, and hydrotherapy. Kinetotherapists were the professionals who worked with patients on therapeutic exercise following the application of a physical modality. Kinetotherapists also had 12 years of general education which was followed by 4 years of university courses that taught movement science with sport application. Additional postgraduate training emphasized either health

care or physical education and gymnastics. Dr Sweeney found that the use of physical modalities for children appeared limited to paraffin and hydrotherapy, although there was some limited use of electrotherapy, ultrasound and infrared light equipment in some settings. She felt that kinetotherapists were the closest professional counterparts to pediatric physical therapy and pediatric occupational therapy in the USA.

Dr Matkin found that speech-language pathologists (logopedics) had been educated in an institute of psychology after completing high school where they generally spent 3 years in general psychology studies and an additional 2 years of specialized study in logopedics. He observed that Romania had no professional counterparts for audiologists, as they are known in the USA. Otolaryngologists and nurse technicians administered hearing tests and followed up on hearing aid recommendations.

In addition to working with the project for AOTA, APTA and ASHA, I also helped World Vision recruit and employ clinical personnel for Romania by providing technical reviews and recommendations of applicants. I participated in the finalization of arrangements for the developmental screening program of ROSES and taught trainers during a three week teaching mission to orphanages throughout Romania to use the Denver II developmental screening test. An important component of my position as consultant was to participate in the dissemination of information for ROSES through public and professional presentations and publications. I was determined also to share the positive aspects of Romania during my speaking engagements to balance the negative images that had been presented by the media.

LATER EASTERN EUROPEAN PROFESSIONAL EXPERIENCE

In 1992, my husband, Howard, and I left our jobs in the USA to work for a year in Romania for the Brooke Foundation. During this year I held a position as director of professional programs and research, which involved coordinating clinical services for the children in the orphanage, teaching a course in pediatric rehabilitation to kinetotherapy students at a private university (Universitatii Mihail Kogalniceanu), continuing research, and developing programs. The Ministry of Health in the Independent Republic of Moldova had also requested workshops in the area of developmental screening, which I provided for them.

During my first visits to Romania in 1990 and 1991, I was informed that I would not be permitted to cross the border to Chisinau, Moldova, because it was then under the control of the Soviet Union. After 1992, the new Independent Republic of Moldova was formed and the Moldovan Ministry of Health was interested in Western consultation. Since the border between Romania and the Independent Republic of Moldova was still guarded by the Soviet Union, my husband and I were subjected to intense questioning and scrutiny before being allowed into the country, despite having appropriate letters of invitation and documentation.

Another change occurring since 1990 was the focus of the service to the children in the two orphanages where the ROSES programs operated, first by World Vision and later by the Brooke Foundation. During the initial 3 years of the ROSES program, the orphanage in Iasi changed from a barren environment with sad understimulated children to a lively educational

and developmental center with children and staff who had new hope and spirit (Fig. 20.7). The Brooke Foundation was developed by Drs Barbara and James Bascom in 1991 to continue their humanitarian work in Romania. Twenty Romanian caregivers had also been hired by Brooke to work with the children. Because of these programs, children no longer spent their days in cribs and the developmentally delayed children with dystrophia were either seen in a therapy room for intervention or had progressed to educational programs. Much of the rocking and self-stimulating behavior was reduced and the children were now integrated for many activities into the community.

Since successful programs of intervention were being implemented in the orphanage for children aged 2 to 4 years, I considered that my efforts could best be directed toward working with the babies in the other orphanage to prevent the kind of developmental delays displayed by the children without such programs. Even the babies of 6 months of age showed signs of delay in the institutionalized orphanage setting. At this time, a study by an American psychologist, Dr Joseph Sparling, with the administrative support of Dr Barbara Bascom, was being conducted to determine whether increased caregivers and specified enhanced activity training would make a difference in the development of the babies who had been randomly selected for the study (Sparling et al 1993). Since I had noticed sensory problems in the older children arising from lack of sensory input (tactile, proprioceptive, vestibular, auditory and visual), I was interested in assessing the infants using a standardized test. The results of the study indicated that all sensory areas were at risk or deficient prior to the addition of the trained caregivers (Haradon et al 1994). Following six months of enriched caregiving, a reassessment showed that there were significant positive improvements in the areas of reactivity to tactile deep pressure, visual-tactile integration, oculomotor control, reactivity to vestibular stimulation and total test responses. No significant changes occurred in the areas of adaptive motor functions.

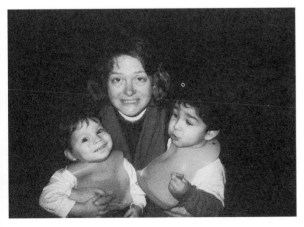

Fig. 20.7 Author Gale Haradon with children from the orphanage.

After being away from Romania for a year, I had anticipated that fewer children would be in the orphanages than previously. Because the policies against abortion and family planning were no longer in effect for the country, I reasoned that fewer families would have children and abandon them to the orphanages. I was tremendously disappointed when the orphanage director informed me that all the beds in the orphanage for the infants were full and there was a waiting list. Poverty, the lack of family planning, expense of contraception and the ready availability of the orphanage to care for children appear to be the reasons for this continued abandonment of the children to the orphanages. The challenge to the orphanage staff is to be able to maintain the new programs and personnel. Diminishing donors and program sponsors for NGO work in Romania necessitated the reduction of funds that had supported the hiring of additional Romanian personnel to work as caregivers for the children. The professional staff are working hard to continue the new programs but it is difficult to do so with limited resources.

Although career path interruptions and financial considerations are factors to consider when working internationally, the opportunities for me were worth taking the risks. An international background has given me the confidence and knowledge to extend occupational therapy programs to other countries and to enable me to be a part of international outreach through professional and university organizations. Continued communication with colleagues in Romania and Moldova is conveniently possible through electronic mail. Development of a pre-post institutional adoption clinic and consultations with international adoption agencies and parents to help with transitions of children from institutions to homes have been a logical extension of my work in Romania (see Fig. 20.4b). This experience has profoundly affected my realization of the impact of public policies on the dissemination of limited funds to programs. Market reforms in Romania have made material goods that were once in limited supply widely available. However, children continue to be abandoned to the orphanages 6 years after the end of the Communist era, and 100 000 Romanian children are reported to continue to live in institutions (SoRelle 1996).

Dedication: I would like to dedicate this chapter to my Romanian colleague, psychologist Melanie Ciuperca, whose sudden death in 1996 left the orphans of Romania without her loving, professional skills.

REFERENCES

Aylward G P 1990 Environmental influences on the developmental outcome of children at risk. Infants and Young Children 2: 1–9

Ayres A J 1972 Sensory integration and learning disorders. Western Psychological Services, Los Angeles

Bridges for Children in Romania 1995 Newsletter, July 17 1995. Bridges for Children in Romania, Suceava, Romania

Brooke Foundation 1993 Annual Report, 1993: program summary projects and descriptions. Brooke Foundation, Washington, DC

Day S 1982 Mother–infant activities as providers of sensory stimulation. American Journal of Occupational Therapy 36: 579–585

DeGangi G A, Greenspan S I 1989 Test of sensory functions in infants (TSFI) manual. Western Psychological Services, Los Angeles

Drotar D 1985 Failure to thrive and preventive mental health: knowledge gaps and research needs. In: Drotar D (ed) New directions in failure to thrive. Plenum Press, New York, pp. 27–44

Haradon G, Bascom B, Dragomir C, Scripcaru V 1994 Sensory functions of institutionalized Romanian infants: a pilot study. Occupational Therapy International 1: 250–260

News from Helsinki Watch 1990 issue of December 29

Provence S, Lipton R C 1962 Infants in institutions. International Universities Press, New York

SoRelle R 1996 Born to be forgotten. In: Houston Chronicle. Internet report April 28

Sparling J 1998 A program of screening and educational intervention in a Romanian orphanage. Conference presentation: 14th International Congress of International Associations for child and adolescent psychiatry and allied professions, Stockholm, Sweden August 4

Spitz R A 1945 Hospitalism: an inquiry into the genesis of psychiatric conditions in early childhood. Psychoanalytic Study of the Child 1: 53–74

World Vision 1990 World Vision annual report. World Vision, Pasadena, CA

21

Cultural and environmental factors in the delivery of rehabilitation services to American Indians

Catherine Marshall
Sharon Johnson

The Indian world is tiny, every other Indian dancing just a powwow away. Every Indian is a potential lover, friend, or relative dancing over the horizon, only a little beyond sight. Indians need each other that much; they need to be that close, tying themselves to each other and closing their eyes against the storms. (Sherman Alexie, *Reservation Blues*)

INTRODUCTION TO AMERICAN INDIAN POPULATIONS

The Indian world *is* tiny. At approximately 2 million individuals, American Indians and Alaska Natives make up less than 1% of the US population (US Bureau of the Census 1994). Even though American Indians are outnumbered many times over by the general population, professionals in rehabilitation must understand that 'there is a need to accommodate the growing ethnic and cultural heterogeneity in America and to acknowledge that many people do not want to give up their ethnicity or culture' (Weddington et al 1995, p. 4). Understanding the needs of American Indians with disabilities should begin with understanding their cultures and histories – the environments in which the peoples of more than 500 tribal nations live (see for example Choney et al 1995). Understanding can begin through experiential activities such as attending a powwow, reading literature such as Sherman Alexie's (1995) *Reservation Blues*, or attending professional development workshops (Makas et al 1997).

The following questions, as well as others quoted throughout this chapter, were asked by participants who attended a professional development workshop sponsored by the state of Minnesota rehabilitation services program and conducted by one of the authors (SRJ). The questions were selected because they represent concerns commonly expressed by professionals in rehabilitation who are learning to work effectively with American Indians. The authors believe that the question and answer format will appeal to rehabilitation professionals eager to learn practical, clinical intervention strategies that can result in appropriate rehabilitation intervention to a population which is typically both under-served and inappropriately served. Responses to the questions are based on one author's personal experiences as a Chippewa and, for both authors, 20 years of professional experience in the field of rehabilitation, including intervention and research with American Indians.

Is it more appropriate to use the term 'Native American' or 'American Indian'?

Whatever makes one more comfortable. The professional would probably want to consider what would make the client more comfortable. 'Preferred term' varies from location to location, tribe to tribe, sometimes reservation to reservation, and certainly person to person. Generally, the term Native American is used more prevalently as one moves south and west through the USA. American Indian is the 'federally correct' term in the USA; probably, the term Native American originated as an attempt by those persons wanting to avoid using the word Indian, which they felt to be a derogatory term. Actually, there is nothing wrong with being an Indian, and nothing wrong with referring to someone as an Indian person. Occasionally, one finds non-Indian Americans born in the USA taking offense with the term 'Native American' because they feel they themselves are Native Americans.

In what ways do different tribal units differ culturally?

Different tribes can be quite similar or as different as night and day. Many of the differences can be found in the spiritual beliefs and the particular reverences members of different tribes might hold, but generally a common thread may be found in their reflections of the order of the natural world – the earth and sky and the elements – components which pervade most of the spiritual thinking. Many of the differences between tribes are determined by geography and location. For example, in the north and east of the USA, water is plentiful; there are many trees, swamps, lakes and rivers. Obviously, in these areas, the means of travel, the foods eaten, the earthly things that are revered will differ from tribal groups living in the southwest where water is scarce, and where cacti take the place of trees. In the words of José Barreiro (1992), editor of *Akwekon Journal*, published through the American Indian Program at Cornell University:

Native peoples of the Americas exhibit both cultural diversity and philosophical consistency. Cultures that have evolved ecosystemically over thousands of years derive not only sustenance and shelter from their specific environments, but their very identities from particular rivers, mountain ranges, coastal and desert regions. Nevertheless, the transcending principles that guide the Native cultures bear a remarkable resemblance to one another. These principles . . . include respect for place, respect for the long-term impact into the future of actions taken in the present, and the glue of kinship, clan and extended family. (Barreiro 1992, p. 4)

Thus while there exists 'philosophical consistency' among Indian people, out of respect for the cultural diversity which also exists among the various nations, it is recommended that rehabilitation professionals focus on learning about the history, values, customs, and culture of the specific nations with which they have the most contact or particular interest (Marshall et al 1996a).

In the authors' experience, members of individual Indian nations are reluctant to accept generalizations in regard to American Indian values and customs. A professional recognition of the diversity of Indian peoples is more appropriate than learning pan-Indian values. For example, while it is generally acknowledged that the family is very highly valued among Indian people, the representatives of several Indian tribal rehabilitation programs cautioned the senior author against developing a CD-ROM training tool that presented the family as a valued support system among Indian people. The planned CD-ROM would present family based rehabilitation research conducted with the Eastern Band of the Cherokee Indians in Cherokee, North Carolina, and the Mississippi Band of Choctaw Indians in Pearl River, Mississippi (Marshall & Cerveny 1994), as well as the results of a nationwide survey focused on family intervention by tribal rehabilitation programs (Marshall & Johnson 1996). The representatives of the tribal rehabilitation programs argued that they were more concerned with the negative effects of over-generalization than they were about educating majority cultural rehabilitation professionals with regard to the importance of family support systems among Indian people.

Concern with over-generalization regarding customs and values may be a reality of many different indigenous peoples throughout the world. For example, in discussing the role of psychology in New Zealand but within the Maori context (Gergen et al 1996), it was noted that 'historically, there is no single Maori culture as a recognizable coherent unit; rather there are many distinctive tribes, each with its own local customs. However, largely for political purposes, a vociferous "Maori" voice was developed to challenge the ever-encroaching British reign' (Gergen et al 1996, p. 499). Similarly, when the senior author asked the indigenous coordinator of rehabilitation research in Mexico to write an article describing his Mixe culture (one of several Indian cultures indigenous to Oaxaca, Mexico), he replied that he would only write about the Mixe culture in Santa María Totontepec, Oaxaca, where he lived – for him to write about the Mixe in universal terms would have been considered presumptuous and an inappropriate generalization of his lived experience (Marshall 1996b).

How are gender roles different in American Indian culture from the White culture? What impact, if any, will this have on the counseling relationship and rehabilitation process?

In general, 'traditional' gender roles may not be too different from a functional perspective – after all, historically, the roles of women and men in the USA typically were defined by the way the land was settled, and also from roles established in Europe. Many Indian tribes were male-dominated hunter/gatherer/warrior groups, and women taking over any of those roles would be looked at as 'non-traditional.' However, as stated earlier, it is difficult to make accurate generalizations across more than 500 tribes. For example, traditionally: 'Iroquois women controlled the property and the possessions and were responsible for child rearing and growing of crops. The men had two duties, hunting and war. The women would sometimes accompany them in both of these pursuits and also had the power to sabotage a war effort by forbidding the men in their family to go to war' (Earle 1996, p. 27). Today, gender roles in American Indian cultures seem to be just about the same as in the dominant culture – changing gradually to a more even distribution of responsibilities, with clear cut lines between men's and women's roles beginning to blur.

Perhaps more importantly, there are role differences between the youth and the elders within American Indian cultures. One encounters tremendous respect for age and elders within Indian cultures – this high level of respect seems to run across all tribes of Indian people and is not simply characteristic of a few. Elders receive respect, even from young and unruly people who might be disrespectful to most others. If the rehabilitation professional is significantly younger than a given Indian client, the professional might want to temper the style of counseling/intervention to show a fair amount of deference to the client's status as an elder. Such behavior modification on the part of the rehabilitation professional would certainly help to form a good relationship with the client.

For Indians who return to the reservation, is the financial 'safety net' waiting to support them?

First of all, among other reasons, due to the investments and natural resources owned by some tribal nations, as well as the talents of individual entrepreneurs, some Indian people are quite wealthy – there is no need or concern for a financial 'safety net.' Other Indian people are quite destitute, while others enjoy a middle-class economic situation. While it is true that the majority of American Indians *do not* live on reservations (US Bureau of the Census 1994), it is interesting that many non-Indians seem pre-occupied with the notion that Indian people could have a life of ease and comfort if they just returned to the reservation(s).

In any case, there is some assistance available to tribal members just by virtue of living on the reservation. They might be eligible for low income housing that is controlled by the reservation. If not, they probably have family or extended family they can stay with. They would still be eligible for county, or local government assistance. Health care is available, as is dental care in most cases, although even on the reservation there may be some distance to travel and that may pose transportation problems. Although some reservations do distribute a share of economic development profits annually, that may or may not be available at the time it is needed, and it is only available randomly across the USA on certain reservations.

PREVALENCE OF DISABILITY AND 'PROBLEM' IDENTIFICATION

The majority of American Indians are young in age (US Bureau of the Censuses 1994). Nevertheless, Indian people have extensive health problems such as arthritis, diabetes and the resulting end-stage renal disease, heart disease, high blood pressure, and orthopedic disorders; many health problems are related to the use of alcohol and traumatic accidents (Nutting et al 1990; Marshall et al 1992a; Marshall et al 1992b; Marshall et al 1990; Weddington et al 1995).

According to summary data published by the National Institute on Disability and Rehabilitation Research (Kraus et al 1996), American Indians, at 21.9% of their population, have the highest rate of disability compared to any other ethnic group in the USA. Specifically, this means that 'an estimated 361 000 American Indians, Eskimos, or Aleuts report a disability' such as those listed earlier (for example arthritis and diabetes); almost half of this number (45%), or 162 000 persons, report having a severe disability (Kraus et al 1996, p. 19). American Indians also 'report the highest proportion of their population age 5 and over needing assistance in activities of daily living, 2.6%' (p. 20).

Rather than focus on these general statistics, given the diversity of Indian nations, rehabilitation professionals might want to dedicate some of their professional development time to better understanding the health risks and disabilities associated with a given tribe of interest or association. For example, there is considerable concern with the health effects of uranium among the Navajo (Erickson & Chapman 1993). As part of the bases for concern, 'an estimated 600 dwellings on Navajo lands are radioactive . . . . The largest spill of low-level radioactive waste in U.S. nuclear industry history occurred on July 16, 1979 . . . [contaminating] a major water source for Navajos and their livestock' (Erickson & Chapman 1993, p. 5). Finally, 'as many as 3000 Navajo men were employed during the uranium boom of the late 1940s through the 1970s' (p. 5). A survey of 50 of these Navajo uranium miners found that 25% had lung cancer, 10% had other forms of cancer, and the majority (66%) had chronic lung diseases; family members also reported having disabling conditions (Erickson & Chapman 1993).

Chronic health disorders and disability levels could be identified and reported for each of the more than 500 Indian nations, as well as for urban Indian communities. Indeed, American Indians experience tremendous health problems and rehabilitation professionals can become frustrated in trying to assist them. This frustration derives from a variety of causes, including mixed messages regarding who can best help, approaches to helping which are not culturally appropriate, attempting to help without sufficient resources, and failure to accurately assess 'the problem.' For example, while it is true that many physical impairments among Indian people result from the abuse and use of alcohol (Marshall et al 1990), rehabilitation professionals should be careful not to ascribe the problems of a client or a group of clients to their ethnicity. Similarly, rehabilitation professionals should be careful to not over-generalize the problems associated with an ethnic population to the individual client. Most unfortunately and unethically, there are rehabilitation professionals, as well as medical practitioners, who cannot separate the word 'drunk' from the word 'Indian,' and will approach any Indian client with the assumption that they are alcoholic (see for example Marshall et al 1992). The more appropriate stance might be to assume that any Indian client has been affected in some way by alcohol addiction – in an immediate family member, in their extended family, in a friend, in their community.

Do Indians have solutions to their own problems? Can they be solved by the White culture? Self-determination? There has been more discussion lately of different ethnic groups having their own solutions to their own problems versus 'imposed' solutions. Is this a form of segregation?

There are several questions here, the most important of which might be, 'Do Indians have solutions for their own problems?' Words such as 'solve' or 'solution' may not be comfortable to some people because these words can connote that a medical 'cure' is needed for a 'disease.' Further, it is not certain that Indian people and non-Indian people would make the same decisions on what constitutes a problem – possibly, the non-Indian culture would identify as problems situations or characteristics that the Indian people think of as virtues. For example, as Lamarine (cited in Choney et al 1995) observed in regard to professionals asking:

'What's wrong with the Indians? Why have Native Americans failed to adapt and flourish in Western society, after all they have had over 400 years to become fully acculturated?' Perhaps we are not finding the right answer because we have been asking the wrong question. A more revealing query may concern why Western society has not adjusted to Native American culture and learned to profit from much of what could be incorporated advantageously into a Western value structure? (Choney et al 1995, p. 79).

Similarly, in terms of problem identification, Harding (1991) has argued:

The development of contraceptives was a technological solution to what was defined by Western elites as the problem of the indigenous Third World peoples. From the perspectives of those peoples lives, however, there are at least equally reasonable ways to define what 'the problem' is. Instead of overpopulation, why not talk about the First World appropriation of Third World resources which makes it impossible for the Third World to support its own populations? Why not say that the problem is the lack of education for Third World women – the variable said to be most highly related to high fertility? After all, just one member of a wealthy North American family uses far more of the world's natural resources in his or her daily life than do whole communities of Ethiopians. Would it not be more objective to say that First World overpopulation and greed are primarily responsible for what Westerners choose to call Third World overpopulation?

Self-determination is key to any type of management of social problems (including health problems) within an ethnic group. 'Is this a form of segregation?' Not really. No one wants someone else to have the power to dictate to them, to set all the rules, to have power of enforcement, to be the 'parent' and they the child. The freedom to run one's own life is absolute bedrock in the USA and we all, no matter what our ethnicity, resent efforts to change that.

'Best' solutions

The previous series of questions typify the frustration and emotion-based concerns that many non-Indian rehabilitation professionals who work with Indian clients may feel – wanting to help but hearing Indian community concerns that the non-Indian is not the best person to be offering that help. There are no 'best' solutions, and certainly not at a total population level. Viewing each person as an individual and finding a way to concentrate on similarities, while both acknowledging cultural differences and providing culturally-appropriate intervention, may be the best place to start for non-Indian rehabilitation professionals. At the community level, rehabilitation professionals should be willing to follow the direction of Indian leaders who are working to better understand and intervene with such diverse epidemic problems as diabetes and substance abuse. For example, as regards psychiatric disorders requiring mental health intervention, 'people of the Seneca reservations attend the local, federal, state, and county mental health programs. But if the problems indicate the need to do so, people may also go to a traditional healer (Earle 1996, p. 28). Earle (1996) was informed that 'the healing practices of traditional Seneca people [are] as follows: first, a person talks to a medicine person who knows how to use traditional herbs and teas to calm a distressed person. The person may talk about signs or dreams which are problematic and the medicine woman may prescribe a ceremony to help' (Earle 1996, p. 28).

REHABILITATION AND AMERICAN INDIANS WITH DISABILITIES

Many forms of rehabilitation exist for persons with disabilities, including vocational rehabilitation, independent living, physical therapy, occupational therapy, speech therapy, mobility training, learning to read Braille, etc. With the exception of the tribal vocational rehabilitation programs (Marshall et al 1993), most rehabilitation programs, including those offered in hospitals and local health clinics, are largely staffed by majority-culture professionals and based on a majority-culture values system, resulting in significant problems of service delivery to persons of minority cultures, including American Indians (see for example Marshall 1994,

Marshall et al 1996c). This is even true of the USA public vocational rehabilitation (VR) program, a federal-state cooperative effort which has existed since 1920; while mandated to serve all persons regardless of ethnicity, problems of access and of appropriate service delivery to American Indians have been documented (see for example Ross & Biggie 1986).

What would be the best approach when doing an initial interview with an Indian client to describe rehabilitation services and at the same time try to understand the client's values and attitudes?

It is important to provide very individualized, one-on-one services to American Indians with disabilities. Rehabilitation professionals want to be able to help Indian people overcome the barriers created by their disabilities in all phases of their lives – from basic activities of daily living to full employment. For example, public VR professionals want Indian people to have appropriate jobs that meet their needs and requirements, and provide as much income as possible. These are basic services that anyone would desire and request. It is difficult to believe that describing rehabilitation in these terms would be offensive to anyone, yet we know there are significant problems in the public VR service delivery to American Indians.

In general, rehabilitation service systems are not unfriendly, but if the professional explaining the available services starts out with a list of things we do not do, will not do, need to have, require before we will serve, it can get very overwhelming for anyone, not just Indian clients. Clients are human beings first and will respond well to warmth, humor, clarity and respect. They will not respond well to officiousness, disrespect, generalities regarding profuse details, or cool disregard. The best approach with an Indian client, regardless of the clinical focus of the rehabilitation professional, is the best approach with any client: understand that they are nervous about a new situation, uncertain if they should be there, unclear about what we do and how we might help them, and provide simple, clear information that will alleviate the stress. Initial interviews are handled differently by the individual counselor or rehabilitation professional, but getting to know a client gradually and letting their story unfold in its own good time is a good habit to get into. Genuine empathy and understanding can go a long way toward breaking down barriers while collecting good usable information.

What types of rehabilitation do American Indians want? It was mentioned that that they do not set their goals high.

Indian people do not always set their sights as high as they might, especially the disabled population. Most likely this has more to do with their feelings of lack of self-worth than anything else. However, this seems to be changing as younger people begin to see more of the world and see it as less threatening. Also, there are now many more opportunities for people to have good, lucrative, professional jobs and still live on the reservation than there were for previous generations. Health care and human service professions are abounding, and the need is constant for well-trained secretaries, bookkeepers, accountants, computer operators, teachers, planners and program managers. Still, barriers, including those to self-esteem, are there. To quote one reservation health care professional: 'If I could do one thing that would be the most meaningful, it would be to find a way to convince the young people that they have value *off* the reservation.' All rehabilitation professionals can contribute to the physical wellness and emotional wholeness that enables Indian clients to experience positive self-esteem, independence in activities of daily living, and economic self-sufficiency.

If a client is involved in a protracted training program due to participating in a variety of cultural activities such as attending family funerals or harvesting wild rice, what service have we really provided when the client does get a job and then gets fired for these types of absences? Aren't we actually preparing the client for another form of failure?

Perhaps the services American Indian clients need most from rehabilitation professionals include helping them to make choices regarding where and how they will follow through on a rehabilitation program or plan. For example, clients are not typically 'fired' for failure to participate as scheduled in a program of rehabilitative physical therapy; however, the physical therapist should make the client aware of the consequences of whatever choice is made. Thus, getting fired from a job because of frequent culture-related absences should not come as a surprise to the Indian person. If it does, then rehabilitation professionals may not have done an adequate job as regards providing role models and rehabilitation scenarios which show cause and effect or as regards counseling ahead of time. With informed choice and knowledge of the consequences, an Indian person may choose not to compromise participation in cultural activities which require several days of 'time away', such as harvesting wild rice or frequent attendance at extended family funerals or healing ceremonies. If such a choice would threaten the successful completion of a program of rehabilitative therapy, or employment, it might be best for the counselor to suggest that the client become self-employed, for example, or work/obtain therapy on the reservation where the individual would lose less time in traveling to and from the various cultural activities.

What have you found that is effective in reconciling the differences between Indian values and employer expectations and requirements when they conflict?

Economic self-sufficiency is often a goal in comprehensive rehabilitation programs and, as discussed in response to the previous question, if a move to the reservation is not desirable or practical, advocacy on the part of the rehabilitation professional is probably the best possible solution when conflicts arise between Indian values and employer expectations. Sometimes there just is not any reconciliation possible, and if the Indian employee wants the job badly enough, the compromise will, more than likely, be on the part of the employee. If an employer is willing to be tolerant of the needs of the Indian person because the employer is gaining a satisfied and loyal employee, that is really good. But not all employers and not all businesses can function in that manner. It can even be difficult for reservation-based businesses to accommodate extensive leave-taking for participation in cultural activities.

For example, the recent development of the casino industry on several Indian reservations has had a singular and significant impact on the employment options of all people living on or near a reservation with a casino. Having a successful casino might be likened to having discovered oil in an otherwise barren desert! Indeed, the casino industry has mushroomed over the years to the amazement of everyone – the reservations, the general public, the state governments, the casino management. Most casinos are expanding to include hotel and conference center facilities, and frequently major entertainment. There are so many jobs available in the service industry category that it is virtually impossible for tribal members to fill all of the jobs – tribes just don't have enough people. Consequently, the casinos have become an employment boon not just for the Indian people, but for all populations in the areas surrounding the reservations where casinos have developed. Casinos have created many jobs and many types of jobs, from accounting and bookkeeping to management and development (see for example Chattanooga Free Press 1997); the building trades are flourishing and towns located near the casinos are feeling the economic benefits of having a large and constant tourist trade. Yet, while trying to accommodate the needs of Indian people with severe disabilities, it has been difficult for the casino managers to meet the needs of having the casinos staffed at all times and still honor the requests of employees for time away from the job to engage in traditional cultural practices.

STRATEGIES FOR IMPROVING REHABILITATION SERVICE DELIVERY

While ensuring that American Indian clients understand the work behaviors demanded by an employer constitutes ethical rehabilitation intervention, expecting that American Indians should behave as dictated by the world views of majority-culture service providers (Choney et al 1995), as well as failing to provide reasonable accommodation for cultural differences, are among those barriers which prohibit appropriate rehabilitation service delivery to American Indians with disabilities. Preston (1995) has observed that 'a human culture is a framework that allows a group of people to comprehend the world' (Preston 1995, p. 24), and that the majority culture in the USA reflects 'a people of action and command, domineering, not usually given to contemplation or doubt' (Preston 1995, p. 23). Thus significant barriers to appropriate rehabilitation service delivery may well relate to the fact that the values of most Indian cultures are in direct contrast to the values of the majority or dominant society (see for example Gergen et al 1996). Rather than action and command, Indian people tend to value patience and deference. Rather than a domineering stance, Indian people tend to value a posture which demonstrates respect. Contemplation or doubt, as reflected in lengthy observation, consultation with elders and other leaders, as well as consensus building before action, would also be highly valued.

Throughout this chapter, the authors have advocated that American Indians with disabilities be recognized both as individuals and as members of an ethnic group whose cultural values differ markedly from those of the dominant society. Appropriate intervention requires a balance of both views. In general, rehabilitation professional should make every effort, at both the personal and the professional level, to understand the cultures of the ethnic minority populations which they may encounter in their spheres of work and to which they should be directing outreach efforts. Strategies for improving rehabilitation service delivery include, first and foremost, acknowledgment of our pluralistic society, acknowledgment of the values of a collective society, and support for indigenous self-determination as reflected in the support of tribal rehabilitation programs.

Acknowledgment of our pluralistic society

As a first step in improving rehabilitation services to American Indians with disabilities, rehabilitation professionals must accept that we live in a pluralistic society and must, themselves, freely experience and participate in pluralistic events and diverse communities (Marshall et al 1996a). Véa (1993) wrote of the benefits of knowing different cultures first-hand:

Mexican or black or Indian kids whose first experience of the white race was the migratory Arkies [people from the state of Arkansas] could never thereafter harbor a categorical hatred of white people. Dirt seemed even dirtier on the faces of blond Arkies ... No Arkie kid ever turned down an invitation to dinner or ever asked what he was eating. Arkie kids ate chitlins and tripe, goat brains or mountain oysters, then sat quietly hoping for more. (Véa 1993, p. 66)

Perhaps most difficult for rehabilitation professionals will be coming to terms with cultures whose values and world views are radically different from one's own – as is the case with the values of American Indians and the dominant culture. Much of the difference in values and world views can be best understood through learning the differences between individualist and collectivist perspectives (Triandis 1994).

Acknowledgment of the values of a collective society

According to Mohawk (1992): 'Most immigrants and their descendants exist largely as individuals in American society. The Indians exist as distinct *groups* and have existed as such since time immemorial' (Mohawk 1992 p. 45). Typically, rehabilitation professionals have not been trained, in schools and universities, or in their homes, to think first of the group. In telling the story of a Yaqui (Indian people historically from Mexico but now generally living in the southwestern USA) family, Véa (1993) described the Yaqui grandfather talking with his grandson: 'I don't hate white people. Taken individually, they are as good a people as anybody else. But together they have a great many problems .... You see, they have no tribe, so if a person across town is hurt or hungry, they feel nothing .... There are some exceptions, though. Your Arkie friends have a sad but enduring tribe ... (Véa 1993, p. 230). Interestingly, while instructing his grandson in the values of a collective society, the grandfather also quickly moves from the values of the tribe to socioeconomic/work values which still reflect allegiance to the group, saying to his grandson, 'You must promise me one thing. If nothing else, promise me this one thing .... You must promise me you will never ever cross a picket line' (Véa 1993, p. 231).

Bhawuk & Brislin (1992) noted that 'concern' is an underlying concept holding together the construct of collectivism, and clarified that 'concern does not refer to affection and worry only; it is rather "a sense of oneness with other people, a perception of complex ties and relationships, and a tendency to keep other people in mind [citing Hui and Triandis]".... *Collectivism recognizes the group, and not the individual, as the basic unit of survival'* (Bhawuk & Brislin 1992, p. 417, italic added). Again, Véa (1993) informs us:

There is no concept of 'poor' for a non comparative, communal society. A Yaqui is only poor when he deals with the whites or the Mexicans. When he is forced to pay taxes on land he has always lived on or when the laws of Arizona require that he buy a tombstone, then he is poor. Then he must reach outside his language for the word. (Véa 1993, p. 31)

Thus in collective societies, the needs of the individual are provided for by the group – there is no embarrassment in being 'poor' or expecting that family and community would assist fiscally in the time of need. Logically, the individual thinks first of maintaining the group (the key to survival).

The family

Within collective societies such as American Indian communities, the basic group unit is the family and 'family' can be a term with very broad meanings. Thus rehabilitation professionals working with American Indians must understand that 'for most Native peoples, family and communal reciprocity are important values. It is not uncommon in family emergencies or ceremonial obligations for a Native person to forego work or school to be with family' (Weddington et al 1995, p. 11; see also Marshall 1995, Marshall & Cerveny, 1994). Generally, at important events such as funerals of family members, including extended family, attendance is virtually mandatory, or at the very least imposes a heavy obligation on the whole family to try to come together.

In regard to the extended family, frequently whole villages are involved in general child rearing and responsibility for one another, so the definition of 'distant' might be very different for an Indian versus a non-Indian person. When interviewing clients or potential clients in treatment centers, halfway houses, and so on, it is so common as to be almost the norm that a woman's or man's children are 'with my sister,' 'staying with my mom,' or 'my aunt (cousin, brother, friend) has my kids until I get back.' If needed, friends in a collective society become family, and with no expectation of financial assistance/reward. However, at the time of illness or death, 'debts' are repaid and Indian people must return to the group to demonstrate their respect and commitment to the family.

Should there be more emphasis on family involvement in the rehabilitation process?

Family involvement is not only desirable when working with Indian clients, it sometimes seems inevitable. Family – and the concept of extended family – can make or break a rehabilitation plan for a client, because the support provided cannot be found anywhere else. In addition, much more attention needs to be given to the family as an inseparable unit in the rehabilitation process. In order for one person in that unit to get healthy, the whole unit's health must be addressed and assistance given wherever possible (Marshall 1995). For example, in discussing diabetes, Nutting et al (1990) noted that 'in designing interventions, too often attention is focused on the individual and fails to recognize that individuals live within and are extensively influenced by their social environment. Interventions that focus on relevant social groups, such as families, households, or individuals within households that regularly eat together, should be tested' (Nutting et al 1990 p. 32).

More information is needed regarding the benefits of involving American Indian family members in the rehabilitation process, particularly with regard to rehabilitation outcomes. Lindenberg (1977), writing more than 20 years ago, concluded a review of family influences on rehabilitation outcome, as well as programs which involved the family in rehabilitation processes, with the following:

> More attention needs to be paid to identifying and studying variables related to outcome, family influences among them. Second, although there is already evidence that work with families influences outcome, it has for the most part been a missing component of rehabilitation practice. The individual is still perceived as a free-standing entity rather than a member of a larger interacting system. Practice remains the captive of a model, which by emphasizing individual counseling, puts the family out of bounds. (Lindenberg 1977, p. 73)

While Lindenberg does not mention cultural influences in her conclusion, it would seem that where families are readily acknowledged as a primary value in the culture, as with American Indians, further research to better understand the role the family plays in rehabilitation outcomes is even more critical.

Support of tribal rehabilitation programs

Support of tribal rehabilitation programs indicates that the rehabilitation professional understands the importance of self-determination and can be responsive to leadership by the people of the community. For example, in the USA, federal legislation exists which enables American

Indian tribes to apply for funding to support their own rehabilitation programs. However, these programs are typically 'short-term demonstration projects that serve as supplements to services provided by the Federal-State [public] VR programs' (Weddington et al 1995, p. 5). While the public VR program has ultimate responsibility to provide appropriate rehabilitation services, and model outreach programs exist which illustrate a state's capacity to appropriately service culturally-different populations (see for example Marshall et al 1993), tribal programs have the potential to fully demonstrate the principles of self-determination and culturally-appropriate intervention within the context of rehabilitation services. Unfortunately, limited funding, extremely short programming cycles, and competitive application processes make providing rehabilitation services through tribal programs difficult at best (Weddington et al 1995). However, continued support of tribal programs is essential, as is continued support for indigenous cultures in their struggles to survive acculturation attempts by dominant societies. American Indians constitute a very tiny proportion of the USA population, but rehabilitation professionals have an ethical obligation to serve them appropriately.

SUMMARY AND CONCLUSIONS

Many forms of rehabilitation exist for persons with disabilities including vocational rehabilitation, independent living, physical therapy, occupational therapy, speech therapy, mobility training, learning to read Braille, etc. Thus all professionals involved in rehabilitation can contribute to the physical wellness and emotional wholeness that enables American Indian clients to experience positive self-esteem, independence in activities of daily living, and economic self-sufficiency. The authors would like to emphasize that rehabilitation professionals should focus on learning about the history, values, customs, and culture of the specific tribes with which they have the most contact or particular interest rather than being content to learn 'pan-Indian' values.

However, having a basis for understanding that many cultures may differ significantly from one's own is an essential first step to working effectively, as well as ethically, with American Indians. Remember that Indian people and non-Indian people would very likely not make the same decisions on what constitutes a problem – very possibly, the non-Indian culture would identify as problems situations or characteristics that the Indian people think of as virtues. As one comes to understand the basic philosophical differences which distinguish collective societies from those which focus on the needs and wishes of the individual, one may have to drastically alter behaviors deemed appropriate by professional training.

For example, if the rehabilitation professional is significantly younger than a given Indian client, the professional may well need to modify the style of counseling/intervention in order to demonstrate deference to the client's status as an elder. Such behavior modification on the part of the rehabilitation professional would help to form a good relationship with the client through demonstration of respect. Similarly, at the community level, rehabilitation professionals should be willing to follow the direction of Indian leaders and support their right to self-determination and leadership. This may be difficult for professionals trained to recognize only the academic credential, but appreciation and recognition of the value of community knowledge forms a critical component of culturally appropriate rehabilitation service delivery.

REFERENCES

Aleie S 1995 Reservation blues. P. Warner Books, c/o Little Brown. Boston, MA
Barreiro J 1992 First words. Akwekon A Journal of Indigenous Issues, Cornell University, Ithaca, NY 9: 4–5

Bhawuk D P S, Brislin R 1992 The measurement of intercultural sensitivity using the concepts of individualism and collectivism. International Journal of Intercultural Relations 16: 413–436

Chattanooga Free Press 1997 Money floods Cherokees' casino; doubts laid aside. Chattanooga Free Press, Monday, June 9, p. B3.

Choney S K, Berryhill-Paapke E, Robbins R R 1995 The acculturation of American Indians: developing frameworks for research and practice. In: Ponterotto J G, Casas J M, Suzuki L A, Alexander C M (eds) Handbook of multicultural counseling. Sage, Thousand Oaks, CA

Earle K A 1996 Working with the Haudenosaunee: what social workers should know. New Social Worker (Fall): 27–28

Erickson J D, Chapman D 1993 Sovereignty for sale: nuclear waste in Indian country. Akwekon A Journal of Indigenous Issues, Cornell University, Ithaca, NY, 10: 3–10

Gergen K J, Gulerce A, Lock A, Misra G 1996 Psychological science in cultural context. American Psychologist 51: 496–503

Harding S 1991 Whose science? Whose knowledge? Cornell University Press, Ithaca, NY

Kraus L E, Stoddard S, Gilmartin D 1996 Chartbook on disability in the United States 1996. An InfoUse report. U.S. National Institute on Disability and Rehabilitation Research, Washington, DC

Lindenberg R E 1977. Work with families in rehabilitation. Rehabilitation Counseling Bulletin 21: 67–77

Makas E, Marshall C A, Wehman P 1997 Cultural diversity and disability: developing respect for differences. In: Wehman P (ed) Exceptional individuals in school, community and work. PRO-ED, Austin, TX

Marshall C A 1994 The assessment of a model for determining community-based needs of American Indians with disabilities: follow-up in Denver, Colorado. Final Report. Northern Arizona University, Flastaff (Available from the American Indian Rehabilitation Research and Training Center, Institute for Human Development, Northern Arizona University, PO Box 5630, Flagstaff, AZ 86011)

Marshall C A (executive producer) 1995 Family Voices (Video Documentary, 40 minutes). American Indian Rehabilitation Research and Training Center, North Arizona University, PO Box 5630, Flagstaff, AZ

Marshall C A, Cerveny L 1994 American Indian family support systems and implications for the rehabilitation process: the Eastern Band of Cherokee Indians and the Mississippi Band of Choctaw Indians. Final Report. Northern Arizona University, Flagstaff (Available from the American Indian Rehabilitation Research and Training Center, Institute for Human Development, Northern Arizona University, PO Box 5630, Flagstaff, AZ 86011)

Marshall C A, Johnson M 1996 The utilization of the family as a resource in American Indian vocational rehabilitation projects (Section 130 projects). Final Report. Northern Arizona University, Flagstaff (Available from the American Indian Rehabilitation Research and Training Center, Institute for Human Development, Northern Arizona University, PO Box 5630, Flagstaff, AZ 86011)

Marshall C A, Martin W E, Jr., Johnson M J 1990 Issues to consider in the provision of vocational rehabilitation services to American Indians with alcohol problems. Journal of Applied Rehabilitation Counseling 21: 45–48

Marshall C A, Day-Davila C A, Mackin D E 1992a The replication of a model for determining community-based needs of American Indians with disabilities through consumer involvement in community planning and change: Minneapolis-St. Paul, Minnesota. Final report. Northern

Arizona University, Flagstaff (Available from the American Indian Rehabilitation Research and Training Center, Institute for Human Development, Northern Arizona University, PO Box 5630, Flagstaff, AZ 86011)

Marshall C A, Johnson M J, Martin W E, Jr Saravanabhavan R C, Bradford B 1992b The rehabilitation needs of American Indians with disabilities in an urban setting. Journal of Rehabilitation 58: 13–21

Marshall C A, Johnson S R, Lonetree G L 1993 Acknowledging our diversity: vocational rehabilitation and American Indians. Journal of Vocational Rehabilitation 3: 12–19

Marshall C A, Johnson M J, Johnson S R 1996a Responding to the needs of American Indians with disabilities through rehabilitation counselor education. Rehabilitation Education 10: 185–199

Marshall C A, Gotto G S, Pérez Cruz G, Flores Rey P, Garcia Juárez G 1996b Vecinos y rehabilitation: assessing the needs of indigenous people with disabilities in Mexico. Final Report. Northern Arizona University, Flagstaff (Available in English and in Spanish from the American Indian Rehabilitation Research and Training Center, Institute for Human Development, Northern Arizona University, PO Box 5630, Flagstaff, AZ 86011)

Marshall C A, Bruyère S, Shern D, Jircitano L 1996c An examination of the vocational rehabilitation needs of American Indians with behavioral health diagnoses in New York State. Final Report Northern Arizona University, Flagstaff (Available in English and in Spanish from the American Indian Rehabilitation Research and Training Center, Institute for Human Development, Northern Arizona University, PO Box 5630, Flagstaff, AZ 86011)

Mohawk J C 1992 Indian economic development: the US experience of an evolving Indian sovereignty. Akwekon A Journal of Indigenous Issues, Cornell University, Ithaca, NY 9: 42–49

Nutting P A, Helgerson S D, Welty T K, Kileen M J, Jackson M Y 1990 A research agenda for Indian health: researchable questions in chronic disease. The IHS Primary Care Provider 15: 29–38

Preston D 1995 Talking to the ground: one family's journey on horseback across the sacred land of the Navajo. Simon & Schuster, New York

Ross M G, Biggi I M 1986 Critical vocational rehabilitation service delivery issues at referral (02) and closure (08, 26, 28, 30) in serving select disabled persons. In: Walker S, Belgrave F Z, Banner A M, Nicholls R W (eds) Equal to the challenge: perspectives, problems, and strategies in the rehabilitation of nonwhite disabled. Howard University, Washington, DC

Triandis H C 1994 Culture and social behavior. McGraw-Hill, New York US Bureau of the Census 1994 General population characteristics: American Indians and Alaska Native areas, 1990 Census. US Government Printing Office, Washington, DC

Véa A, Jr 1993 La Maravilla. Plume, New York

Weddington J R, Sanderson P L, Johnson V A, Rice B D 1995 Report from the study group on American Indian rehabilitation programs: unmet needs. Twenty-first Institute on Rehabilitation Issues. Arkansas Research and Training Center in Vocational Rehabilitation, University of Arkansas, Fayetteville

22

Culture and its impact on the rehabilitation program: a Palestinian perspective

Jo Simister
Ahmed Younis

INTRODUCTION

This chapter will first present unique features of the culture of the Palestinian people living in East Jerusalem, the West Bank and Gaza Strip and the relationship of that culture to the provision of health and rehabilitation services. This is followed by a discussion of the inherent limitations of foreign involvement in the development and implementation of those services. Unless otherwise referenced, the information given in this chapter is the result of personal experience, observation and knowledge within the family and community.

It is estimated that of the 2 million Palestinians living in East Jerusalem, the West Bank and Gaza Strip, about 56 000–62 000 people have various disabilities requiring rehabilitation services. Of these, about 12 000 received injuries as a result of the *Intifada* (the Palestinian uprising against the 30-year Israeli military occupation) (Abdel-Shafi 1992, Giacaman & Daibes 1989, Khader 1996). As is typical for a developing country, most persons with a disability (PWD) are young: 46% are 14 years old or younger (FAFO 1993). Therefore, there are proportionately large numbers of children requiring rehabilitation services, especially for cerebral palsy, congenital conditions, and developmental delay (YMCA 1994, Barghouthi & Daibes 1993).

A holistic approach to rehabilitation for Palestinians requires an understanding of the cultural background that influences individual rehabilitation needs in order to develop and use the potential of the community. Tylor (1871, quoted by Leach, 1982, pp. 38–39) gives one of the classic definitions of culture as 'that complex whole which includes knowledge, belief, art, morals, law, custom and any other capabilities and habits acquired by man [sic] as a member of society.' Keesing (1981) describes culture as 'systems of shared ideas, systems of concepts and rules and meanings that underlie and are expressed in the ways that human beings live.'

The rehabilitation process should address the needs of the patient in society and facilitate reintegration into the normal environment. Wade (1995) defined social integration as 'the individual's ability to participate in and maintain customary social relationships.' In Palestinian society these tend to be gender-related and centered on the extended family, education, work, and marriage.

The foregoing concepts stress the sharing of ideas and understanding about how people live, and it is here that the effectiveness of any rehabilitation program can stand or fall. To benefit from the skills and knowledge being offered, the receiver of rehabilitation services must respect the one offering them, and also feel that they are respected in turn.

When considering the culture and rehabilitation of Palestinian people, it is also essential to consider the geopolitical situation, particularly as it affects access to hospitals and other special facilities. The two larger sections of territory (the Gaza Strip and the West Bank) are separated by a tract of Israel, and free passage between the two is not yet possible, nor can Palestinians pass freely into Arab East Jerusalem. All of the major rehabilitation facilities for Palestinians are located in the West Bank or East Jerusalem.

Palestinian society has witnessed an upsurge of international interest in rehabilitation projects over the last decade. In 1987, the *Intifada* erupted, with immediate implications for rehabilitation. The daily TV views of stone-throwing Palestinian children and youths caught in street confrontations with Israeli soldiers captured attention world-wide. Many medical and paramedical personnel volunteered their services alongside others lacking professional skills in

rehabilitation but moved by humanitarian concerns (Simister, research in progress).

The *Intifada* has precipitated many changes within Palestinian society. Most notable in the rehabilitation field has been the change in attitudes towards disability. Many young Palestinians have received seriously disabling injuries, highlighting the needs of *all* PWD, a previously 'invisible' sector. The *Intifada*-injured were mostly young men, from all backgrounds; many had already received an education, making them an articulate and active group (Gaff 1994).

Education is particularly highly regarded as the key to future freedom and prosperity now that 40% of Palestinians (60% in the Gaza Strip) are refugees (FAFO 1993, Morgan 1989). The educational level of Palestinians is the highest of any country in the Middle East except Israel, with 17 per 1000 of the general population in higher education (Khader 1996).

THE PALESTINIAN FAMILY AND COMMUNITY

People from non-Arab cultures are often confused about the relationship between religious and other aspects of life in Arab countries. Many believe incorrectly that 'Arab' is synonymous with 'Muslim' and that Arabic cultural values are therefore Islamic religious values. Palestinians are predominantly Sunni Muslim, but Palestinian society has its own unique traditions and conventions and its own interpretation of Islamic values. In particular, to confuse Palestinian culture with Islam is to ignore a strong Christian influence. Approximately 6.7% of Palestinians belong to various churches, mostly Greek Orthodox or Roman Catholic (Sabella 1994).

Although many aspects of Palestinian culture are influenced by religion, there is often confusion over whether something is done for religious purpose or some other reason. In fact, many customs and behaviors have more in common with other Mediterranean groups (Greece and Turkey) than with other Arab groups (Saudi Arabia and the Gulf States). The incoming health professional should beware of stereotyping the prevailing social attitudes as Islamic, whatever that might be perceived to be: the norms can vary widely from one village to the next, and from family to family.

Palestinian society is also a curious mix of developing and developed. Its proximity to Israel and individual family links outside the country have led to a high level of material prosperity for some people. Most homes have a range of domestic appliances, for example, and there is access to and expectation of high-technology in medical care. However, some of the more remote villages still have no telephone, potable water, or electricity, and per-capita income is very low, especially in the Gaza Strip (Khader 1996). There is a high incidence of Third World diseases, particularly parasitic infestations and kidney problems resulting from poor quality water supplies, alongside many health problems of the First World, including rising numbers of cardiac complaints and cancer (UPMRC 1987).

The Palestinian community is generally collectively oriented rather than individualist, so group well-being takes precedence over individual choice. Conservative family values are transmitted from generation to generation, forming a stable structure that has survived the traumatic events of the last century relatively intact. The involvement of an individual in any activity is not simply a personal matter but part of the family's identity and status in the community. Therefore personal behavior and demeanor within the community setting can have serious consequences. Concepts of family pride and shame are very strong, and give rise to discussion of behavior and sanctions against those who have wronged the family. Typical transgressions include adultery, theft, selling of family land and property, and the drinking of alcohol, all of which threaten the reputation, dignity and cohesion of the family. The importance of 'proper' behavior also applies to 'foreigners' – anyone from outside the community – including rehabilitation workers.

The Arab family is generally patrilineal, patriarchal, extended, patrilocal, endogamous, and occasionally polygamous. Several patrilineally extended families form a larger social and power unit called a *hamula*, often living as neighbors in the same quarter of a town. They usually cooperate in such enterprises as building a home, paying marriage expenses and harvesting (Geraisy 1994). Family or *hamula* members are mutually responsible for the protection and security of each other, and this includes the protection and care of members with disabilities. It would not be unusual to find that many family members actively participate in the rehabilitative process.

Relationships in an extended family are not always calm, and when there is a problem senior members will gather together to hear the grievances and discuss solutions. Sometimes the extended family will bring great pressure to bear on individuals or nuclear branches, especially if the good name of the whole family is concerned, as in the matter of marriages and social behavior. The extended family gains its status and position in society through the numbers and quality of male members and their material standing. However, it is possible for a small family without great wealth to be well-esteemed, for example if their members are respected for their education and wisdom (Younis 1998).

The nuclear family is becoming more common, especially in urban areas. However, in most cases, the family is still thought of as the extended group, spanning three or four generations, with different branches living under the same roof or in neighboring dwellings. This is particularly the case in the rural villages, in the Old City quarters of the major towns, and in the refugee camps.

Although the patriarchal pattern is increasingly being challenged, the father (or, in his absence, the eldest son), is usually the head of the family and the breadwinner. He is chief decision-maker regarding friends and socializing, marriages, education, and health and rehabilitative care. The mother's traditional responsibilities are to care for the family (including PWD), prepare meals, keep the house, and look after the children. Daughters normally assist with domestic activities.

A mother becomes more powerful by producing children, especially males. Two goats will be slaughtered to celebrate the birth of a son and one for a daughter as a'qeqa, or protection for the newborn. The first son is particularly important because the new parents will take his name, becoming 'mother of' and 'father of' so-and-so.

Until recently, a child born with a disability would very likely be kept out of sight and take little active part in family life, though receiving love and care (Younis, paper for the Global Disability meeting of the Save the Children Fund, April 1994, unpublished). Now disablement is less of a stigma than previously, and the birth of children with disabilities is less regarded as a matter of family shame; the same trend applies to disabilities resulting from accidents or other misfortunes, although a son with a disability might be perceived as more tragic than a daughter with a disability.

However, the presence of individual frail members needing special protection can still be a strain (financial and otherwise) and a source of embarrassment (Younis, paper prepared for the Global Disability meeting of SCF, April 1994 unpublished; Younis 1998). With the integration of some children with disabilities into school, and a significant amount of disability affecting already educated people, participation in society is now more common. However, access to integrated schooling and rehabilitation services (other than a local clinic possibly with some physical therapy) is largely a matter of circumstance and luck. Opportunities will be much fewer if there are no services locally and the family has little money. More effort will be made in the case of (male) heads of families who have become disabled in later life and therefore have responsibilities, but the situation for women is less encouraging. It is more difficult for women to live an independent life anyway, even if they are from the more liberated and educated sectors of society.

The main leisure activities center on the family and hospitality: visiting, eating, drinking tea and coffee, smoking, talking. Exchanging visits with neighbors, family, and friends is key because there are almost no public restaurants, sports facilities or clubs, especially in the villages and refugee camps. Much of the talking is discussion of community affairs, politics, and recounting anecdotes, and there is no exclusion of members of the family on the grounds of disability.

Particularly welcome in social gatherings are those injured in defense of their faith or community, and the high-profile attention they have received has affected the integration of people with many other kinds of disabilities. However, someone with a conspicuous disability will be at a disadvantage in social settings and may well feel too shy to participate. The young often feel particularly self-conscious, but older people are used to being deferred to respectfully.

Marriage confers respectability on mixed social relationships, which otherwise are difficult to experience in conservative families and community settings. In the more traditional Palestinian communities, marriages are not contracted directly between the couple but by negotiation between representatives of the families. There has, however, been an increase in the number of consensual marriages in recent years, shifting the criteria on which spouses are chosen from scrutiny of family background towards compatibility and personal qualities (Sayigh 1989). Several marriages among PWD are a result of friendships developing in the rehabilitation center, though the non-disabled spouses' families needed time to accept this in some cases (Daoud 1996, lecture to physical and occupational therapy students, Bethlehem University, December). However, it must be admitted that a severely disabled woman will not find it so easy to find a marriage partner, presumably because it is more difficult for her to fulfill society's expectations (Younis 1995).

In the development of a collective response to rehabilitation, Palestinian community leaders are influential. Formerly these leaders were respected persons from prominent local families, possibly active in the mosque or other forum. Recently, they are as likely to have a prominent role in the wider political, educational, or social sphere. These leaders have an important function in maintaining social justice and order, mediating disputes between families and individuals, and brokering marriage and other contracts. Although many of these leaders are very concerned about the welfare of the people in their area and may personally accept people's disabilities, they do not always have a realistic knowledge of the limitations imposed by a disability. Nevertheless, it is extremely difficult to introduce anything new into the local community without the approval of these leaders, or at least their knowledge, and therefore they should be included in the planning of community rehabilitation programs (Younis 1995).

BELIEFS ABOUT HEALTH AND HEALING

Rehabilitation professionals would be wise to learn about the local cultural beliefs about health and healing. The concepts of health, wellbeing, peace and serenity are closely related in Arabic, and usually expressed in the word *salaam*. *Salaam* is used extensively in greetings and everyday expressions and is usually translated simply as peace. The word is from the same root as *Islam* and *Muslim*.

Islam sees health and disease in the integrated context of the spiritual, ecological, and social environment. The entire life is guided and directed towards wholesomeness and longevity, with the emphasis on prevention. Individuals and societies are seen as located within the context of nature, society, and humankind, within a oneness and unity of all creation (Khan 1986).

The sick and disabled are excused observance of the five obligations of Islam if they have difficulty performing them. These obligations include profession of faith, prayer, fasting, pilgrimage and almsgiving. *Surah* (chapter) 24, verse 61 of the *Qur'an* says, 'There is no fault in the blind, nor in one born lame, nor in one afflicted with illness' (Ali 1938), which directly disputes any superstition that disability is a sign of the displeasure of God. However, some people do continue to think in this way, or at least will greet such events with phrases such as 'God willing' or 'God is generous.'

There is quite an extensive historical pharmacopoeia (the apothecary was originally an Arab development), and the words alcohol, elixir, and syrup all derive from Arabic (Moloney 1985). The use of various herbs is quite widespread, and various household substances are used as first aid. For example, hemorrhages may be treated with a compress of coffee grounds; cuts from rusty nails or other corroded objects are given a heat treatment by touching the area with a smoldering cloth; scorpion and snake bites are treated by bleeding the area immediately, possibly sucking and spitting out the contaminated blood (Younis 1998).

Herbal remedies are used for treatment of abdominal and chest pain, abscesses, respiratory problems and in obstetrics. Examples include using hot baked onions as a dressing for an abscess (or a compress of pepper leaves if the abscess is new), infusions of fenugreek, ginger and honey or of chamomile and cumin for coughs, thickened mixtures of fenugreek, cumin and anise for promoting lactation, infusions of sage or cumin and honey for colic pain in children. When a newborn child fails to gain weight, infusions of fenugreek or other herbs are used. Sesame seed oil or menthol are rubbed on the chest in cases of breathing difficulty. Olive oil is widely used to soften and soothe skin complaints (Simister, unpublished work 1997; Younis 1998). Bonesetting and strains and sprains are all still treated by types of splinting and a method of plastering using egg, grated soap and flour, possibly with the addition of sweet smelling herbs. The bonesetter will not usually reduce the fracture, and often the splinting is very tight, causing a greater risk of vascular problems or malunion of the bones (Younis 1998).

Massage (an Arabic word from *masa'*, meaning to touch) is used for headaches, abdominal and back pain, and joint injuries by people who have inherited the skill through generations: the practicing member of a family usually passes on the skill to one of the offspring with the same gift, and thus particular families gain a reputation for this healing art. Children's spasms with fevers due to fright are treated by massaging the pubic area with olive oil (Younis 1998). Newborn babies are frequently massaged with olive oil during the first weeks of life, in combination with manipulative movements, and often the child will be swaddled for a few hours every day for the first few weeks (Odeh 1995). One of the most frequent ailments treated is Bell's palsy, either by slapping the face with slippers covered in poultry excrement, or pressing the side of the face underfoot (serious damage has been known to occur from this). Manipulation is used for back pain. Treatment usually includes covering the body with warmed oil and blankets, followed by manipulation and traction of the whole spinal column (Younis 1998).

An ancient and still widely used method of pain relief throughout the Arab world is cautery, administered by the local wise man or *hakim* over the site of the pain as a counter-irritation. This use occurs even amongst educated families, chiefly for headaches and sciatic pain. Cupping (inverting a warmed vessel over a painful area to relieve pressure through suction), hot sand bags and hot water bottles are used extensively in treatments of back pain, dysmenorrhea and any soft tissue injury. Cold water is used for recent injuries and burns (Younis 1998).

Another widely used traditional method of healing could be termed spiritual because it is administered by a *mushawith* (magician, charlatan or quack) and involves recitations of verses of strange words, burning of sweet smelling herbs and wearing of amulets containing illegible words as protection against the devil, the cause of disease. The *mushawith* will also prescribe actions such as slaughtering a sheep or a male turkey. Being of a superstitious nature, all of this is forbidden by Islam and in some countries could lead to imprisonment (Younis 1998).

Many people believe in magic and the evil eye. These are sometimes thought to cause a disability. People attempt routinely to divert this power by proverbs and small actions. For example, no-one should ever be complimented on their beauty or possessions. Spells can be detected by a *sheikh* (religious leader or teacher),

who will also perform exorcisms in accordance with Islam, using readings from the *Qur'an* and prayers. The *sheikh* will never do any harm, but the *mushawith* will cast harmful spells for a large fee (Younis 1998).

Treatment by reading the *Qur'an* is also known following the example of the Prophet Mohammed who used soothing actions and readings to cure pain. There is a *Qur'an* treatment unit at the Disabled Association in one of the West Bank towns (Qalqilia), where patients with epilepsy are treated by playing tapes of the *Qur'an* very loudly through headphones. Treatment using the *Qur'an* is also used for children with mumps (still regarded as a dangerous disease because of its possible effect on fertility): the child is taken to the *sheikh* to have a verse from the *Qur'an* written on his face (Younis 1998).

Although many people now have access to modern methods of treatment and facilities, albeit with difficulty, many of the treatments and attitudes of the past concerning health persist, especially in remote areas. Many people continue to consult a traditional or spiritual healer as a first resort, especially for chronic diseases and permanent disabilities. Others will consult these alternative healers if they are not happy with the modern doctors' approach (i.e. the prognosis is not hopeful, there is no improvement), often traveling long distances and paying much more than to a doctor. All consultations are complicated by the fact that very few doctors or healers will say outright if the condition is unlikely to improve (as is typical with many kinds of disabling impairments), but will delay the bad news by holding out hope of a cure. When no cure appears, the opinions of other healers are sought.

REHABILITATION SERVICES FOR PALESTINIAN PEOPLE

Rehabilitation services have suffered from fragmentary funding and organization, mainly because of too few knowledgeable or suitably qualified personnel at all levels. The field has been dominated by non-governmental organizations, given the lack of governmental structure over the last decades (Barghouthi & Giacaman 1990). Although the newly-constituted Palestinian National Authority (PNA) now has partial responsibility for health and social welfare, lack of funding will force continued reliance on international and voluntary aid for the foreseeable future (PHC 1993). The organizations active in the rehabilitation field now range from local committees and cooperatives formed by parents and friends of PWD (and PWD themselves) through the larger charitable institutions that have founded the major rehabilitation centers, to international organizations that provide funding, usually via local partner organizations (Younis 1998; Younis, paper prepared for the Global Disability meeting of the SCF, April 1994, unpublished).

International support

The reliance on international funding continues to include foreign personnel, especially for training programs in unfamiliar skills. These workers will probably be selected for their professional expertise and though they might have visited the region, or at least have a strong impression of its identity from a biblical or tourist point of view, this knowledge is likely to be 'generally uninformed, diffuse and tangential' (Bowman 1992). If at all possible, it makes sense for foreign workers to acquaint themselves with the living conditions, expectations, and social norms of the community in which they will be working. This is a prerequisite to respecting these values meticulously in a non-judgmental way, harmonizing the therapeutic approach with the aspirations of the client.

International support tends to be contingent on the national priorities, history, and concepts of that funder's origin. For example, the bachelor's level physiotherapy program recently implemented by Bethlehem University with funding from British sources and British professional leadership was founded on a British curriculum modified to fit into an American educational model. Similarly, the Swedish-funded initiatives to improve the orthotics

workshop at the Princess Basma Center used Swedish expertise and technology and imported Swedish equipment; their rehabilitation program for people with spinal cord injury in Abu Raya Center was originally in Swedish translated into English, though intended for Arabic speakers.

Problems

International organizations and their local partners bring a global perspective to bear in project planning, presumably motivated by a genuine concern to bring the best benefits possible to the people. But sadly the best efforts frequently backfire: equipment is not used to optimum advantage, people do not come to the facilities, staff feel that somehow their work is missing its mark. What has happened?

Some of the problems arise from the policies of the funders. For example, the major need is for operating costs. However, the constitutions of many development aid organizations forbid them to fund these costs, as opposed to expensive and extensive imported equipment. This equipment, a long time in transit from the donor country, may well arrive damaged. But few funding proposals include maintenance or training in maintenance, so costly yet potentially useful items lie unused. Sometimes indeed, the terms of the donation state that international expertise must be used, e.g. Japanese kidney dialysis machines that only Japanese engineers may maintain.

Another problem associated with international funding is the time lag between a proposal and its acceptance. A proposal to fund a desperately needed audiology diagnostic center in Gaza was submitted to the European Union (EU). Approval came 3 years later, by which time two other centers were running in the suggested location. Changing the location, type of center, or type of service would require another proposal, resulting in further delays before it could be implemented.

Another difficulty is the physical terrain of the Palestinian communities. The developed world's expectation of a rehabilitation program that includes, for example, 'Western'-style wheelchair management and driving a car is not valid. Locomotion is difficult even for the able-bodied in the crowded and sand-logged refugee camps of the Gaza Strip: the streets are often very narrow and frequently have an open sewage channel down the center. The hilly villages of the West Bank have steep tracks impassable to wheelchairs and multi-level houses built into the slopes. In the Old City quarters of ancient urban centers such as Jerusalem and Nablus, centuries-old houses have been extended in piecemeal fashion and now have awkward access, with twists and turns and many flights of steps.

Other problems are intrinsic to the Palestinian sociopolitical situation, whereby concerted health planning has been almost impossible. Organizations operating in the Palestinian community often lack coordination and often take a 'splintered, single issue approach to health problems which are increasingly complex and often inter-related' (Abdeen 1992, p. 2). The maldistribution of services also remains a problem.

Furthermore, Palestinian society is in social and political transition, and needs and priorities are changing perceptibly (Simister, unpublished work 1995). A project begun in 1988 (early *Intifada*) needed a thorough evaluation and review in 1993 (beginning of transition from Israeli to Palestinian authority) and will need to be assessed again in the future as the political situation evolves. This will be especially true if the program is creating a major change in conditions, such as has occurred in training people in the rehabilitation professions. As an example, international physical therapy personnel coming to the area during the *Intifada* revolutionized ideas of what could be achieved through this style of treatment and brought demands for other kinds of therapy. As a result of their influence in practice and training, there is a newly established Palestinian physical therapy profession with some 270 physical therapists (Younis and Dawson, unpublished work 1991). On the other hand, only a handful of speech, audio or play therapists, special educators, or other rehabilitation professionals exist (see Ch. 30).

The case of occupational therapy is different again. A few international occupational therapists have worked in the Palestinian community, and there is a diploma-level training program in neighboring Jordan, which takes a quota of Palestinian students. However, the Palestinian Ministry of Higher Education has challenged plans to implement a local bachelor's level program in occupational therapy. According to the ministry, the school is not staffed by qualified personnel according to the World Federation of Occupational Therapists, and it is not valid for the current Palestinian situation. This itself shows an encouraging dimension of empowerment of the receiving community, in that they now feel able to insist on development projects of internationally recognized standards and national validity.

SUMMARY

Rehabilitation aims to facilitate a PWD's participation in normal everyday life to the fullest extent that the person desires. Much of Palestinian everyday life consists of community and family customs which the health practitioner should recognize as central to the clients' self-esteem and standing in the community. A token nod towards the life values of the patients is not sufficient. The caring professional must understand the people's concerns, their mode of life, their religious and moral values, and the basics of their social structures, in order for advice and treatment to be meaningful. Also, a purely biomedical (functional) approach to rehabilitation is out of place, as is a purely psychosocial approach: both should be united.

Direct transfer of knowledge from one culture to another is unlikely to be valid, and therefore foreign consultants are strongly advised to cooperate closely with local professional leaders in their field, and particularly not to work in the community alone. However, they should also recognize that local advice will probably be subjective, depending on the individual concerns and interests, and therefore discretion should be exercised in balancing different opinions. It is important to remember that in many situations no clear national policy exists and no reliable assessment of needs has been made.

It is important to develop a rehabilitation sector that is affordable and sustainable, and appropriate to the physical and social–political realities. The individual beneficiaries of rehabilitation programs understand their opportunities and limitations most clearly, because they are living at the interface between project planning and the constraints of what is practical in the real life situation. They should be fully involved in the planning and implementation of rehabilitation programs.

Finally, a rehabilitation program must recognize the impact of cultural values on the rehabilitation process itself and use these values to involve the family and community fully. The designers of any community program should hold these values in their minds, because the program's successful outcome will depend on working with, and not against, these values in its development (Younis 1995).

REFERENCES

Abdeen Z 1992 A health strategy for the Occupied Territories. Proceedings of the 'Palestine for Peace' Conference, Brussels, Sept 28–Oct 1, 1992. Network of European NGOs in the Occupied Territories, Jerusalem

Abdel-Shafi K 1992 General social services in the Occupied Palestinian Territories. Proceedings of the 'Palestine for Peace' Conference, Brussels, Sept 28–Oct 1, 1992. Network of European NGOs in the Occupied Territories, Jerusalem

Ali A Y 1938 The Glorious Kur'an: translation and commentary, 3rd edn. Sheikh Muhammed Ashraf, Lahore

Barghouthi M, Giacaman R 1990 The emergence of an infrastructure of resistance: the case of health. In: Nassar J R, Heacock R (eds) Intifada: Palestine at the crossroads Praeger, New York

Barghouthi M, Daibes I 1993 Infrastructure and health services in the West Bank: guidelines for health care planning. Health Development Information Project in cooperation with the World Health Organization, Ramallah, West Bank

Bowman G 1992 The politics of tour guiding: Israeli and Palestinian tour guides in Israel and the Occupied Territories. In: Harrison D (ed) Tourism and the less developed countries. Wiley and Sons, London

FAFO 1993 Report 151: Palestinian society in Gaza, West Bank and Arab Jerusalem: a survey of living conditions. Fagbevegelsens Senter for Forskning, Utredning og Dokumentasjon, Oslo

Gaff A 1994 The human rights of persons with disabilities. Al-Haq, West Bank

Geraisy S F 1994 Socio-demographic characteristics: reality, problems and aspirations within Israel. In: Prior M, Taylor W (eds) Christians in the Holy Land. World of Islam Festival Trust, London

Giacaman R, Daibes I 1989 Towards the formulation of a rehabilitation policy: disability in the West Bank. Bir Zeit University, West Bank

Keesing R M 1981 Cultural anthropology: a contemporary perspective. Holt, Rinehart and Winston, New York

Khader N R 1996 Socio-economic and health profile of the Palestinian Arab inhabitants of the Old City of Jerusalem. Society for Austro-Arab Relations, Jerusalem

Khan M S 1986 Islamic medicine. Routledge and Kegan Paul, London

Leach E 1982 Social anthropology. Fontana, Glasgow

Moloney G E 1985 A doctor in Saudi Arabia. Regency Press, London

Morgan R 1989 The demon lover. Norton, New York

Odeh J 1995 Congenital dislocation of the hip: the influence of certain factors including the practice of swaddling. A study in the village of Biddhu. Bulletin of the Palestinian Child Society 1 (3): 249–256

Sabella B 1994 Socio-economic characteristics and the challenges to Palestinian Christians in the Holy Land. In: Prior M, Taylor W (eds) Christians in the Holy Land. World of Islam Festival Trust, London

Sayigh R 1989 Palestinian women: triple burden, single struggle. In: Khamsin (ed) Palestine, profile of an occupation. Zed Books, London

Simister, J. Research in progress, concerning international development workers in the Palestinian community, registered with the University of Ulster, UK

UPMRC (Union of Palestinian Medical Relief Committees) 1987 An overview of health conditions and services in the Israeli Occupied Territories. Union of Palestinian Medical Relief Committees, Jerusalem

Wade D T 1995 Measurement in neurological rehabilitation. Oxford University Press, Oxford

YMCA/Beit Sahour Rehabilitation Program 1994 Palestinian disability survey: West Bank. East Jerusalem YMCA, Jerusalem

Younis A A 1995 The influence of a traditional society on the emergence of a rehabilitation program for spinal cord injured people. Proceedings of the 12th Congress of the World Confederation of Physical Therapists, Washington

Younis A A 1998 Social reintegration of spinal cord injured people in Palestine. Doctoral Thesis, University of Ulster, UK

23

Upgrading physical therapy education in Vietnam

Elizabeth Kay
Nguyen Thi Huong
Nguygen Thi Minh Chau

INTRODUCTION

The Vietnam Project began in March 1993 as a cooperative effort between Health Volunteers Overseas (Washington, DC) and the Vietnamese Ministry of Health (MoH), with funding from the United States Agency for International Development (USAID). Its goal is to improve rehabilitation services in Vietnam. This five and one-half year project is a national multi-disciplinary effort that includes the disciplines and specialties of orthopedic surgery, physiatry, rehabilitation nursing, and physical therapy. This chapter focuses on the physical therapy portion of the project and describes an intervention to upgrade physical therapy in a developing country through the education of local professionals.

The thirteenth most populated nation in the world, Vietnam's population has grown rapidly (2.2% per year), its per capita income is low ($240/year), and the child malnutrition rate is high (42%) (UNICEF 1994). About 40% of the Vietnamese are under the age of 15 years (World Bank 1993) and 80% live at subsistence level (Tue 1993). Compounding the health care problems created by poverty, Vietnam's health care system has had to deal with the large number of people injured by war.

NEED FOR REHABILITATION IN VIETNAM

The Ministry of Health (MoH) estimates that 5–6% of Vietnam's 65 million citizens (4 million people) have a disability (Q P Lung, personal communication 1993). Of these people with disabilities, the MoH estimates that 55% have motor impairments, 34% are deaf or blind, 8% have mental retardation, and 3% have other types of disabilities. The most common causes of motor problems are polio, cerebral palsy, cerebral vascular accidents, and trauma that results in fractures, head injuries, spinal cord injuries, and amputations. Some of these pathologies are regional in distribution (for example, respiratory problems are more common near the coal mines in the central regions, and vehicle accidents are mostly limited to the biggest cities). The MoH estimates that 1 400 000 Vietnamese, including war veterans, need but are not receiving rehabilitation for their disabilities.

The MoH estimates may be high, however. Detailed data on disabilities collected by community based rehabilitation (CBR) projects operating in 52 communes in five districts of Quangnam-Danang province are of interest for verifying national estimates. The population in the five districts is 198 155 people of whom 7029 (3.55%) have disabilities and 1466 (20.86% of the disabled) are reported to be in need of rehabilitation (V N Se, personal communication 1993).

This disability rate, well below both the World Health Organization estimate of 10% and the MoH estimate of 5–6%, suggests that Vietnam's incidence of disability has been overestimated, a phenomenon that has been discussed by other authors (Miles 1986, Marfo 1995). A more reasonable estimate of the number of Vietnamese with disabilities who require rehabilitation is probably about 550 000. Using Quangnam-Danang's finding that 41% of the people with disabilities had difficulty with moving, the national estimate for those needing rehabilitation to improve movement is probably about 225 000 – less than one sixth of the MoH estimate but still a sizable challenge for Vietnam's health care system.

Despite the large number of people with amputations from the war, polio and cerebral palsy are the main causes of movement prob-

lems in Quangnam-Danang. However, a child immunization program has been quite successful and 92–94% of all children in Vietnam have been immunized. There were only two new cases of polio treated in the province in 1993, although treatment of the polio sequelae will remain a problem in Vietnam for many decades.

THE VIETNAM PROJECT

Project management

The Vietnam Project is being implemented through the joint efforts of four major working groups: the Washington, DC, staff of Health Volunteers Overseas (HVO), HVO staff in Hanoi, an American technical advisory group (TAG), and the Vietnamese rehabilitation steering committee to the MoH. The HVO-Washington staff administers the grant funds, completes all grant reports, and coordinates all US-based activities and communications. The HVO-Hanoi staff is responsible for all communication and for organizing all activities in Vietnam. The TAG, made up of volunteers representing each of the disciplines and specialties included in the grant activities, sets project objectives, recruits and coordinates volunteers, and plans the content of activities. The Vietnamese rehabilitation steering committee suggests grant activities, as well as the locations and participants suitable for those activities, and assists with obtaining government permissions and approvals. Any disagreements about activities or priorities are generally resolved through direct discussions between members of the two advisory groups, but HVO-Washington staff make all final decisions. This administrative structure has proven quite efficient and is useful for providing input from the Vietnamese and the American rehabilitation professionals.

Project implementation

The project has been divided into two phases. The first phase, lasting a year and a half, focused on developing the team approach and the professional skills of the project's orthopedic surgeons, physiatrists, nurses, and physical therapists. In response to a request to update professional education to improve management of patients in several diagnostic groups, the program started with a series of multidisciplinary workshops. The 1–2 week workshops covered the medical, surgical, and rehabilitation management of patients with:

- orthopedic injury due to trauma
- neurological damage secondary to stroke or brain injury
- amputations
- spinal cord injuries
- cerebral palsy
- rheumatoid arthritis and other connective tissue diseases
- burns (pediatric and adult).

Four themes ran throughout the workshop series:

1. the application of all skills and knowledge to community-based rehabilitation as well as to central and provincial-level hospitals
2. the use of realistic and appropriate functional goals
3. a focus on generic treatment theories and techniques, with an emphasis on practicing assessment and problem-solving skills
4. generalization of all problem-solving and treatments skills to other diagnostic groups in addition to the one focused on at the particular workshop.

The workshops were useful in teaching basic knowledge and skills, but the multidisciplinary focus also proved invaluable for getting doctors to interact with therapists and nurses as colleagues rather than technicians who worked under their orders. The modeling of professional interactions and team roles by the visiting doctors, nurses, and therapists contributed to redefining the role and status of therapists at least among the rehabilitation professionals. For the physical therapists, the formation of relationships with colleagues from other regions of Vietnam was another important outcome.

While more diagnoses could have been addressed in the workshop phase, HVO decided that the project had met the goals of teaching basic patient management and introducing the team concept. The TAG felt that it would be more beneficial to redirect the project towards needs specific to a profession or specialty. In physical therapy the transition from team workshops to these activities for members of individual professions was preceded by a meeting to establish priorities. Participants included the head teachers and teachers from the three physical therapy schools in Hai Duong (north region), Danang (central region) and Ho Chi Minh City (south), clinicians from hospitals in the north, central, and south regions, and two HVO physical therapist volunteers. The issues and problems identified at this meeting were used for planning the next 4 years of this project. Table 23.1 summarizes the issues, problems, and suggested solutions that were identified through collaboration of the Vietnamese physical therapists and the HVO physical therapist volunteers. It also summarizes the progress that has been made through 1996 in dealing with these issues.

The inclusion of therapists, and the educators of therapists, from a variety of regions and work environments was important for gathering information on how to improve physical therapy services in Vietnam. The issues were identified by having the participants work in small groups that were varied for each task. Information on the most common medical diagnoses seen by physical therapists was collected by region because regional variation had been mentioned as a concern and it seemed best to start with groups of people who were familiar with each other. Although this was not a controlled system of data collection, it was interesting that all of the physical therapists saw a similar variety of patients regardless of the region they worked in. Furthermore, the physical therapy problems presented by these patients appeared to be virtually identical. Due to the similarity of medical diagnoses and physical therapy problems seen in the three regions of Vietnam, the professional knowledge and skills that need to be learned are uniform throughout the country.

Table 23.1 Overview of issues, problems, recommendations, and progress*

Issues	Relevant problems	Suggested solutions	Progress (March 1993–June 1996)
1. Inconsistent and inefficient physical therapy treatment with inadequate focus on functional outcomes	Need to know how to work effectively on a rehabilitation team for patients requiring more complex care	Team workshops on select diagnostic groups	Six workshops were held on different diagnoses
	Physical therapists need a course to update their knowledge, decision-making skills, and practice	Develop and offer an update course for physical therapists	The manual for a 2-week update course was completed. Three pilot courses have been run by HVO volunteers and five have been run by Vietnamese teachers
2. Weaknesses in service delivery	Many provincial or district hospitals lack positions for physical therapists	Encourage hiring of physical therapists at all provincial and district hospitals	See No. 6 below
	People often lack transportation and funds to get care at even the district level	Fund physical therapy rooms and equipment at hospitals and facilitate CBR	Some local efforts to convince health services to fund
	Therapists do not always know how to work effectively with CBR workers	Increase cooperation with CBR training and programs	Increased cooperation with CBR training programs. Head physical therapy teachers at Schools No. 2 and No. 3 are regional CBR coordinators
3. Lack of standardization of credentials and training of people working in physical therapy	Many graduates of physical therapy are unemployed or under-employed Assistant doctors, nurses, and others are hired to provide 'physical therapy'	Ministry of Health should establish credentials needed for those hired as physical therapists. Those working as physical therapists prior to 1990 should be accepted, but all others should need to be graduates of Schools No. 1–3	No progress made to date with the MoH, but teacher(s) at School No. 3 are working with the heads of hospitals and rehabilitation departments to increase jobs and to encourage the hiring of physical therapy school graduates only
4. Educational preparation of physical therapy students	Curriculum content and length	Consultant assistance to design new curriculum Focus training on physical disabilities Increase program to at least 3 years	Workshop to develop a new bachelor's degree curriculum was held July 1996
	Education is only at the diploma level	Discuss changing from a diploma to a bachelor's degree program	Permission granted by MoH and MoEd to Hanoi Medical College for bachelor's degree
5. Teacher preparation	Need for higher academic credentials	Teachers need a minimum of a bachelor's degree and ideally a master's degree	College level bachelor's degree offered part-time in Ho Chi Minh City. Plan to discuss other programs with MoH and MoEd. Physical Therapy Overseas to assist with instruction
	Need for improved knowledge of teaching methods	Instruction in teaching methods with guidance in applying them	Course offered at School No. 3 in Ho Chi Minh City
	Need for increased knowledge in theory and practice of physical therapy	International intervention to assist the teachers of physical therapy	Workshops and update course experiences. Donation of audio-visual equipment and books

Table 23.1 Overview of issues, problems, recommendations, and progress* (contd.)

Issues	Relevant problems	Suggested solutions	Progress (March 1993–June 1996)
6. Need to recognize knowledge base of physical therapy is different from, although related to, training and practice of physicians	Doctors do not have knowledge or skill base to direct physical therapy education	Prepare physical therapists to direct their own educational programs by having a knowledge of the scientific basis of physical therapy	Workshops provided some knowledge as did the donation of books. However, HVO participation in implementing new curricula, more books, and requests to other organizations to assist are essential
	Doctors in hospitals need to have a better understanding of the benefits of physical therapy	Provide Vietnamese doctors with training on the need for rehabilitation and the role of physical therapists	Team approach modeling and message in workshops. Workshop for physiatrists included relationship with physical therapists
7. Difficulties advancing physical therapy	Need to lobby for and implement above	Organize a national physical therapy organization	Tentative approval of rehabilitation leadership but government freeze on formation of new organizations
		Vietnam National Rehabilitation Association (VINA RHEP) and steering committee representation	Physical therapist representative named to VINARHEA executive committee and steering committee
		Join the World Confederation for Physical Therapy and the international community of therapists	WCPT contacted but can not join until national organization is authorized

* The progress listed above includes all changes that have occurred and are not all the direct result of HVO involvement.

OBSTACLES TO ADVANCING PHYSICAL THERAPY IN VIETNAM

Many issues interfere with providing suitable and efficient physical therapy in Vietnam. These include an inadequate knowledge of functional assessment and treatment, a lack of standardization in the credentials of people who work as physical therapists, multiple sociopolitical and environmental problems that limit the delivery of physical therapy, the low status of physical therapists, the limited educational credentials of physical therapists, inadequate teacher preparation, an outdated curriculum in physical therapy education programs, and a lack of understanding among the Vietnamese about physical therapy. All of these issues are interrelated, but the most critical ones are the knowledge and skill levels of the practicing therapists and the need to improve the accessibility of services to better utilize these skills. The education of new therapists is a secondary concern: some of those issues, such as teacher preparation, would be addressed when updating the knowledge and skills of the current therapists. The process of participating in workshops and developing an update course will also prepare the teachers to take a more active role in determining what curricular changes are needed. Political issues, such as the advancement of the profession and getting the MoH to allow only the graduates of the three physical therapy schools to call themselves physical therapists are long-term goals that will take continued effort. Given these priorities, the physical therapy portion of the project's second phase started

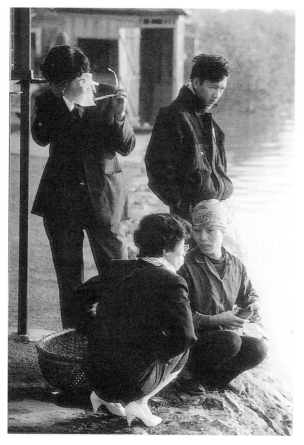

Fig. 23.1 Traditional bargaining in Vietnam is done squatting, making this an important position to train during rehabilitation (Nguyen Minh Chau, BS, PT, bargaining in the Haiphong).

with a focus on updating patient management skills.

For the two decades preceding 1993, an international embargo isolated all of Vietnam from the Western world. Prior to 1973, the USA had been influential in medical and dental education in South Vietnam, although Canadians ran School No. 3 in Ho Chi Minh City from 1972 to 1975. In 1993 medical education and care in the southern and central portions of Vietnam were still very American in style. The teachers from Schools No. 2 (Danang) and No. 1 (Hai Duong) were mostly educated at School No. 3 during the 1980s, providing some uniformity in education and practice throughout Vietnam. However, the therapists in the North had been heavily influenced by ties to Eastern Europe during the 1980s and early 1990s. Hence, physical therapists in the North use more heat, electrotherapy, massage, and hydrotherapy, with a concomitant reduction in exercise and functional training, than is practiced in the southern and central regions of Vietnam.

Despite any historical differences, there are many common needs. Since the therapists had been educated as technicians, it was decided that they would benefit from learning clinical decision-making skills as well as evaluation, goal setting, and treatment planning for functional outcomes (Fig. 23.1). Treatment skills need to be enhanced in some areas, but most therapists have at least basic treatment skills that just need to be used more effectively. The HVO workshops in phase one began this educational process.

Updating therapist knowledge

A group of Vietnamese physical therapist educators and clinicians from the three regions of Vietnam worked with experienced physical therapist educators from HVO to develop a 2-week 'update' course. Two weeks is the longest that clinicians can practically be away for a course. The course is participatory and flexible enough to accommodate the varying knowledge levels and skill needs of the physical therapists throughout Vietnam. It emphasizes direct patient care. Because the model is self-sufficiency through educating local professionals, the project prepared Vietnamese teachers to teach the course in their own regions of the country. The Vietnamese teachers designated to teach the update course attended one course to learn content and provide input regarding its suitability, a second course as an assistant to HVO volunteer instructors, and a third as the course instructor with an HVO assistant. Vietnamese will teach all subsequent courses.

A manual was developed to provide structure and uniformity to the courses. It also provides some reference information because language and finances make it difficult for the therapists, especially in rural areas, to have access to professional books and materials.

Employment

Although the update course is a step towards making physical therapy services more relevant to Vietnamese people with disabilities, multiple problems limit the availability and effectiveness of physical rehabilitation in the country. For example, many provincial and district hospitals lack positions for physical therapists, and even when rehabilitation departments exist the positions are often filled by assistant doctors and nurses who are not educated in rehabilitation. Hence, although only about 700 graduates of the three physical therapy programs are actively interested in working in physical therapy, unemployment is a big problem. This is especially remarkable in that there are no Vietnamese occupational therapists. To match the employment needs of the physical therapy graduates with the rehabilitation needs of people with disabilities, it is important to convince officials at the MoH and the health services to employ physical therapists in the rehabilitation departments of hospitals. It has been suggested to the MoH that it limit the practice of physical therapy to graduates of the three physical therapy programs and individuals who had been working as 'physical therapists' since 1989. This does not exclude the training and hiring of technicians to provide some supervised care, or the training of CBR workers, but it would guarantee that professionals provide therapy.

Although no progress has yet been made with government regulation, Nguyen Thi Huong, director of rehabilitation at School No. 3, has identified unemployed graduates in areas without physical therapists. Her efforts to educate hospital administrators in the South about the importance of including physical therapy have

been successful in creating jobs at Duc Trong District Hospital (Lam Dong Province) and the Rehabilitation Center in Vung Liem District (Vinh Long Province). Credit also goes to Handicap International (HI) which supported these new departments and positions by donating equipment and supplies. Key to the success in both efforts was the identification of unemployed therapists who lived in the districts with inadequate rehabilitation services, the personal intervention by a respected and experienced Vietnamese physical therapist, and the willingness of a donor to respond to local initiatives.

Because of the large number of unemployed therapists (Table 23.2), increasing the effectiveness and employment of therapists is more important than increasing the number of graduates. A trend at the central level to redirect rehabilitation resources away from professional services to non-professionals in community based rehabilitation is a concern. While the therapists recognize that the MoH strongly supports the concept of CBR to meet the needs of people with disabilities, especially in the rural areas, there is concern that CBR is being considered a replacement for physical therapy services. It is essential to convince the MoH officials that an effective CBR program requires competent professionals to provide complex care when it is required. However, it is also recognized that therapists need to learn the knowledge and skills to support CBR. All physical therapy goals and activities need to be consistent with the existence of CBR and the needs of the community. Because the head physical therapy teachers at Schools No. 2 and No. 3 are also regional coordinators for CBR, they have been instrumental in incorporating CBR principles and instruction on appropriate technology into both the update course and the diploma curriculum.

Physical therapy education

All three MoH-run physical therapy programs are two and a half years long and grant a diploma at graduation. However, the effectiveness of these programs is of concern; the teachers and graduates think that the curriculum is

Table 23.2 Employment and unemployment of therapists

Region/School No.	Employed in physical therapy	Unemployed or work outside physical therapy
North/School No. 1	53%	47%
Central/School No. 2	12.5%	87.5%
South/School No. 3	40%	60%

outdated and insufficient in depth. The three programs share a curriculum that was originally written in 1978 and last modified in April 1989. Authored by physicians from the areas of medical training and rehabilitation, it does not represent input from physical therapists – an issue that concerns many Vietnamese rehabilitation experts.

Before curricular changes can be initiated, decisions need to be made about the role of the graduate. The therapists feel that graduates in Vietnam should be able to provide comprehensive treatment for people with movement problems. This would require the curriculum to move from a focus on performing treatment with modalities and manipulation to a focus on functional goals and the exercise, mobility training, and training in activities of daily living (including vocational and avocational pursuits) that are needed to meet those goals. Foundation courses in biomechanics, lifespan changes, the neurosciences (especially motor control), exercise physiology, and the scientific basis of movement and exercise all need to be introduced to provide the theoretical basis for physical therapy evaluation and treatment. Given the volume of information that needs to be introduced to the curriculum, there is a consensus that the minimum length of study should be increased to 3 years. Furthermore, international consultation from physical therapists is encouraged to assist the effort of the MoH and the directors from the three programs to develop a curriculum that includes the knowledge and skills taught in more developed countries, meets internationally accepted standards, and prepares graduates to provide effective treatment that meets the needs of Vietnamese with physical disabilities.

The diploma level, as opposed to baccalaureate education, has immediate advantages in Vietnam. A 3-year diploma would allow for improvements in professional preparation for clinicians without significantly increasing the education costs or the number of graduates. Having a diploma also makes the graduates more likely to accept the present pay scale for physical therapists in Vietnam. Given these advantages, diploma-level education is expected to continue in Vietnam. However, fundamental changes in content and length raise the issue of changing the physical therapy educational program to the baccalaureate degree level. Independent physical therapy practice is a necessity in Vietnam because physician supervision is impractical given the shortage of physicians outside of the urban areas and physicians' lack of knowledge about physical therapy. Independent practice is more consistent with a university degree, and university graduates should be more cost-effective despite the increased costs of educating and employing them. Cost-effectiveness would be achieved as university graduates practice more independently and take over supervisory roles. However, it is not unusual in developing countries for higher paying foreign businesses and non-profit organizations, as well as overseas recruiters, to lure university graduates with a bachelor's degree away from the profession or country for which they were educated.

In March 1996, the MoH and the Ministry of Education and Training authorized Hanoi Medical College and Nam Dinh Medical High School to jointly offer the first baccalaureate program in Vietnam. The degree program is intended to educate teachers and hospital department heads. A workshop to start the development of a baccalaureate curriculum took place in July 1996. Modifications to that proposed curriculum were made in December 1998 in order to meet new government regulations.

Teacher preparation

Teacher preparation is an issue whether physical therapy is taught at the diploma or the baccalaureate level. Only two physical therapy teachers (both from School No. 3) have completed more than diploma-level education in physical therapy and both received their college degrees in Vietnam. Most teachers have graduated from the very school that employs them, so they have had limited opportunities to learn different knowledge or skills. Schools No. 1 and No. 2 have physicians who teach theory, but even these teachers lack advanced education in their areas of instruction. The physicians also lack education in physical therapy making it difficult to link theory to the practice of physical therapy. Hence the teachers' problems include academic credentials, knowledge in the movement sciences, physical therapy evaluation and treatment skills, inadequate exposure to different teaching methods, and instructional resources, including audiovisual aids and books.

One solution is to persuade the MoH to offer physical therapists the same opportunities as physicians to attend courses in Vietnam and abroad. Currently, physicians get nearly all foreign invitations. Establishing priorities in physical therapy are also essential so that foreign visitors and donors can be better coordinated to meet the priorities identified by the Vietnamese. For example, physical therapy lecturers from different groups and countries need to be directed towards teacher development in the areas the teachers have identified. Both the MoH and the Ministry of Education and Training denied a request for a one-time master's degree program for educating teachers using foreign volunteers, but it is still possible that some of the Vietnamese teachers will have an opportunity to get advanced degrees overseas. School No. 3 has offered a course on teaching methods, and HVO has used all project workshops as opportunities to expose the participants to different teaching methods and styles. Finally, some audiovisual equipment, books, and other educational materials have been donated to the schools, but more donations are still needed.

Recognition of physical therapy in Vietnam

Physical therapy in Vietnam changed to some extent between 1993 and 1997, but more shifts at the national level are still needed and will require active local leadership and a professional association. A government-imposed freeze on new professional organizations has prevented a national physical therapy associa-tion from forming. This has made Vietnamese therapists ineligible to join the World Confederation for Physical Therapy (WCPT), although they have made progress towards joining the international community. Two Vietnamese physical therapists attended the 1995 WCPT Congress with the assistance of HVO, but in general, funding for international travel is inadequate and will affect future participation.

Physical therapists have also made important strides at the national level. The steering committee to the MoH and the executive committee of the Vietnamese National Rehabilitation Association (VINAREHA) have both added a physical therapist member. At the end of 1995, the physician, nurse, and therapist members of the association elected a physical therapist as the vice president for the southern region. Such changes are big improvements for therapists, who had been considered technicians and worked under strict doctors' orders only 3 years earlier.

IMPORTANT LESSONS LEARNED

The HVO/USAID Rehabilitation Project in Vietnam has produced and facilitated many changes in physical therapy, but it also illustrates nine important lessons for future projects.

1. First, sustainability requires that local existing or potential leaders be identified, developed, and given ownership of the project, or its goals, over an established time frame. These key people need to have their leadership and management skills developed, and then they must get the authority to lead. There is a dichotomy in developing countries in that physical therapists may not have the academic credentials for high-level jobs, but once in possession of credentials they may gain responsibility much faster than their counterparts in more developed countries. Neither scenario allows much opportunity for development through mentoring or peer support. Volunteers can effectively provide this support,

but it is important that the volunteers have the appropriate experience, credentials, and abilities for this role.

2. Sustainability requires hosts who are not only prepared to manage the project but feel that it is worth continuing. Make sure that the planning process is inclusive, meaningful to the participants, and in compliance with the regulations of the host country. If a broad base of clinicians, teachers, and decision makers participate in the planning process, they can identify potential problems, explain desired outcomes, and gain a stake in the success of the project. In Vietnam, officials from the Ministry of Health, Ministry of Education and Training, the National Rehabilitation Association, and the school directors all played critical roles in authorizing or supporting different parts of the project.

3. The third lesson concerns critical mass, defined as the smallest number that can achieve an objective or sustain itself. This concept is important because it suggests that it is better to invite two or three therapists from a hospital rather than individual participants from more hospitals. While MoH officials found it more fair or equitable to spread the invitations to as many hospitals as possible, a single person tends to be less successful at effecting change in themselves or their hospital than a group of people who can use each other to reinforce what they have learned. Hence, long-term change occurs more easily by educating groups of therapists.

4. Program success depends on realistic project goals and activities. Both hosts and donors need to avoid being overly optimistic or idealistic, at least in the short term. For example, the Vietnamese therapists need to understand that it is futile to put too much effort into planning to have all physical therapy education in Vietnam move to the baccalaureate level because Vietnam lacks teachers and job opportunities for graduates. Volunteers need to be realistic about the level of professional skills, the level of economic development in Vietnam, and the accessibility issues that the people with disabilities, and hence the therapists, face in Vietnam.

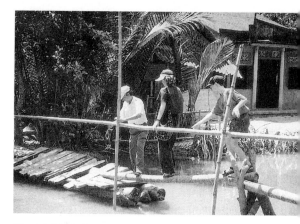

Fig. 23.2 Monkey bridges such as this one create a challenge for people with physical disabilities in the Mekong Delta.

Monkey bridges (single logs that straddle rivers) (Fig. 23.2), inaccessible buildings, uneven surfaces, and bicycle or motorcycle transport are everyday realities in Vietnam. More jobs including homemaking, require manual labor.

5. Cooperation is essential in several respects For example, the Vietnam project utilizes volunteers educated in different countries, and with ties to different treatment philosophies and specialties, yet all of the volunteers worked to coordinate their teaching around the needs identified by an active group of Vietnamese physical therapists. Cooperation between organizations is equally important. Because Handicap International was developing CBR programs, HVO could concentrate on professional development.

6. Respect for colleagues is important. It takes time to understand which differences in practice are necessary local adaptations and which are due to deficits in professional education. Difficulties with communication and variation in skill levels can further confuse the visiting therapists' understanding of what needs to be taught. Respect the host therapists enough to ask them to explain their work conditions, as well as their professional strengths; they acknowledge their weaknesses when they invite your participation in the project. Respect for all colleagues not only improves working relation-

hips but also prevents the hosts from having to choose between their colleagues from other countries and non-governmental organizations. The volunteer organizations benefit from cooperation as it allows all groups to share the cost of effecting a meaningful long-term change.

7. The best volunteers are 'experts' who learn as much as they teach. Volunteers need to be aware of some local pathologies, health care models, patient treatments, financial realities, and patient beliefs. Polio and 'Honda foot' (a complex ankle fracture caused when two motor bikes pass too close) are examples of common pathologies in Vietnam that are unfamiliar to the visiting therapists. CBR is widely used in Vietnam, but the model is relatively new to the volunteers. Since physical therapists in Vietnam are responsible for training CBR workers and assisting with CBR, it is important that the volunteers be aware of this model. Unfamiliar treatments encountered by the volunteers are mostly related to traditional medicine practices, including acupuncture. Another difference is the general lack of funding for health care in Vietnam; the local therapists need to know how to assist the patients and their families with acquiring or making appropriate aids and visiting therapists often need to defer to their 'students' in this area (Fig. 23.3).

8. It is essential that volunteers understand the local beliefs or culture that affect patient and family compliance. For example, some Vietnamese believe that disabilities are due to an error that the person committed in their past life. Although this belief appears to be decreasing, it may cause patients and family members to be fatalistic and unwilling to participate in rehabilitation. Others seek Western medicine because they believe that medicine or massage will provide a quick fix. Patients expect to play a passive role in their rehabilitation, and volunteers often find this frustrating. Another pervasive belief is that respect and responsibility are shown by caring for relatives with disabilities. For example, it is the role of children in Vietnam to show respect for their parents by taking care of them. If an older person has difficulty moving, it can be difficult to

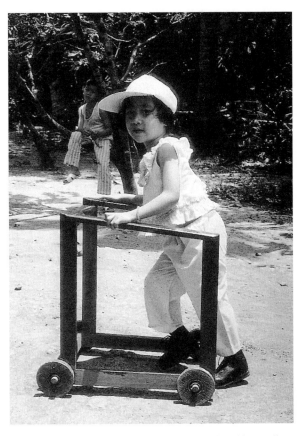

Fig. 23.3 A 5-year-old Vietnamese girl walks with a walker made by the CBR worker and therapist in her village.

get their grown children to encourage physical independence because that is interpreted as a lack of respect. Stressing that therapy will help the patient rejoin or contribute to their family is one strategy for presenting rehabilitation in a way that is compatible with this belief.

9. The final lesson is to have patience! The challenges have probably existed for a long time. Patience is especially important for short-term volunteers, who must accept that they are part of a longer process. Change is generally slow everywhere, but in developing nations the inertia can seem insurmountable. Bureaucracy, a lack of money, and the great need to educate can be formidable obstacles. However, it is worth the time it takes to get things done right. Anticipate a time frame that is realistic for achieving programmatic and personal goals.

CONCLUSION

The HVO Vietnam Project demonstrates how to use short-term volunteers to educate local professionals. On the negative side, there is a potential lack of continuity between the short-term volunteers, inconsistency in the materials they present and the way they present them, and a need for each new volunteer to develop their own reputation. However, even these disadvantages can be minimized by a strong, dedicated coordinator who keeps in close communication with the people in the host country and the volunteers.

This model has four major advantages. It benefits from the input of a large number of volunteer therapists who can bring expertise, ideas, resources, and energy to the project. It is sustainable: the Vietnamese educated during the project are professionals capable of taking over the educational process started during the project. It is appropriate: the training was done in the same environment and with the same patient problems that the participants work with every day. It includes a relatively large number of professionals who can directly benefit from the program. The project in Vietnam illustrates one way to utilize education of local professionals by short-term volunteers to upgrade that profession and the services its members can provide.

REFERENCES

Marfo K 1995 Care of children with disabilities in developing countries. In: Wallace H M, Giri K, Serrano C V (eds) Health care of women and children in developing countries, 2nd edn. Third Party Publishing, Oakland, CA, pp. 550–561

Miles M 1986 Misplanning for disabilities in Asia. In: Marfo K, Walker S, Charles B (eds) Childhood disability in developing countries. Praeger, New York, pp. 101–128

Tue N X 1993 Speech delivered by delegation of the Ministry of Labor, Invalids, and Social Affairs of Vietnam at US NGO conference on Vietnam, Cambodia, and Laos Virginia, June 17–20, 1993

UNICEF 1994 The state of the world's children, 1994. UNICEF/Oxford University Press, Oxford

World Bank 1993 World development report 1993: investing in health. World Bank/Oxford University Press, Oxford

24

Appropriate prosthetics and orthotics in less developed countries

Lawrence Golin

INTRODUCTION

Among the most challenging aspects of transferring appropriate rehabilitation techniques to the less developed countries (LDCs) of the world is the permanent establishment of a self-supporting, non-government orthotic and prosthetic center. Yet this challenge must be met. In spite of the recent advances in controlling crippling diseases, the rate of disablement continues to increase. M. R. Rousseau, citing International Labor Organization (ILO) statistics, says that 'the present population of physically disabled is estimated to be nearly 500 million. In the next century, this population is expected to be 700 million, of which a vast majority of these will come from third world countries' (Rousseau 1996).

Disabled persons in LDCs will not have the luxury of having ambulatory aids, prosthetics, orthotics, or corrective splints provided by third-party payers such as are found in more developed nations. By and large, these individuals will be indigent poor, unable to afford enough food and clothing, much less an ambulatory aid, even if such aid would increase their ability to function and find work. These factors constitute a vicious cycle of poverty, disablement and more poverty. Furthermore, these financial pressures seem to make it impossible that any orthotic-prosthetic center would maintain itself as a self-supporting business.

However, government-owned orthotic and prosthetic centers are constantly beset with problems of inadequate funding, lack of initiative, bureaucracy, and high costs of operation. Moreover, because they have been taught to follow Western methods, these centers frequently supply culturally inappropriate orthotics and prosthetics. 'Salaries are low, there is a great shortage of materials: the workshop staff so often has to search and scrap things in the black market in Dhaka' (Pluyter 1989). Still, financial constraints do not usually close government orthotic and prosthetic centers. Even though these workshops may be minimally productive and run in the red, governments would lose constituent support if they were closed down.

In recent years, non-governmental organizations (NGOs) have tried to fill the gaps where civil administrations have failed. By and large, these agencies are directly accountable to donors, more efficient, and goal-oriented. Yet, they also have their problems. As long as a foreign advisor is present and dedicated to the work, cultural imperatives make it necessary that the advisor's foreign ideas be treated with respect. Too often after the advisor leaves, no culturally accepted administration or indigenous planning is set up, and the project is not sustainable.

This chapter, based on one expatriate's 30 years' experience working in Bangladesh, will describe how a local artificial limb and brace shop has been developed and addressed these issues.

BANGLADESH

Bangladesh, one of the world's poorest and most crowded countries, exemplifies the challenges that might face any expatriate seeking to work in a LDC. An independent nation since 1971, it is part of the Indian sub-continent, located at the head of the Bay of Bengal and sandwiched between Calcutta, on India's eastern border and the Indian state of Assam. It borders Burma (Myanmar) to the south. Within its 144 000 square kilometers (about the size of the state of Wisconsin in the USA), 125 million people are crowded together. The population is increasing at the rate of 2.5% per year – 538 people per hour (US Department of State 1987).

About 90% of the people live in rural areas with limited access to modern health facilities. In 1992, the infant mortality rate was 97 per 1000 live births and the life expectancy at birth 53 years (UNICEF 1994).

In Bangladesh, the world's second largest Muslim country, 83% of the population is Muslim. Hindus constitute a sizable (16%) minority, and there are a small number of Buddhists, Christians, and animists (US Department of State 1987). The literacy rate is 35%, with the rate for boys far higher than that for girls. The average yearly wage is about US$125 per annum (Haroon Diary 1996).

People with amputations

The cause of amputation depends, in large measure, on a country's stage of development and whether it is at peace or war. In war zones and post-war zones, the greatest number of amputations result from fighting and landmine explosions. Landmines have been responsible for hundreds of thousands of amputations, most notably in Vietnam and Cambodia. In developing nations not at war the 'motor-cyclification' of transportation, coupled with overloaded buses, trucks, trains, and animal-drawn carts, cause an ever increasing number of traffic accidents that often result in amputations. Leprosy, tumors, and snakebites also can lead to amputation (Staats 1995).

It is estimated that 4–7% of Bengalis with a disability – 60 000–130 000 people – have an amputation of a lower extremity. Many of these amputations occurred during the war for independence in 1971. The others are primarily due to trauma associated with traffic-related injuries. The rate of new amputations in Bangladesh is about 10–15 000 cases every year (Pluyter 1989).

In Bangladesh, disablement is further compounded by the attitude of society towards persons with a disability (PWD). A disability is not always associated with a specific reason (i.e. punishment for sin), but it is understood as an act of God's will. This is why so many PWD are not encouraged to seek physical rehabilitation (Pluyter 1989).

Disability in Bangladesh is generally associated with the begging profession, and the concept of 'alms for the poor' is well entrenched in the culture. Thus, many amputee beggars are not rehabilitated with an artificial limb because they would lose their major source of income. Nevertheless, a person with an amputation does not easily decide to resort to begging for a living. It definitely lowers a person's status and often limits the opportunity for personal relationships such as marriage: a beggar is a social outcast and lacks the ability to support a family.

It is within this type of cultural context that a proposal has been made to help amputees in a new and different way. In no way is it suggested that this program should be strictly adhered to in all circumstances if one is attempting to develop an appropriate prosthetic and orthotic center. Rather it is a model of what could be done. The program outlined here, while only in its formative stages of development, has a very good chance of succeeding where other efforts have failed.

A HISTORICAL PERSPECTIVE: ESTABLISHING A REHABILITATION PROGRAM

However difficult the present rehabilitation picture, it is still harder to imagine the even worse conditions that existed in 1967, when I first came to what was then called East Pakistan. At that time, there were a couple of trained physical therapists, no occupational therapists, no prosthetists or orthotists, and no rehabilitation centers for PWD. In fact, before 1972, only one fully trained orthopedic surgeon was working in the whole country (Olsen 1973, Golin 1982).

The overall health situation was very bad, and in 1959 a child of a resident expatriate died from a simple bowel obstruction. The father searched for a surgeon from Akyab in Burma to Dhaka in the heart of East Pakistan. Along this line of 400 miles, he could not find one person who could help his suffering daughter (Olsen 1973). This tragedy led several North American doctors and nurses to establish the Memorial

Christian Hospital (MCH) in Cox's Bazar District in 1966 (Olsen 1973). Even with the development of this small, 40-bed mission hospital, there still was no place where an amputee could get a prosthesis, no place where a child with polio or rickets could get walking calipers, and no place where a patient with a contracted limb could get relief (Golin 1982).

In 1968, prospects for PWD began to improve. At this time, a physical therapist, Valerie Taylor, came from the UK to train physical therapy assistants at Chandraghona Christian Hospital near Kaptai Lake. I was one of her students. Taylor instilled in her students the desire to do something to help the many persons with paraplegia who had come to the hospital.

Taylor understood the meaning of appropriate technology, whereby local supplies are fabricated into simple, low-cost, yet useful aids. For example, she took simple splints made of plastic pipe and applied them to patients' legs to provide stability in their knees and ankles. Toe springs were used to keep the ankles dorsiflexed. With this help, many learned to walk with ambulatory aids.

Understanding the need for a rehabilitation facility, Taylor expressed the desire to some day establish a home for rehabilitating persons with paraplegia. This desire was eventually fulfilled in the establishment of the present well-known NGO, the Center for Rehabilitation of the Paralyzed, in Savar, Dhaka; it is the only one of its kind in Bangladesh. This 200-bed rehabilitation center for persons with spinal cord injuries has become a standard of success in the area of cross-cultural cooperation.

I learned much from this simple training. In 1968, although I lacked formal training in physical therapy, I sought to duplicate what had been done in Chandraghona by opening a physical therapy department at Memorial Christian Hospital. I began with an 8 ft by 10 ft cubicle. In this tiny space was room for one treatment table, one baker unit, one set of folding parallel bars, some home-made sand bags, and a pulley suspension unit hung from an overhead fan hook in the ceiling. An inverted hospital bed hung from the ceiling made a 'Guthrie Smith' exercise apparatus, and a rudimentary whirl-pool was made from a cable-driven propeller attached to a grounded-wire electric motor. This simple equipment completed the department and cost about US$500 in today's money. Even with this limited facility, PWD could receive some therapy.

The war for the liberation of Bangladesh started in early 1971 and continued until the end of the year, when Golden Bangladesh was declared free and independent. More than any one act, the liberation war brought the terrible plight of the maimed and paralyzed to the conscience of the Bengali people and to the whole world. Thousands of freedom fighters lost their limbs or were paralyzed from spinal injury. Seeing the need, the 'Father' of the nation, Prime Minister Sheikh Mujibur Rahman (whose daughter, Sheikh Hasina Wazed, is now prime minister), sent an urgent message to the world in 1972, requesting help rehabilitating these people (Golin 1982).

This impetus led to the creation of the first rehabilitation hospital and orthotic-prosthetic center in the country. Under the leadership of a retired missionary orthopedic surgeon, Dr Ronald Garst, the Rehabilitation Institute and Hospital for the Disabled (RIHD) was established in Dhaka in 1974. It is actually a 450-bed orthopedic hospital with a small rehabilitation department. From this hospital, in the mid 1970s, 24 young men and women earned BSc degrees in physiotherapy, and 30 young men learned to make limbs and braces. Unfortunately, by the late 1970s the school had closed because the government refused to recognize the therapists and prosthetists as professionals and did not open paid positions in the national health system for the graduates. As many as could emigrated to other countries, especially the physiotherapists who, although never recognized as licensed physical therapists by the World Confederation of Physical Therapy, were more marketable because of their university degree (Golin 1982). Fewer than a handful of that group of graduates remain in Bangladesh today.

In 1972, I left Bangladesh for my homeland, the USA, to enroll in physical therapy studies.

After receiving a certificate in physical therapy from the University of Pennsylvania in 1973, I returned to Bangladesh in 1974. Shortly thereafter, the International Council of Churches gave MCH a grant of US$3000 to build an artificial limb-and-brace shop. MCH hired one of the trainees from RIHD to work in this new shop, which began in 1975 by making plastic-molded shank, solid-ankle, cushion-heel (SACH) limbs, as well as braces made from cast-off prosthetics and orthotics that were sent as relief supplies from the USA.

It took several months before someone could be found who would be willing to wear one of the fabricated limbs. In an act of desperation by the prosthetist, a man with an amputation who was just visiting the hospital was asked if he was willing to be fitted with a limb. That patient, after receiving his limb, was never seen again. Moreover, it had been noted that amputees provided with limbs consistently reverted back to using crutches. The culture could not accept the idea that someone could possibly walk again after having lost a limb: people were used to using a stick, crutch, or homemade peg leg. Also, a prosthesis might cost the equivalent of a year's wage; it was simply not affordable and the notion of being given an appliance did not enter people's minds. Prosthetics was so new an idea, so foreign to the Bengali way of thinking, they could not accept it. This idea began slowly to change when a prominent local businessman was fitted with an artificial limb. When he proved its usefulness by driving his motorcycle with it, amputees began coming to the hospital at a rate of about one person per week.

It soon became obvious, however, that the Western-style technology (i.e. a plastic-molded SACH foot prosthesis) is not suitable for the culture, climate, or topography of Bangladesh. The Western-type limb requires a leather shoe and a sponge-rubber SACH heel. These parts would wear out in a few weeks in the wet rural areas where most Bengalis live. A poor farmer, unable to buy even a new pair of shoes, would hang the prosthesis on the wall and revert back to using crutches or a peg leg (Upadhyaya et al

1987). Just as important, the SACH foot does not allow the amputee to squat, which is the way people in South-Asian cultures sit. People squat when socializing, eating, toileting, or working in the fields.

Slowly, there was a realization that appliance compatibility must match lifestyle. The differences in the chair-sitting culture of the West and the floor-sitting culture of the East necessitated an alternative prosthetic design. However, an attempt at using cast-off orthotics or braces made from bamboo or steel rods with wooden clogs also failed. They were not durable and were too heavy and unattractive. Alternative materials had to be imported at extremely high cost. Something had to be done to make a product lower in cost and at the same time useful within Bangladeshi society.

JAIPUR FOOT PROSTHESIS

In 1974, Drs P. K. Sethi, M. P. Udawat, and S. C. Kasliwal of Sarai Man Suigh Hospital and Rehabilitation Center (SMS) in Jaipur, India, published a paper, 'Lower limb prosthetics for amputees in rural areas,' describing the development of the Jaipur foot. They had fabricated an intriguing footpiece using readily available, vulcanized tire and microcellular rubber. These materials were fitted into a sand-casted aluminum mold (see Fig. 24.1) and heated so that the fabricated foot imitated the anatomy of the human foot, including the tendons. Ordinary village people reportedly accepted this Jaipur foot, for it allowed them to carry out their normal activities, including barefoot walking even in water or over rugged terrain.

Another technical advancement was the idea of using aluminum as a prosthetic shank hammered into the shape of the stump and molded into a patellar tendon weight-bearing socket. With this prosthesis, a person with an amputation could squat and sit cross-legged, which is impossible with the conventional artificial limb. In addition, the aluminum shank makes it possible to revise the socket after normal shrinkage of the amputee's stump. Expensive resin plas-

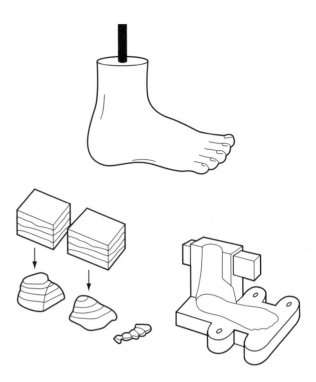

Fig. 24.1   The Jaipur foot (adapted from Pluyter 1989).

tics, polyvinyl acetate sheeting, plaster of Paris bandages, and complicated jigs are not needed to fabricate these sockets. Furthermore, the aluminum shanks are much lighter in weight and can be made by village tin workers at a far faster rate (several per day) than traditional 'Western'-style prostheses (Golin 1991).

In the summer of 1983, Dr S. C. Kasliwal, chief project director at SMS in Jaipur, invited me and one of the prosthetist-orthotists to learn to make the trans-tibial prosthetic aluminum shank. Returning to Bangladesh, we carried Jaipur foot pieces in our suitcases (consequently having to prove to Bangladesh customs that we were carrying artificial limb foot pieces, not gold or smuggled drugs). We brought artificial foot pieces across the Indian border for several years until we found money to purchase a vulcanizer and footpiece dies for MCH. In spite of these troubles, these foot pieces, added to the homemade aluminum shanks, made the prosthesis far more acceptable to people with amputations.

In 1992, a group of prosthetists from MCH went to Sri Lanka, to the Colombo Friend in Need Society, to learn to make the footpieces themselves using dies made in India. The Colombo Friend in Need Society had started a successful Jaipur foot program under the instruction of a US prosthetist, who had been taught by Dr Kasliwal in Jaipur (Colombo Friend in Need 1988). This successful non-governmental project continues to give free artificial limbs to the victims of Sri Lanka's civil war. It is financed almost entirely from donations given by the people of Sri Lanka.

At almost the same time, MCH received a grant of US$10 000 from the Australian High Commission in Dhaka to purchase a sterilizer-vulcanizer unit from India. In addition, a US$3000 grant from the Royal Netherlands Embassy financed the purchase of the footpiece dies from India. These dies had to be bought in India and shipped with the sterilizer unit to Chittagong. An attempt to make footpiece dies locally proved unsuccessful. The technology is beyond the skill of the local artisans, and Sethi (1995) believes that it is unrealistic to expect each limb-fitting center to produce its own Jaipur feet. Rather, believing that large-scale production is necessary and appropriate, he has prevailed on a rubber factory in India to begin commercial production. In Bangladesh, the prosthetists still depend upon the Indian dies.

Finally, in June 1993, the first Jaipur Foot Artificial Limb Center in Bangladesh was formally dedicated at MCH. Since then, an average of two people with amputations have been fitted with limbs every week. In 1996, a satellite limb center, the Immanuel Artificial Limb Center, opened in the country's second largest city, Chittagong, staffed by a new prosthetic trainee. It was officially dedicated by the first secretary of the Australian High Commission.

Western professionals have questioned the efficacy of the Jaipur foot artificial limb, wondering if non-professional prosthetists can produce an artificial limb with a good fit or function to its wearers. Is it possible to develop and produce a new technology while still maintaining high quality? To answer this question, a study was done in 1995 of 30 individuals who had received Jaipur foot artificial limbs at a free artificial limb camp in Patiya, Chittagong, in February 1992. Of the 30 people who received these limbs, 23 were still using them 2 years later. Most of these people were leading active, normal lives, reinforcing the idea that prosthetic durability is a critical issue. However, for some the footpieces were wearing out after 2 years, and the wearers could not afford to buy new ones at 450 taka (about US$12) (Golin 1995). Durability needs to be improved. Although the rubber foot can be patched up at a local tire shop, ongoing efforts are underway to produce a polyurethane version of the Jaipur foot (Sethi 1995).

In effect, the Jaipur foot prosthesis seems to be appropriate to helping many poor people with amputations return to a more normal life. On the other hand, even its extremely low cost (about US$40 in Bangladesh for a below-knee prosthesis) is not low enough to assist the very poor. Something further must be done.

Orthotics

Alongside the introduction of the Jaipur foot to Bangladesh, there have been attempts to develop culturally appropriate orthotics. Improvements began when calipers were made from aluminum window frames and ship plate (see Fig. 24.2). Further improvements were made in 1993 when polypropylene beads became available. This material makes it possible to fabricate a plastic ankle foot orthosis (AFO) by fashioning the heat-treated plastic over a plaster of Paris mold of a person's foot. All that is required is an ordinary oven heated to 70°C, a pie pan to place the beads on, and about 30 minutes. The melted material is malleable and can be formed into an orthosis over the impression of the foot. This orthosis is especially effective for children with diplegic spastic cerebral palsy, after serial casting. It seems to maintain the range of motion in the ankle quite well.

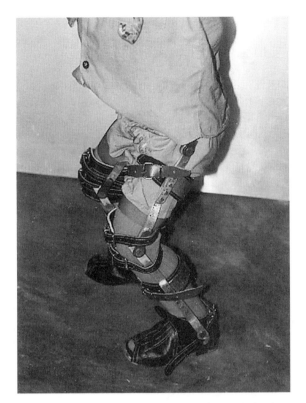

Fig. 24.2 Rickets HAFKO made of aluminum window bar. The shoe is made in our own workshop. Rickets is endemic in our area.

A PLAN FOR INDIGENIZING A NATIONAL PROSTHETIC-ORTHOTIC CENTER

The development of any culturally appropriate, self-sustaining NGO in an LDC is more likely to be successful if certain principles are considered. These include:

1. Most likely, foreign funds will be needed to initiate a project. Because financial resources are so critical at the national and individual level in LDCs, an outside source must provide initial costs. Finding alternative, government-to-government or NGO funding can be difficult, but it is possible. In Bangladesh, because the goal was to produce something concrete at a low cost, obtaining small grants for this project was feasible. Two nations provided funds for the first Jaipur Foot Artificial Limb Center. When the Immanuel Limb Center in Chittagong was built,

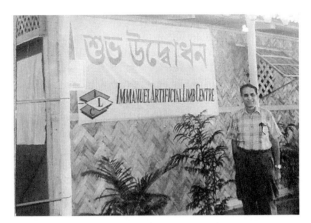

Fig. 24.3 Author Harry Golin in front of the Immanuel Limb Centre, Chittagong.

it could have started up with a modern prosthetic workshop with foreign assistance on purchased land. Instead, the workshop was constructed using bamboo and a tin roof, with the barest essentials, for about US$2500 (Fig. 24.3). The center was built on a piece of land rented from a very supportive person. It has become a simple starting point from which something larger can be built later. This structure can be easily maintained at an affordable cost. Yet a good working relationship has developed with the original funders, and there is an expectation that these same nations could be called upon in the future if there is an urgent need.

2. Foreign expatriates will likely be needed to assist with developing the project. Expatriate personnel are frequently called upon to help implement a program for PWD in LDCs. Their expertise is needed to develop an appropriate basic curriculum, train national workers, update worker skills, and outline a program that could be continued after the foreigner leaves.

In many respects, this is an enormous undertaking. The expatriate must be sensitive to the sociocultural realities of the host country and the persons with amputations. The cultural and language barriers between the foreigner and national occasionally cause conflicts and misunderstanding. The foreigner should try to be observant and respectful of the local culture and people and should try to learn the national language.

The expatriate must have a solid understanding of what is feasible in a country facing great economic limitations. The danger is that the foreign adviser will want to set up things the way they are 'back home', for example, expending money for expensive equipment and foreign training of national workers. It is completely impractical to want to reproduce the advanced prosthetic and orthotic technology of the developed world. If the product's price is too high, then the majority of clients will not come for services. It is the story of supply and demand but on a more critical scale. Many times, the product ends up subsidized with foreign funds. This ends up defeating the purpose of indigenization.

The expatriate must be willing to stay long enough for the project to have a solid start. In my experience, 2 years would be a basic requirement, but 4 years is preferred. Before the expatriate advisor leaves, the entire workshop should be registered as an official NGO with the national government. This ensures the legal continuation of what has been established.

3. National workers are trained within their own culture and using cost-effective local materials. Skilled artisans can perform manual labor of excellent quality. Sethi (1995) reports that when comparing schooled, urban-educated diploma holders in rehabilitation engineering with apprentices from the artisan class, the quality and quantity of output of the Jaipur foot favored the artisans. Additionally, he reports that the patients were more satisfied with the 'non-formal' group.

Although originally some Bangladeshi trainees were sent to Sri Lanka and India, these countries are still easily accessible to Bangladesh by surface transport and have very similar economic and cultural conditions to it. If workers went to a place like Singapore, which is far more industrialized and where almost all materials and supplies are available, they would likely be tempted to rely on imports instead of buying them on the local market. Also, the workers surely would suffer from culture shock.

4. A relationship should be developed with local organizations and people. It is necessary to collaborate with doctors and other professionals and lay people in the community. These people will probably become members of a managing board for the fledgling organization and be the source of referral of patients.

Also, a relationship should be developed among local service organizations to pay for the cost of limbs and braces for the poorer patients. The gap between the wealthy and the poor is no more evident than in the LDCs. Lion's, Kiwanis, and Rotary clubs are examples of service organizations of well-to-do business people who are eager to help those that are willing to help themselves. It is usually these types of organizations that support programs to help the poorest PWD. Until the appearance of the Immanuel Artificial Limb Center in Chittagong, there were few opportunities for humanitarian aid to PWD. Since its founding, service organizations have been very eager to help and have hinted that they might be even more energized if vocational training were offered to the clients in addition to the prosthetic limbs.

It has been the experience of both the Viklang Samiti in Jaipur and the Colombo Friend in Need Society that when they provided limbs free of charge, local donors came forward to pay for their entire operation. In contrast, in Bangladesh there is an attempt to cover the cost of manufacturing from proceeds accumulated by selling a product with an additional subsidy from service organization funding. It is a belief that everyone should pay something towards their appliance, even if it is a very small amount. The fear is that if something is given away, many would regard the gift as having no value. The prosthesis or orthosis would be put on the shelf and not maintained.

5. The workshop must be managed reasonably well. The logistical complexities of the center must be managed well, with attention paid to personnel, budgeting, scheduling, space, supplies, and more. A system of checks and balances should be developed within the workshop and everything within it inventoried monthly. Cost analyses must be developed to determine the cost of making each item produced. A manager who is also a national prosthetist-orthotist would be accountable to the board of directors at every level of this operation.

A salary structure needs to be developed so that workers are paid sufficiently and not tempted to accept gratuities. Gratuities are the way of the East, but they are the doom of any enterprise. As soon as gratuities are accepted, the quality of the work depreciates and demand is made for more money. As a result, the product is made at a cost no one can afford. With fixed prices displayed publicly everyone knows where they stand.

Hiring PWD is encouraged. It provides the opportunity for people with amputations to see role models. Also, since jobs for PWD are limited, there is an incentive to work hard and be honest.

CONCLUSION

A great challenge awaits anyone who seeks to aid in the establishment of an orthotic-prosthetic center in an LDC. Generally, there are two very different and often conflicting approaches: the top-down approach of using high technology imported from the West or the simplistic approach of traditional, primitive technology. But, as Sethi (1989) points out:

A distinction is not being made between science and technology. We are confusing expensive gadgetry with good science. This often is not so. It requires some very sophisticated thinking to arrive at a simple solution. It is much easier to work out a complicated and expensive solution. . . . Expensive gadgetry often possesses impressive 'symbolic value' as opposed to 'use value' (Sethi 1989, p. 118).

This chapter has given an example to show that even in the most difficult of situations, something can be done to alleviate the problems of PWD. It has outlined a culturally appropriate program that will preserve the continuance of any advisor's efforts.

Still, one question remains to be answered. Why would anyone desire to enter into such an undertaking? That question is left to you to answer. In my case, being part of a Christian mission organization, my colleagues and I have a command from Scripture that draws us to this task.

REFERENCES

Colombo Friend in Need Society 1988 Annual Report. Colombo Friend in Need Society, Colombo, Sri Lanka, p. 1

Golin L 1982 Physical therapy and physical rehabilitation in Bangladesh. Proceedings of the 9th International Congress WCPT, Stockholm, Sweden, p. 658

Golin L 1991 Dramatic improvements in prosthetics and orthotics in the developing world. Proceedings of the 11th International Congress WCPT, London, England, p. 664

Golin L 1995 The efficacy of the Jaipur foot prosthesis in the developing world. Proceedings of the 12th International Congress WCPT Washington, DC, USA, p. 1123

Haroon Diary 1996 Dhaka, Bangladesh, p. 4

Olsen V 1973 Daktar diplomat in Bangladesh. Moody Press, Chicago, pp. 83–84

Pluyter B 1989 Artificial limbs in Bangladesh. National Hospital Institute, Utrecht, Netherlands, p. 1

Rousseau M R 1996 Rehabilitating the disabled. Weekend Independent Newspaper, Dhaka, Bangladesh, 26 July 1996, p. 5

Sethi P K 1989 Technological choices in prosthetics and orthotics for developing countries. Prosthetics Orthotics International 13: 117–124

Sethi P K 1995 The Jaipur experience. Report of the International Society of Prosthetics and Orthotics (ISPO)

Consensus Conference on Appropriate Prosthetic Technology for Developing Countries. Phnom Penh, Cambodia, June 5–10 1995. ISPO and USAID, pp. 89–94

Sethi P K, Udawat M P, Kasliwal S C 1974 Lower limb prosthetics for amputees in rural areas. In: Weil M F, Enna C (eds) Surgical Rehabilitation Leprosy. Williams and Wilkins, Baltimore, MD, USA

Staats T B 1995 The rehabilitation of the amputee in the developing world: a review of the literature. Report of the International Society of Prosthetics and Orthotics (ISPO) Consensus Conference on Appropriate Prosthetic Technology for Developing Countries. Phnom Penh, Cambodia, June 5–10 1995. ISPO and USAID, pp. 67–72

Upadhyaya M, Sharma C, Sharma S 1987 Modification of the below knee prosthesis of aluminum shank with Jaipur foot by high density polyethylene shank. Proceedings of the 6th North Zone Annual Conference of Orthopedic Surgeons, Patala, Punjab, India, p. 2

UNICEF 1994 The state of the world's children. Oxford University Press Oxford

United States Department of State, Bureau of Public Affairs (1987) Background notes, Bangladesh. Washington DC, USA, p. 3

25

Paper technology and community based rehabilitation: cultural adaptation in Zimbabwe

Harry Finkenflügel

INTRODUCTION

In kindergarten and primary school, most children learn how to make dolls and toys from papier-mâché, but these days papier-mâché art also appears in exclusive shops and at exclusive prices. In Zimbabwe, this well-known technique was rediscovered as a very useful method to make all kinds of household utensils, aids and appliances for children with a disability. Rehabilitation workers have realized that paper technology products can be used or even sold, that paper and cardboard are available and that this technique is easy to learn.

Over the years, paper technology has become an integral part of the training of rehabilitation technicians and of community based rehabilitation (CBR) programs in Zimbabwe. It has proved to be a good example of 'resources for rehabilitation that are available in the community,' which is a key phrase in definitions of CBR (Helander et al 1989). CBR is a complex process and this chapter will illustrate how one appropriate and culturally adapted technology can strengthen it.

COMMUNITY BASED REHABILITATION IN ZIMBABWE

Before 1980 health services in colonial, and later minority-ruled, Zimbabwe (then called Rhodesia) were highly centralized and segregated. With independence in 1980, the new government devised a plan to expand and decentralize health services in order to increase accessibility to all people. From 1980 on, the Ministry of Health (MoH) has stressed that a network of interrelated rural, district, provincial and central health services is essential for the development of health care in this southeast African nation of 11 million people. Health workers at the provincial level have an important role in the training and supervision of health workers at the district and rural level.

Within this framework, the MoH established a nation-wide network of rural health centers, district hospitals and provincial hospitals. At the same time, the ministry emphasized professional development. Training schools for nurses, rehabilitation technicians (RTs), environmental health technicians and other health workers were revitalized or started. At the University of Zimbabwe, medical doctors (and later also physical and occupational therapists) were trained.

One large group this decentralized network would serve were people with disabilities. The National Disability Survey (Ministry of Labor and Social Services 1982) revealed that approximately 276 300 people (of an estimated population then of 7.5 million) suffered from physical or mental conditions that had progressed to the stage where adequate functioning was no longer possible. At that time only the three central hospitals (in Harare, Chitungwiza, and Bulawayo) and six provincial hospitals had a rehabilitation or physiotherapy department. Moreover, because a substantial number of therapists had left the country in 1980, these departments operated on an under-utilized and intermittent basis.

The 2-year training of RTs started in 1981. A cadre that could be trained locally and in a relatively short time to staff the rehabilitation departments in district and provincial hospitals was required. RTs, who could carry out basic rehabilitation skills, typically worked in a scarcely equipped department or the wards, and they also became involved in hospital outreach programs. It was realized that the RTs could take the lead in setting up CBR projects. As a result, the training became more family – and community – oriented (Finkenflügel 1991).

By 1988, the infrastructure within the MoH was sufficiently developed to support the development of community-oriented rehabilitation service. Eight districts (one in every province) were prepared to start a CBR pilot project (Ministry of Health 1990). The main aims of these projects were to provide rehabilitation services at the community level and to serve as a training project for RTs and other health workers in the provinces.

All eight CBR pilot projects started with a 4-week workshop. Part of this workshop was a door-to-door survey. Volunteers visited, in total, 104 000 people and identified 4556 persons with a disability. RTs screened about 80% of them under supervision of occupational therapists and physical therapists. In total, 1614 persons with a disability that could benefit from rehabilitation services were registered (Ministry of Health 1990). Most of these people were not coming to the rehabilitation departments in the hospitals or to the hospital's outreach program. They could only be reached in their own communities. However, looking at the number of people identified as needing service and noting the limitations of personnel and transport, it was not possible for the RTs to visit all clients. It was also impossible to provide enough aids and appliances. Clients either had to come to the hospital or the RTs had to travel widely to measure, fabricate, fit and adjust these appliances.

To fill the gap between the RTs based in district hospitals and the newly identified rural clients, Village Community Workers (VCWs) and volunteers were educated in basic rehabilitation principles. Thus, CBR in Zimbabwe can be best described as the final step in the decentralization of rehabilitation services. Because of this, the people in the community, including the VCWs and volunteers, depended heavily on the health workers of the district hospital.

Rehabilitation workers soon realized that a community had to rely more on its own strengths, possibilities and resources if the projects were to be sustainable. They organized workshops for the VCWs and volunteers who assisted with the initial survey, initiated community rehabilitation committees and worked on ways to use locally available, low-cost materials in rehabilitation.

In Zimbabwe, materials like leather, metal strips, wood and rubber are available but expensive, and require special tools and skills to be utilized appropriately. Paper and cardboard proved to be good alternative materials for those children that need adapted chairs, special toys or aids. Paper could be collected from shops, hospitals and government agencies. Fortunately there is hardly any competition for the use of paper and card. In any community with a few shops, a clinic or a few government agencies it is easy to find enough paper to make a chair, toy, aid or whatever else might be needed. For these reasons, paper technology has been introduced as part of vocational training and as an income-generating activity for persons with a disability. The basic technique is simple and items like chairs can be made by almost everyone, although skills must be developed to make items that can be sold.

PAPER TECHNOLOGY

In the late 1970s, Bevill Packer, a sociology lecturer in a Zimbabwe college of education, had to teach art. He realized that after graduation most teachers would go to schools in rural areas. These schools operated on a very basic budget: there was no way they could afford materials for art classes. Packer and his student-teachers decided to work with no-cost materials. Paper and cardboard, often in combination with plastic bottles and other waste materials, became the most popular materials. After retiring in 1982, Packer further developed the idea of low-cost paper based technology. It was no longer considered 'art' but an appropriate way of making items that could be used in every household. He made chairs, tables, trays, baskets, toys, puppets, dolls houses, solar cookers, etc.

Rehabilitation workers became interested in making adapted chairs, corner seats, hearing aids and toys for children with a disability.

Paper technology was also introduced in vocational training. People with a disability learned to make things that not only improved their skills but could also be sold at the local market.

No fancy tools are needed for paper technology. A bowl, a stirring stick and a knife will do. The products can easily be adjusted and reinforced if necessary. The appliances can even be repaired and remodeled within the community. The technique is simple and can be taught to any family or community member.

Paper technology is now part of the curriculum for RTs and occupational therapists. This enables the rehabilitation workers to gain a good idea of the possibilities of paper and card. It also equips them to transfer this knowledge and skill to the people in the communities.

Principles and examples

Packer (1988) gives numerous examples of some basic techniques in his book *A Manual of Appropriate Paper Based Technology*. The book is quite useful, but keep in mind that paper technology is not an academic exercise; the only way to learn is to do. It might be wise to make a few things for yourself and your family. This will not only equip you with the necessary skills but send the message that you take it seriously. From my own experience, I learned that my students (RTs) were happily surprised to see that my own children used paper technology chairs and played with a paper technology wheelbarrow. It is important to show that appropriate technology is not second rate technology: it is good enough for the clients with a disability in the rural areas, and it is good enough for rehabilitation workers in the towns, at work and at home.

Whether making an adapted chair, an ear trumpet, a toy or a bowl, the basic materials and principles are the same. As Packer stresses, paper technology articles must be:

- strong
- useful
- attractive
- very cheap to make (ICTA 1988).

The only costs are for flour to make paste and varnish for finishing. Almost every type of paper can be used. Scraps of paper can be soaked, ground and mixed with leftover *sadza* (cooked maize meal) to make mash. Sheets of paper can be pasted together, torn into narrow strips and layered to make, for example, bowls or trays, or to strengthen stools, chairs or tables. Thin card (i.e. shoe boxes or posters) can be laminated to build such things as heavier types of furniture or a base for adapted chairs or prone tables.

When tearing paper or card, note that all paper and card has a grain direction. There is always one direction (often top to bottom in newspapers) that can be torn easily and straight. The other direction will be more difficult to tear in a straight way.

Making paste is simple but must be done with care. Lumps in the paste will make it difficult to produce an attractive article. The easiest way is to make paste from plain flour (not self-rising). Mix a little flour thoroughly with cold water until it is like cream. Add boiling water rapidly while stirring. The paste is ready when it changes color and thickens. Two heaping spoonfuls of flour will do for one liter of water. Another way to make paste uses left-over *sadza*: break it into small crumbs and mix it with boiling water. The paper and card get soaked with paste. It gets strong as it dries. To make sure that the laminated surfaces or layers will dry up in the way planned, pressure is applied to all pasted papers. For pressure use wooden boards weighted with bricks or stones, or plastic bags full of sand. To keep things together use nylon strings (cut from old nylon stockings) or bicycle tubes.

Once the paste is applied another principle that one must remember is to make use of the stretch and shrink of paper. All paper and card stretches when wet and shrinks when dries. By alternating the grain direction, laminating successive courses and applying pressure when needed, the drying and shrinking process will result in a strong piece.

To start: getting familiar with the material and the techniques

Paper technology articles often start from a fixed shape (e.g. a bowl, a plate, a tray) or a constructed model.

Making a bowl. First, cover a bowl with sheets of thin plastic to keep it separate from the paper and paste. Next, take three pieces of paper (newspaper) and smear paste on each of them. Lay them on top of each other so the paper is now three layers thick. Tear these three-layer pages in strips (along the grain), about 2 cm wide. Place the bowl downwards (Fig. 25.1) and layer the bowl with the strips in such a way that it gets completely covered. It is important to avoid air bubbles between the layers. Once

a. Turn bowl upside down and cover it with thin plastic sheets

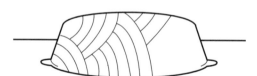

b. Cover the bowl up with 3-layer paper strips

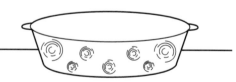

c. Decorate the replica with magazine pictures or paint it

Fig. 25.1 Making a bowl. a. Turn bowl upside down and cover it with thin plastic sheets. b. Cover the bowl with 3-layer paper strips. c. Decorate the replica with magazine pictures or paint it.

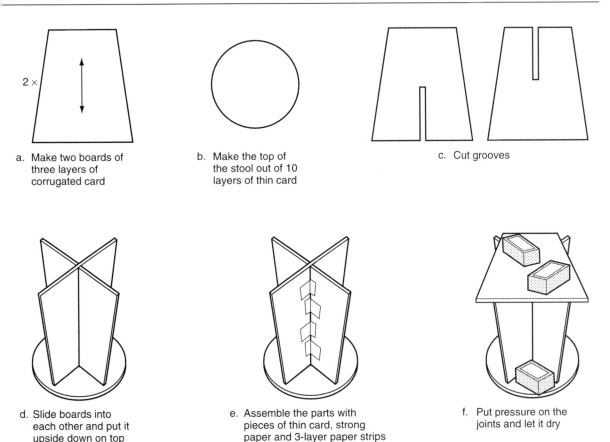

a. Make two boards of three layers of corrugated card

b. Make the top of the stool out of 10 layers of thin card

c. Cut grooves

d. Slide boards into each other and put it upside down on top

e. Assemble the parts with pieces of thin card, strong paper and 3-layer paper strips

f. Put pressure on the joints and let it dry

Fig. 25.2 Making a stool. a. Make two boards of 3 layers of corrugated card. b. Make the top of the stool out of 10 layers of thin card. c. Cut grooves. d. Slide boards into each other and put it upside down, on its top. e. Assemble the parts with pieces of thin card, strong paper and 3-layer paper strips. f. Put pressure on the joints and let it dry.

enough layers have been applied to the bowl, separate the replica to allow for drying. After it is dry, cut the edge with a knife or scissors. To smooth the edge, soften the replica with paste and mold it again.

There are different ways to decorate the replica. It can be painted or covered with a layer of colorful pieces of paper or with pictures. To make sure the article will last, varnish it. Although these bowls can be used as household items, they are often used as show pieces because of the attractive decorations.

Making a stool. Start with a construction made of corrugated card. Depending on the size (and the use) of the stool, paste together two sets of three to five layers of corrugated board, to make the base pieces (Fig. 25.2). Use about 10 carton

cards to make the top of the stool. Cut identical pieces and stick these together. Let the base boards and the top dry, applying pressure to make sure they stay flat.

After drying, cut grooves in the boards (half way up or down) and slide them into each other. Place the stool upside down and join all parts together with pieces of card or paper. The best thing is to start with pieces of thin carton cards and a strong type of paper (cement bags, millie meal bags, etc.). Finish off with a few layers of three-layer paper strips or pieces. Let it dry again and apply pressure on the joints.

With the stool nearly finished, make sure that it stands flat. If it is rocking, smear paste on the edges to make it soft and rub the stool on a flat and rough surface (e.g. a cement floor). The

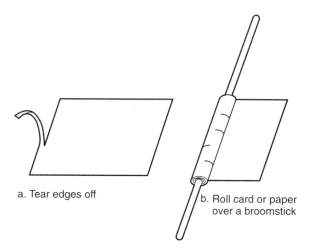

a. Tear edges off

b. Roll card or paper over a broomstick

Fig. 25.3 Making a tube. a. Tear edges off. b. Roll card or paper over a broomstick.

stool is now ready to be decorated or painted and varnished.

Making tubes. Paper technology tubes are remarkably strong. These tubes can be used as furniture legs and rails, axles in toy-cars or push-chairs, and many other items.

First, apply paste to paper (preferably thin card, but newspaper will do as well). Next, tear off cut edges and roll the paper with the grain over a pasted broomstick or PVC-tube. Use as many layers as needed. End with a few pieces of paper to make sure the card sticks well. Twist and pull the stick or PVC tube and take it out. Let the paper tube dry.

Case studies: paper technology and rehabilitation

Paper technology can also be used to make appropriate adaptive aids for children and adults with disabilities. In many low income environments, using paper technology may be the only feasible alternative available.

A corner seat for Farayi. When introduced to Farayi in his family's traditional round hut, the mother informed the RT that Farayi cannot sit, crawl or walk. His joints and muscles are very tense and he needs complete care. Although Farayi cannot talk, he understands his mother when she talks to him.

The RT classified Farayi, the fifth child in a family with six children, as a child with cerebral palsy. After discussion with the mother it was decided to make a corner seat. This type of seating would improve Farayi's posture and body position while enabling him to sit independently.

After Farayi's brothers and sisters were sent out to collect paper and card, the RT prepared the boards, using corrugated carton. A week later, the boards were put together, and the RT

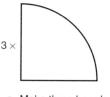

$3 \times$

a. Make three boards (quarter of a circle) out of corrugated card

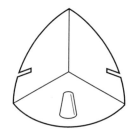

b. Assemble these three boards in to a corner seat. Cut grooves inside boards to fit a table. A block is placed between the legs to maintain position

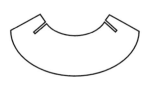

c. A table will help the child to correct posture and will be used for playing

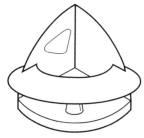

d. Extra paper is added at the right side board. The whole chair is tilted by adding a strip under the sitting board

Fig. 25.4 Making a corner seat for Farayi. a. Make three boards (quarter-circle) out of corrugated card. b. Assemble into a corner seat. Cut grooves in the side boards to fit a table. A block is placed between the legs to maintain position. c. A table will help the child to correct posture and will be used for playing. d. Extra paper is added at the right side board. The whole chair is tilted by adding a strip under the sitting board.

asked to have Farayi sit in the chair to see if it would give him the right posture. Together with the elder children, the RT strengthened the chair joints and told the mother that after a few days she could start using it.

At the technician's next visit, Farayi was sitting in the chair for many hours a day. To correct his posture, a bit more corrugated board and paper strips were pasted at shoulder height on the right board. Also the whole chair was tilted a bit more so Farayi could keep his head in a properly aligned position (Fig. 25.4) One of the daughters volunteered to decorate the chair nicely. She used a lot of magazine pictures and colorful pieces and turned it into a real work of art.

A chair out of a box and a canvas strip for Kundai. Kundai (4 years old) and her mother attended a workshop on 'children with cerebral palsy' organized by the rehabilitation workers of the provincial hospital. Kundai has cerebral palsy with hydrocephalus. During home visits, the RT would go through exercises with the mother and evaluate the progress of the child.

The mother supported Kundai's sitting position with pillows, but it was difficult to maintain a good position. After discussion with an occupational therapist, it was decided to make a seat with a canvas strip similar to a hammock (Figs 25.5a, 25.5b). A suitable box was found and cut into the right shape. The box was reinforced with pieces of card and paper, and two tubes were made out of thin card and newspapers. The laundry and linen section of the hospital provided a piece of canvas. Kundai's mother decorated the chair with the help of the other mothers in the workshop.

Mr Nkombe's ear trumpet. Mr Nkombe's wife was one of the VCWs who assisted in the CBR pilot projects. After completing a survey in her area, she asked for assistance for her 62-year-old husband who has difficulty in hearing. He had been seen by a doctor at the hospital but nothing could be done for him, as hearing aids are not available. When the RT talked to Mr Nkombe he puts his hands behind his ears, thus suggesting the need for an ear trumpet. With a bowl, a cream carton and clay, the model of the trumpet was made. After covering it with a piece of thin

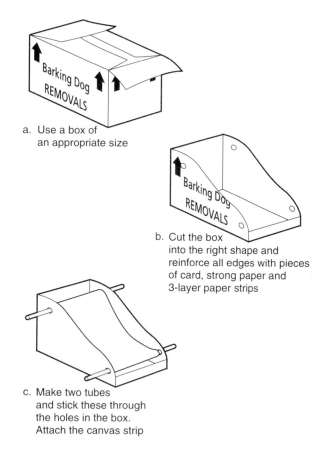

a. Use a box of an appropriate size

b. Cut the box into the right shape and reinforce all edges with pieces of card, strong paper and 3-layer paper strips

c. Make two tubes and stick these through the holes in the box. Attach the canvas strip

Fig. 25.5a Making a chair for Kundai out of a box and a canvas strip. a. Use a box of an appropriate size. b. Cut the box into the right shape and reinforce all edges with pieces of card, strong paper and 3-layer paper strips. c. Make two tubes and stick these through the holes in the box. Attach the canvas strip.

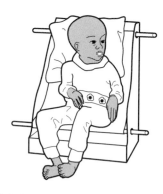

Fig. 25.5b Kundai sitting in her chair.

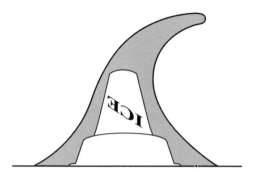

a. A model of the eartrumpet is made out of a bowl, carton and clay

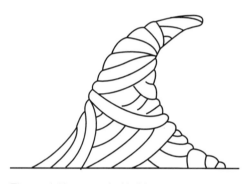

b. The model is covered with 3-layer paper strips

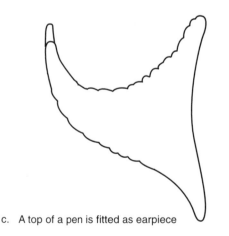

c. A top of a pen is fitted as earpiece

Fig. 25.6 Making an ear trumpet. a. A model of the ear trumpet is made out of a bowl, carton and clay. b. The model is covered with 3-layer paper strips. c. A top of a pen is fitted as an earpiece.

plastic, it was laminated with three-layer newspaper strips. The ear trumpet was then removed from its model and fitted with an ear piece made from a pen top. Mr Nkombe assured us that this aid was quite helpful.

A therapeutic activity for people with mental disability. Children and young adults with a mental disability come to Kukura Neshungu, a community day-care center in one of the townships of Mandondera to sing, play and be trained in activities of daily living. At the request of the volunteers, some of the young adults were taught how to make simple articles, such as small stools and bowls, from paper and card.

In this case, the guidance of the volunteers was essential in order to complete a project. At the start, the volunteers had expected the people attending the day-care center to be able to make items that could be sold. However, they soon realized how difficult this would be. Although the basic technique is simple, it takes physical exercise and emotional patience to make paper technology 'art' that can be sold. Nevertheless, the clients were very proud to take their project home to show that they were able to make something unique.

A means of involving fathers in rehabilitation. The care for children with a disability in Zimbabwe is almost completely in the hands of women. In each of the eight pilot projects, only a few men (fathers and uncles) were the caregiver of a child with a disability. In an attempt to involve fathers in the rehabilitation of their child, RTs in one of the CBR pilot projects organized a workshop just for them. In these workshops, fathers made a toy, a chair or a prone board for their child. By doing so, they learned to think about the difficulties their child had to face and possibilities for adaptive equipment. Paper technology was introduced as a valuable and affordable construction method. Often there was disbelief ('it will never be strong'), but by working with paper and card the men became enthusiastic. A lot of energy was spent 'to make things look nice': the fathers did not want to make 'disabled' aids for their children with a disability.

Paper technology as an income-generating project

In Gweru, paper technology bowls and trays hold a prominent place in one of the tourist shops. The shop owner explained that women both with and without a disability provided these items. Among them is a woman with a long psychiatric history. She lives in the rural area with her sister's family and contributes to the family income by making beautiful trays, which her sister takes into town to be sold. On the trips back home, the sister brings more empty boxes that can be turned into trays (Fig 25.7).

CONCLUSION

In one chapter it is impossible to give a complete overview of all the possibilities of paper technology. Hopefully this has given enough ideas on how to work with those who have very limited resources to improve the quality of life for people with a disability. CBR is built on the strengths of the community, and with paper technology the community gains an additional tool with which to further develop potential. One of the main advantages of paper technology is that rehabilitation workers are not making aids *for* the clients but are working *with* the caregivers and the clients. Caregivers need to gain the confidence and the skills to repair these aids and to enlarge or renew them, for example, when a child grows up.

It is significant that paper technology is also used to make toys, stools, chairs and tables for family members that are not disabled. Paper technology is not something for a special group of people, and this contributes to the acceptance of paper technology items for people with a disability.

Paper technology has now been introduced in sheltered workshops in developing and developed countries. Professional artists also make use of this technique but have not taken over the market (probably because of the labor-intensive work). Paper technology is a good example of how a low-cost, well-known technique can be reinvented and explored to be appropriate, affordable, and acceptable in the field of rehabilitation.

Acknowledgments I would like to thank Mr Bevill Packer and Mr Timothy Gono for introducing me to paper technology and with whom I had the pleasure to teach the rehabilitation technicians.

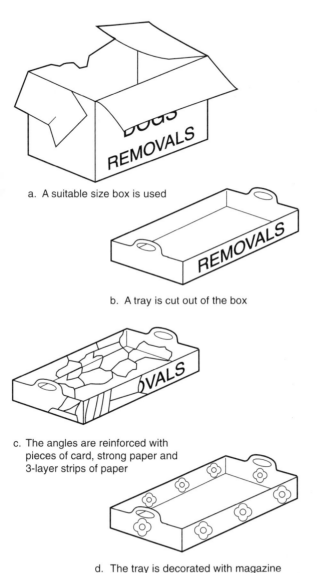

a. A suitable size box is used

b. A tray is cut out of the box

c. The angles are reinforced with pieces of card, strong paper and 3-layer strips of paper

d. The tray is decorated with magazine pictures, gift paper or is painted

Fig. 25.7 Making a tray out of the bottom part of a box. a. A suitable sized box is used. b. A tray is cut out of the box. c. The angles are reinforced with pieces of card, strong paper and 3-layer strips of paper. d. The tray is decorated with magazine pictures or gift paper, or painted.

REFERENCES

Finkenflügel, H J M 1991 Help for the disabled – in hospital and at home. World Health Forum 12: 325–330

Helander E, Mendis P, Nelson G, Goerdt A 1989 Training in the community for people with disabilities. World Health Organization, Geneva

ICTA 1988 Appropriate aids and equipment for disabled people in Africa. Report from a seminar in Harare, Zimbabwe, March 20–26 1998. Stockholm

Ministry of Health Rehabilitation Unit 1990 A report on eight community-based rehabilitation (CBR) pilot projects. Harare, Zimbabwe

Ministry of Labor and Social Services 1982 Report on the national disability survey of Zimbabwe. Ministry of Labor and Social Services, Harare, Zimbabwe

Packer B 1988 A manual of APT, appropriate paper-based technology. IRED, Harare, Zimbabwe

Wolf-Vereecken M J 1993 Cerebral palsy children in Africa: early identification and intervention. Tool, Amsterdam

Cross-cultural research

Biomedical practitioners should not make assumptions about the meaning of disability or the role of rehabilitation based solely on their own perspectives. Historically, there has been relatively little research to discern the meaning of disability and rehabilitation cross-culturally, especially by rehabilitation professionals, and relatively few examples of publication in the literature typically read by those professionals. Section 4, 'Cross-cultural Research', provides examples of qualitative and quantitative research that can aid in the development of cultural competence by increasing the understanding of particular populations. This section adds to the knowledge base in this field and encourages cross-disciplinary and cross-cultural research, especially by practicing clinicians who have never before ventured into this arena.

Cross-cultural Rehabilitation: an International Perspective should generate many questions that the clinician would like answered to better understand the nature and meaning of disability and rehabilitation in different environments. In this way, the likelihood of achieving cultural proficiency is increased. That is, the degree of cultural competency whereby culture is held in high regard and the need to conduct research, disseminate the results, and develop new approaches that might increase culturally competent practice is recognized.

The first two chapters in this section focus on the patterns of health beliefs and behaviors of families with disabled children in rural Jamaica, an upper-middle-income country in the Caribbean that is in the midst of transition from a Third World, developing nation to an industrialized nation. The study population are participants in a community based rehabilitation (CBR) program, the 3D Project: Dedicated to the Development of the Disabled, founded by Marigold Thorburn.

Chapter 26, 'Health beliefs and behaviors of families with children who are disabled in rural Jamaica', by Ronnie Leavitt, defines the medical care systems and explanatory models of these individuals whose culture is influenced by African, European, and North American traditions. Leavitt complements Groce (Ch. 4) by giving a more detailed description of attitudes toward children with a disability (CWD), the cultural adaptation by the family, beliefs about the cause of disability, and healing practices, for one specific population.

This research has three main conclusions:

1. It appears that CWD are not particularly stigmatized at the household level. Nevertheless, societal stigmatization and apathy do exist. As a result, these children are not being prepared to integrate fully into Jamaican society.
2. This population has adapted their cultural belief systems and actual behaviors to match their material realities. That is, it would appear that people who have a disability, and their caretakers, have demonstrated 'contextual accommodation'.
3. There is a range of variation of beliefs and behaviors with regard to disability and rehabilitation, supporting the concept of intracultural diversity.

It has been generally presumed that PWD are stigmatized at the family level and that they are a burden. These findings, however, do not support the notion of family stigmatization, and several of the other chapters also point to PWD participating in household and community activities, albeit sometimes after an intervention such as CBR. As for being a burden, 'contextual accommodation' indicates that adaptation is quite attainable. With regard to specific beliefs and behaviors regarding disability and re-

habilitation, the conflicts with Western views are explicit yet not insurmountable and have implications for developing services and working with a community to achieve shared goals. Clearly, there is a wide range of variation in different cultures, and there have been no definitive answers to questions regarding stigmatization of PWD or what interventions are likely to be more successful in helping to achieve full participation of PWD into society.

In 'Barriers to successful implementation of community based rehabilitation in Jamaica', Marigold Thorburn draws conclusions from a series of research studies within 3D Projects during the late 1980s and 1990s. Thorburn has pursued the impact of particular human variables on the implementation of CBR, noting the philosophical and methodological difficulties inherent in attempting to evaluate a CBR program. For example, the question is raised, is it more important to show progress in the developmental status of a child, or is it more important to know the wider impact of CBR on the family? Thorburn addresses research that primarily focuses on the parents' involvement with the 3D Project. Specifically she addresses the impact of knowledge about disability, severity of disability, child rearing roles, experiences of families with health services, community attitudes toward disability, and more.

One finding, with very practical implications for the practicing clinician, repeated by Stout and O'Toole (Ch. 15) and Jelsma and Zhanje (Ch. 28), is that it might be unrealistic and unfair to ask an already busy and burdened caregiver for an intensive time commitment to rehabilitative efforts. Thorburn cites a situational analysis of disabilities and rehabilitation in the Caribbean, where the informants identified their priority needs as things like transportation, income-generating projects, respite care, job placement, mobility aids and self advocacy; not early intervention or CBR. (Possibly, this is because people do not know about the concepts of CBR, or possibly it is deemed less relevant.) It is quite obvious that finding out the priority areas of need for a particular population would be a primary goal. What is less obvious to those not already used to practicing in a cross-cultural environment is that the goals may be quite different than ones identified by the therapist.

Thorburn concludes with strategies to minimize the identified barriers, especially those geared toward increasing parental involvement in the CBR process. For many years Thorburn has believed that, along with home based training, the efforts of parents in educating and supporting new parents of CWD or other family members of PWD are the most critical components to successful implementation of CBR.

Taken together, Chapters 26 and 27 help to document the varied responses to disability at the individual family level and by the larger community within the Jamaican culture. They also exemplify how one set of research questions can generate many more research questions and how an understanding of disability and rehabilitation in a particular sociocultural context can be a process that requires many years of study by many professional disciplines.

'Impact of the Harare parents' groups for children with a disability and their parents: are caregivers satisfied with the service?', by Jennifer Jelsma and Maude Zhanje, also addresses the critical issue of parental involvement in CBR. Chapter 28 describes the inner-city neighborhood based Parents' Groups (PGs) that evolved as an outreach component of the Children's Rehabilitation Unit (CRU) in Harare, Zimbabwe, as a means to maximize meager health resources while providing a good quality service.

Some of the results are particularly germane to understanding the sociocultural context in which rehabilitation occurs. In contrast to the work described in Chapter 26 by Leavitt, Jelsma and Zhanje report that 26% of the caregivers reported a significant life change (i.e. a breakdown in their marriages) as a result of having a child with a disability. All of the respondents reported strained family relations. At the same time, the effect of the extended family appears to be ambivalent. Previous studies (including those reported on by Thorburn) noted that the cultural practice of encompassing the extended

family within a close knit unit may be helping to maintain the mental health of the caregivers. Yet, in this study, the extended family is often perceived to be a negative influence on family relations. Nevertheless, this group overall had low levels of stress associated with coping with their children.

Also important (and seen in the work by Leavitt and by Masin) is the sometimes apparent co-existence of mutually incompatible differences between the explanatory models of the clients and the practitioner. In addition, there is the difference between perceived knowledge regarding disability and actual knowledge. Often misconceptions abound. Surely, improved education regarding the cause of disability and the setting of realistic goals for a particular PWD is an area that needs continued attention in much of the world.

The biomedical model has been severely criticized for encouraging the professional to take charge. That does not mean, however, that the role of the professional is insignificant. In this study, the caretakers strongly expressed the desire for more individualized treatment sessions by a rehabilitation worker. Although the principle of 'empowerment' is critical for PWD to lead a full and satisfying life, Jelsma and Zhanje ask if all parents wish to be empowered with regard to providing therapy for their children? It is possible that parents wish the professional to be the professional, so that they might do the parenting. The authors conclude that concerned rehabilitation workers cannot impose a CBR philosophy on a society that still has a conventional understanding of the provision of medical and rehabilitation care. This consideration would be fundamental when trying to adapt CBR to either a developing country or an industrialized nation. But, in reality, alternatives may exist where there are professionals, but what happens when there are no – or very few – professionals?

Helen Masin, in Chapter 29, compares two specific ethnic groups in one geographic urban area in the USA. 'Cross-cultural parent education and early intervention: Cuban and African-American families in Miami, Florida, USA', specifically addresses maternal knowledge of and attitudes toward physical therapy during an early intervention program. This research fosters cultural competence by providing specific knowledge of the clients' way of life and greater insight into the impact of ethnicity on a rehabilitation intervention.

Masin begins by describing public policy in the USA regarding early intervention for CWD. This discussion might be useful for clinicians working in other countries where legislation supporting the rights of CWD has been less forthcoming. Masin stresses the notion that services must be family-centered (as opposed to only child-centered) and that therapists must understand family dynamics and culture.

Although similarities exist between the African-American and Cuban-American clients, the results of this research point to several differences that may be accounted for by cultural variables associated with ethnicity. For example, the Cuban-American mothers stressed the importance of *personalismo*, that is, the idea that it is important for a therapist to develop a personal relationship with the family as opposed to a purely 'professional' relationship. For their part, African-American mothers seemed more concerned by their child's lack of motor development. This is associated with an emphasis, in the African-American culture, on motor skills and childhood independence. Masin also reminds us that both of these groups differ in some respects from most of the practicing therapists in the USA, whose cultural value systems are more aligned with the Euro-American tradition. Clinicians must be sensitive to these differences.

Chapter 30, 'Professional development, personality and self-esteem of Palestinian physical therapists', differs from the preceding chapters because it describes research related to the practicing professionals rather than PWD. Dawson is interested in how a professional body can develop in a nation that does not have a well-established history of that profession, an inquiry also posed by Kay and her colleagues (Ch. 23) and Nelson and Rubi (Ch. 19). Chapter 30 pro-

vides a window through which to get a picture of how the physical therapy profession is practiced in a particular environment, in this case a politically unstable environment with limited resources and opportunities. Issues identified by Dawson (such as limited scope of practice, cultural barriers to Western-style evaluation and treatment procedures as well as to the idea of continuing education, and the lack of public knowledge about what physical therapy can do) are also common to most other developing nations where professional development has been limited.

Dawson also explores the personality and self-esteem profiles of Palestinian and Irish physical therapists to see how these may interrelate with professional development. Based on questionnaires, she found statistically significant differences for some personality characteristics and degree of self-esteem between the two groups. Although certain aspects of a therapist's character may be universal because of the humanistic nature of the job, other characteristics necessary for practice are culturally based and differ between countries. Dawson proposes that if these can be identified, that knowledge might prove useful to the process of professional development and also aid individuals who are considering cross-cultural work to overcome the problems associated with culture shock and ethnocentrism. The discussion of these variables and their relationship to culture complements material from Chapter 2, 'The concept of culture', Chapter 8, 'Cross-cultural communication', and Chapter 22, Culture and its impact on the rehabilitation program: a Palestinian perspective'.

To summarize, Section 4 provides examples of cross-cultural research in the fields of disability studies and rehabilitation. Further study validating conclusions from these studies needs to be done within additional cultural environments. Moreover, the quest for additional information to facilitate an understanding of the meaning of disability and rehabilitation throughout the world and professional cultural competence remains a high priority.

26

Health beliefs and behaviors of families with children who are disabled in rural Jamaica

Ronnie Leavitt

This chapter describes and analyzes the patterns of health beliefs and behaviors of families with children who are disabled in rural Jamaica. These data are part of a larger study that includes:

1. An ethnographic description of the 3D Project : Dedicated to the Development of the Disabled, which is a community based rehabilitation (CBR) project.
2. An analysis of the issues and problems associated with a CBR program in a low income, rural environment.

This study defines the culture of disability and rehabilitation for a particular population. Knowledge of this information has facilitated more effective care and the development of an appropriate cultural response by the 3D Project. It could be replicated in other nations and cultures, and it is an example of how one can combine the theoretical and practical domains of a rehabilitation science, such as physical or occupational therapy, public health, and medical anthropology. This chapter summarizes material found in *Disability and Rehabilitation in Rural Jamaica* (Leavitt 1992).

INTRODUCTION

This research is an effort to define the medical care systems and explanatory models of families with disabled children who live in a developing nation and have limited access to formal medical services. Medical anthropologists Fabrega & Manning (1979) define medical care systems as 'the constellation of beliefs, knowledge, practices, personnel, and facilities and resources that together structure and pattern the way members of a sociological group obtain care and treatment of illness' (Fabrega & Manning 1979, p. 41). Others, such as Foster (1976), use the term comparative ethnomedicine, defined as 'those beliefs and practices relating to disease which are the products of indigenous cultural development and are not explicitly derived from the conceptual framework of modern medicine' (Foster 1976, p. 774). In either case, in most Third World nations, 'modern' or 'Western' medicine is intertwined with 'indigenous' or 'folk' medicine, and it is likely that there is functional continuity between the two systems. This results in medical pluralism, the existence and use of many different health care alternatives within societies.

One process through which medical ethnography analyzes local health care systems has been developed by Kleinman (1980). He sees the health care system as a special kind of cultural system that includes such elements as patterns of belief about the causes of illness, decisions about how to respond to specific episodes of sickness, and the actions taken in order to effect a change. The beliefs and behaviors exhibited by an individual are influenced by macrosocial and bioenvironmental factors. Specifically, Kleinman has developed the theory of an explanatory model (EM) in order to analyze this kind of cultural system: 'EMs are the notions about an episode of sickness and its treatment that are employed by all those engaged in the clinical process. The study of patient and family EMs tell us how they make sense of given episodes of illness, and how they choose and evaluate particular treatments' (Kleinman 1980, p. 105).

EMs attempt to explain five major questions for specific illness episodes. These are: etiology; time and mode of onset of symptoms; pathophysiology; course of sickness; and treatment (Kleinman 1980). The answers to these questions are formed and employed in response to a particular illness.

Kleinman's EM is a microscopic, internal, clinical view of the patient's cultural health care system. However, an EM is certainly presumed to be influenced by social institutions (clinics, hospitals), social roles (healing, sick role), interaction settings (home, doctor's office), and economic and political conditions. Thus, it is necessary to analyze EMs in a concrete setting.

Other medical anthropology theorists have also researched and tested specific models, within specific cultural settings, in order to explain certain health beliefs and behaviors. Yet, this important theoretical domain has hardly been looked at with regard to disability.

JAMAICA: THE NATION AND ITS PEOPLE

Jamaica, the largest English-speaking Caribbean island, is part of the West Indies. The topography consists mainly of coastal plains and mountainous regions, although it is Jamaica's beaches that are most famous and attract a large number of tourists. The parish and city of Kingston is the seat of government and commerce. Since Jamaica became independent from Britain in 1962, relative political stability has been the norm (Gleaner 1985).

The estimated population of Jamaica is 2.5 million people, with 34% under 15 years of age; 54% live in cities (UNICEF 1994). Approximately three-fourths of Jamaicans are pure Negro, with most of the others of mixed race. Social stratification exists, but it is secondary to skin color and economic differences. Within the household, a low rate of formal marriage and high rates of economic instability and mobility for males result in a great deal of migration and thus the relative absence of males within the household. This often leads to female-headed households (Paterson 1982).

Jamaica is classified as an upper-middle-income country, with a free market economy and a dominant private sector. The per capita income in 1992 was US$1380 (UNICEF 1994), but there is considerable inequality in the distribution of wealth. In addition, while Jamaica is moving from a Third World, traditional, agricultural society to a modern, more technical one, it is not yet as economically stable or as prosperous as countries in the industrialized world.

Health care and health status

The health care delivery system and health status of the people in Jamaica are also in transition. The relative incidence of acute communicable diseases is decreasing and those chronic diseases most often seen in the elderly are increasing. The infant mortality rate in 1992 was 12 per 1000 live births and the life expectancy was 73 years (UNICEF 1994). Primary health care programs are the focal point for health activities with health centers throughout the country. A limited secondary and tertiary system also exists. The private sector is restricted to the middle and upper class. Health personnel are in short and declining supply due to the large numbers of professionals who emigrate.

In Jamaica, concern for the plight of people with disabilities has always been a low priority. Although a few individuals have been active in this cause, it took the World Health Organization (WHO) International Year for Disabled Persons (IYDP) in 1981 to bring forth significant activity. Rehabilitation services had historically only been available in Kingston, mostly at the Mona Rehabilitation Centre, with virtually no services in rural areas. During the 1980s and 1990s, this began to change with the advent of programs oriented to CBR. The 3D Project, which attempts to provide comprehensive services to children with single or multiple disabilities, has contributed significantly to the now available services that some people with disabilities can access. (See Ch. 27).

Health beliefs and behaviors

With regard to health beliefs and behaviors, there appears to be cultural variation among groups on the island, and changes are inevitable with continued modernization. Certain African beliefs are maintained, although in modern times European and North American culture seems to be the dominant motif in the media,

educational and health care systems, and in the religious arena. The African heritage is reflected in much of the current Jamaican culture and folk medical belief systems. In particular, the Jamaicans' belief in African forms of witchcraft and animism is relevant to the issues addressed in this research (Morrish 1982, Cassidy 1982, Brathwaite 1978, Walker 1986).

Obeah, or the practice of witchcraft, was transmitted by African slaves to Jamaica and remained their own esoteric possession, not to be shared with their masters. *Obeah* (also seen as *Obi* or *Obia*) is 'essentially a magical means whereby an individual may obtain his personal desires, eradicate ill health, procure good fortune in life and business, turn the affections of the objects of his love or lust towards himself, evince retribution or revenge upon his enemies, and generally manipulate the spiritual forces of the cosmos in order to obtain his will' (Morrish 1982, p. 41).

The *obeah* man or woman (synonymous terms are balm-man, bush-doctor, do-good man, four-eyed man, *buzu*, *guzu* or *zuzu* man, shadow catcher, professor, and knife and scissors man) keeps his 'things' in his *obi* place. These 'things' are composed of such materials as blood, feathers, parrot's beak, grave dirt, rum, and egg shells, and his 'bush' is a concoction of medicinal herbs. (There is, as expected, great suspicion toward people inquiring about *obeah*.) It is reportedly practiced and believed in by large numbers of people, even though it is forbidden by law.

Other categories of 'professional practitioners' are the 'spiritualist,' 'Mayalist' (from the African word *Maye* meaning sorcerer, or wizard), 'psychic,' or 'mother,' the latter two being females who guide their clients on general matters (Robertson 1982).

Strongly linked with the practice of *obeah* is the belief in 'duppies' ('bugaboo' and 'jumby' are terms also used). The concept of 'duppy,' meaning ghost or spirit, was originally derived from the Ashanti belief in the *saman* and *sasa* elements in the human being. The *saman* was the ghost that was the form in which the dead could become visible upon earth. The *sasa*, in contrast, was the invisible spiritual power of an individual that caused a spell to be worked on someone so that they might suffer. Today, both terms are covered by the word duppy.

The duppy is frequently blamed for things that go wrong or are evil. Duppies can be visible and invisible, and they can work through people, animals, birds, and plants. Duppies 'feed' upon bamboo root, fig leaves, and the gourd-like fruit of a vine called duppy pumpkin. Mushrooms, sometimes referred to as duppy caps or duppy umbrellas, are associated with duppies. Duppies live and play around the silk cotton tree and are especially fond of the night. They are thought to be unpredictable, sometimes helpful and sometimes harmful. *Obeah* ritual is often concerned with the duppy. The *obeah* may sometimes cause a problem by 'putting' the spirit sickness on a person, or the *obeah* may 'work it off.'

Related to these topics is the general domain of Jamaican folk medicines. Again, the dominant origin of the folk medicine practices are West African (Robertson 1982, Lowe 1972). The treatments can be as simple as the use of a bush tea for a cold, avocado to lower high blood pressure, and pawpaw to get rid of a boil, or as complex as the treatment by an *obeah* man employing many of the previously mentioned materials. Most 'bushmen' are not *obeah* men but rather spiritualists who believe that herbs can strengthen the physical body and therefore help to ward off ailments. Often, the spiritualist believes in the necessity of supporting the healing herbs with religious ceremony, charms, fresh air and sunlight, or other foods such as cock soup, or roasted animal testes.

In addition to these folk medical beliefs, a multitude of superstitions relate to foods and health. Some of these are (Campbell 1974):

- Liver makes the baby's tongue heavy
- Condensed milk gives babies worms
- Cornmeal porridge turns back the teething water into the infant's stomach and this causes diarrhea
- If babies drink goat's milk they will have a big forehead
- Cocoa and chocolate rot bones

- Crayfish makes you foolish
- Ripe banana in combination with butter is poisonous

The following folk tales are representative of a body of Jamaican folklore that is important for its impact on the particular sample population studied during this research. These tales, regarding babies, were shared by a group of eight women who worked with a Peace Corps volunteer who happened to be pregnant (Thams 1986).

- Newborn babies should have a red ribbon tied around their left wrist to ward off evil spirits. Duppies are afraid of red.
- Newborn babies should sleep in a red nightshirt to ward off evil spirits and 'nigger mouths,' or people will talk a lot of nonsense to the baby.
- A Bible, opened to the 23rd Psalm, should be laid by the baby's head when he is sleeping.
- Place an opened pair of scissors or a horseshoe over the bedroom door where the baby sleeps to keep away evil spirits.
- When walking outside with the baby do not walk backwards as this will allow for spirits to play with the baby.
- Evil spirits will follow you home if you take a baby out at night before his christening.
- Put asafetida (a mixture of beeswax and roots) in front of the baby's hair to keep away cold and evil spirits.
- Do not let menstruating women hold a baby or it will get stomach cramps.
- Do not eat pear (avocado), ackee, rice or peas when nursing as they will upset the baby's stomach.
- If a pregnant woman has sex with a man other than the baby's father, the baby will be handicapped.
- Do not leave baby clothes hanging on the line after 4 p.m. as the spirits will run on them.
- When a baby's navel stump falls off, the mother must bury it outside under a young plant to ensure that the baby will grow strong and healthy.
- Do not cut a baby's hair before he can talk or he will have problems talking.

METHODS OF RESEARCH

This ethnographic study combines the concepts from general anthropological theory, the culture of a North American physical therapist, and, as much as possible, the Jamaican population under study. Thus, it uses both an emic (insider's) point of view and an etic (outsider's) point of view. To provide an ecological, or holistic approach, this ethnography includes the broad features of the 'cultural landscape' as well as the small details of the culture of the families with children with disabilities in rural Jamaica. The specific tools of research were participant observation, unstructured key informant interviews, and structured interviews with families participating in the 3D project.

The research site was St Catherine parish, Jamaica. The families in the sample population were participants in the 3D Project. Structured interviews were completed for 81 families. A majority of the interviews took place at the homes of the participants. Key informants were the community rehabilitation workers (CRWs) who provided services to the families; most of these workers were also mothers of disabled children (Fig. 26.1).

The interview schedule was constructed to elicit a range of descriptive data associated with the key theoretical domains under study: stigma, adaptation, and health beliefs and behaviors. In coding the data, 103 variables were constructed for the numerical analysis. Ethnographic descriptive materials and quotes were excerpted directly from tape-recorded interviews and field notes.

RESEARCH RESULTS

Characteristics of the child with a disability

There were 46 male and 35 female children in the study groups. The average age was 7 years, the mode was 4 years, and the median 5 years. The relatively young ages of the participants was encouraging: early intervention maximizes function and minimizes complications or secondary handicaps. The largest category of children were mentally retarded (including Down Syndrome) (N=30) or classified as multiply disabled with cerebral palsy (CP) and mental retardation (N=22). In nearly all the cases, the impairment was prenatal or perinatal. The children were classified as having a moderate (N=48) or severe (N=33) disability (Fig. 26.2). It

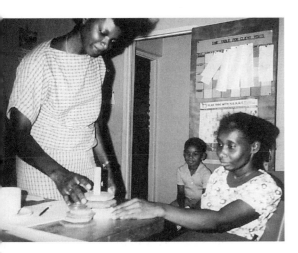

Fig. 26.1 Community rehabilitation workers in 3D Projects, Jamaica. Role playing early stimulation activities. Photo courtesy: Ronnie Leavitt.

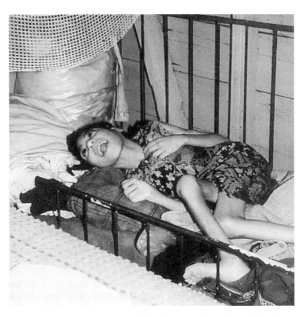

Fig. 26.2 Participant in 3D Projects. Although not ideal, living at home is the most appropriate place for this severely disabled child. Photo courtesy: Ronnie Leavitt.

is assumed that children with minimal impairments or disability would not enroll in the 3D Project. Nine of the 31 children between the ages of 6 and 17 years were enrolled in a school program.

Material (economic) conditions

The families who participate in the 3D Project are generally very poor. Very few of the participants had a regular source of income. For each case in this study, a composite of several material item variables was used to determine an overall economic indicator. Families received one point if they owned a working material item, such as a radio, gas stove, refrigerator, television, or telephone. Housing structure was also considered (Fig. 26.3). For example, points were given for indoor toileting, indoor cooking, a tile or cement floor, and cement walls. The range of economic status scores was from 1 to 15. The mean was 7.4, the mode 5, and the median 7.

Social and structural characteristics of the family and household

Two-thirds (N=55) of the primary caretakers for the children with a disability were the mother of

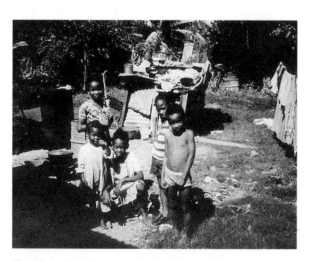

Fig. 26.3 Participants in 3D Projects, Jamaica. Impoverished living conditions. Photo courtesy: Ronnie Leavitt.

the child. The second largest group (N=14) were females one generation removed, usually grand mothers. Other caretakers were aunts (N=5) fathers (N=5) and paid helpers (N=2). The aver age age of the caretakers was about 37 years.

There was a wide range of household organi zation types, with the most common being sin gle female with child and other adults presen (N=21), followed by a married couple with chil and no other adults present (N=16). The tota number of people in a household averaged 6.5 In all, 75% of the households had a male pres ence.

The informants overwhelmingly expresse strong religious convictions, although many d not regularly attend church. Religion and spiri tuality are reported to play an important part i the lives of most Jamaicans, especially as means of withdrawing from everyday socia and economic deprivation (Morrish 1982).

Perceived stigma

The concept of stigma was measured by direc observation and reported comments by th informants. Statements reported by the infor mants used to measure degree of stigma wer concerned with how often they took the chil with a disability out of the house compare with non-disabled children, and what friend and neighbors said about and to the child.

Forty-seven informants reported that, to thei knowledge, no neighbors, friends, or famil members said negative things about their child Rather, the neighbors seemed to be quite fond o the child in question. Thirty-two informant reported hearing negative comments, but mos believed they were isolated incidents, usuall coming from one person. The informant typi cally added, 'I don't pay them attention.' Thos who reported negative comments have a signifi cantly lower score on the economic item scale.

In 55 cases, it was reported that caregiver took the child with a disability outside of th household in a manner similar to non-disable siblings. Taking a child with a disability outsid was highly associated with the child's age, th degree to which the child is handicapped, an having maximized activity of daily living (ADL) skills. There was a significant tendency for these children to be younger, moderately disabled and otherwise performing whatever ADL skills possible, and having fewer children less than 9 years old in the household. These findings seem reasonable.

Of the 26 cases when the child was not taken outside of the house, 13 caretakers specifically stated that the reason was because it posed a physical burden for them. In other words, the child was too heavy to be carried. (Only three children in the study population had a wheelchair.) Some other reasons are that the child has no shoes, the child holds the caretaker back, the child is teased by others, or the child is 'rude' (i.e. naughty). In at least some of these 13 cases, it appears that stigma may have been a factor in the child not being taken outside in a manner similar to other children.

Although stigma was not present in most instances at the family and local community level, children with disabilities are not being prepared to integrate fully into Jamaican society. They are rarely able to attend school and they are not prepared for any future vocation.

Cultural adaptation

Several variables measured the degree to which families appeared to have adapted to having to care for a child with a disability. Questions asked of the caretaker included ones related to their major concerns and possible life-style changes.

For the most part, the presence of a child with a disability in the household did not lead to significant life-style or economic changes for the families. Thirty-seven informants reported no life changes, 20 reported a psychological complaint such as 'worry' or 'fretting' over the child, 16 complained that they could not go out as much as they wished, and six complained of not being able to look for a job. Thus, a total of 22 informants reported some economic or life-style change, and 57 of 81 informants reported no such changes. It appears that caretakers of children with a disability have demonstrated 'contextual accommodation'.

Health beliefs and behaviors

Health beliefs regarding causation of disability

The range of variation in the beliefs of the caretaker concerning the cause of the child's disability is considerable. Typically, the informant would preface their remarks with 'I don't know, but maybe,' or there was some ambivalence evident. For example, the informant might say, 'I believe such and such, but my mother (or husband, neighbor, etc.) thinks such and such'.

There was also a range of variation in the probable validity of the responses. That is, from the point of view of a medically educated Westerner from a developed nation, some responses were scientifically sound and others were unlikely. Examples of probable valid naturalistic causes of disability include: jaundice, prolonged and difficult labor, a history of German measles and a chromosomal abnormality. Examples of probable invalid naturalistic causes of disability include: lack of proper diet (stated by a mother who has a child with Down syndrome); 'nerve shock' or other examples of 'fright'; and when the informant believed the problem was hereditary, yet the child appeared to be brain damaged from meningitis or cerebral palsy.

Examples of responses that are oriented toward naturalistic belief systems include the following:

Fits damage the brain . . . . I am sort of curious, because I have four of them at home and he's the only one that born in the hospital, so sometime I sort of think – what really happen – I don't know . . . . People tell me maybe spirit troubling him, but I don't really think that.

Like how I have the children fast and the food me eat. Maybe I did need more nutritious food [she names liver, fish, cheese, greens, etc.]. Me had a problem with me big daughter . . . sent her to buy shoes and she run away with a guy and she never come back until long after the baby born. I was very worried.

Long time it take to born . . . . The after birth is coming before . . . . I had lots of clots . . . . The brain no grow, it's no the head, it's the brain.

The doctor say the child had jaundice. I ask why. He say because of sweets – maybe I eat sweets when I was pregnant.

Jaundice at birth and she premature. The hospital didn't have the facilities for the jaundice, to burn it out, so the jaundice damage her.

In contrast to these beliefs are those in which the caretaker believes in a supernatural cause for the child's disability. It is quite possible that informants under-reported their belief in supernatural causes:

The duppy . . . well, because babies are small, people who pass off like to play with them. That's what cause the life of my last baby . . . . When you leave baby alone, the duppies play with him. The duppies want to give assistance.

When me seven months, I saw a duppy and was frightened. Also, the house family lived in was over a graveyard.

I believe in normal sickness with some addition of evil. The devil throw some sensation on her at the school.

Evil play with her . . . . The spirit lady said it because me was nicer to my father than my mother, and it is me father's duppy.

Describing a dream, the mother says:

I heard somebody call me, and I say stupidness, and the girl replied name of man – he not live around here. I dream about Adescalene's father [who is dead] and he said he was going to show her something – then he pitched across the bed in my vision. Adescalene took sick in me vision in the middle of the night and she wake up sick having fits.

The Kumina Queen (a religious leader), who is the 'adoptive mother' of a retarded boy says:

It's a kind of spiritual order . . . the mother leave him at night and when she coming back for it nobody there to look about the baby. Spirit come and fingle it [plays with it or caring for it] . . . me give the child sugar and water and the spirit no like that . . . the father says spirit feed him – him sick and vomit up some green things [the child vomits up the bad spirit food].

Whether the caretaker believed in a natural or supernatural cause, there appeared to be a strong religious component to the belief of many of the caretakers:

I just believe God make him and he make everyone of us to his own likeness.

Well, maybe he [God] would [have caused the child's disability], he know that I can cope. Because I don't think he going to give you more than what you can manage.

Sickness is not our fault. God gave it to us. We have faith in God.

God gave him to me – because the other children is good. He must know the reason. God caused it.

In contrast, a few people did not believe that God had any connection to their child's problems no matter what they believed was the cause:

I don't believe that God make him sick like that. Me say is me the problem come from since me was young.

I don't believe God ever give you anything that is bad. If you are sick it's just maybe a natural thing.

God don't make anyone sick. Sickness is from the devil.

Forty-nine caretakers believe that their children are disabled due to natural causes. Seven informants believe that the disability is due to a supernatural cause. Fourteen informants were ambivalent in their feelings as to why the child is disabled, and eleven informants claimed that they had no idea why the child was disabled. More specific details concerning the sample's beliefs regarding the cause of their child's problem are seen in Table 26.1.

There is a significant relationship between those caretakers who profess to have a very strong belief in God and those who believe in the possibility of a supernatural cause. Also, there is a strong tendency for those who believe in the possibility of a supernatural cause of the disability to use a variety of traditional healing practices. Supporting data are detailed below in the discussion concerning health behaviors.

There were no other statistically significant findings with respect to beliefs concerning the cause of the child's disability. Cause was not significantly related to such things as the caretaker's age, level of education, degree of cosmopolitan contact, the household's economic status, the child's diagnosis or degree of impair-

Table 26.1 Beliefs concerning the cause of the disability

Cause of the Problem	Frequency
Natural causes	63*
Birth trauma or prematurity	17
Childhood disease or accident	14
Mother had problem**	11
Hereditary or genetic disease	7
Jaundice/blood incompatibility	5
Psychological problem	3
Food ingestion	3
Unknown	3
Supernatural causes	21*
Evil spirit/devil	9
'Duppy'	8
God's will	4
Unknown cause	11

* These numbers denote the total number of informants who believed in a particular type of cause and those that were ambivalent. Some individuals named two possible causes of the child's disability.
** Examples include high blood pressure or rubella during pregnancy.

ment, or variables associated with perceived stigma or adaptation.

Current behaviors and traditional healing practices

An important area of investigation was the use of traditional healing practices. Fifty informants reported that they use one or more healing practices not suggested by medical personnel or the CRWs in order to improve the child's condition. Thirty-one informants claim to not use such practices. (Once again, it is presumed that, if anything, these data represent an under-reporting of the use of traditional healing practices.) By virtue of the fact that each member of this sample was registered in the 3D Project, the use of these practices does not preclude the use of cosmopolitan medicine and community health programs.

Example of statements concerning the use of indigenous healing practices for the treatment of a child with a disability are:

They say using olive oil you can help the joints to souple.

I use baths a whole lot of times, in the night, put wash pan of water over here, and put two sticks and cross them – let it stay overnight, and bathe him in the morning.

To keep away the spirits the child is dressed in red clothes.

Me boils coconut oil and mix with olive oil – use it to anoint her legs. They say it help the stiffness.

Catch water from six in the evening and let it sit all night and get night dew. Wake him at five in the morning and sop [beat] him legs in it.

I put milk in the bath, and no talk with anyone until after the bath.

Bathe her in Old Man Beard bush.

Dig a hole to the level of the waist. Bury him in it for one hour, remove him and stand him.

Me use grapefruit juice and brandy to wet his mole [brain]. It helps to keep his brain steady.

Yes, I wouldn't hide you that [going to a mother lady], cause I had to try all that because I see and get the vision and maybe it can be a different inferior spirit come along and hurt her.

The mother lady sent me to the bush doctor shop. Get some kind oil to use on her and bush to boil.

Religion appears to be as important a factor in influencing the caretaker's behavior with regard to treatment practices as it was in influencing the caretaker's belief system:

When the child does not have a duppy sickness the mother takes her to a doctor. But when it is a duppy sickness, 'You get a different power to deal with that. Me lay my hand on him and pray . . . I know when they [the duppies] come and run them . . . I rebuke the spirit and he have to go . . . Only I is safe to do it, because me only one who feel the holy ghost. I is a Christian . . . I speak unto God . . . speak in tongues . . . It happens at the moment and I interpret the word. The Lord will keep away the duppies.

In everything we have to think of God and so we have to pray, for she could not talk but now she is say 'no.'

God is able to do all things. I leave him in God's hands.

I think God have a different plan for him. I'm praying to see that plan when it come through. I love him [the child] very much – what hope for him I'd like to be around when that hope come through. God will make him better in a way he can help himself.

I know the Lord can heal him ... don't know if my faith is strong enough. You need great faith ... Darvey [the child] no have faith.

Give God praise, I can't praise, I can't stop giving ... that day [when the Pastor prayed for the boy], you should be there ... it was a glorious time ... and therefore I know the blessing from the Church follow him ... God is a healer ... you must seek earthly help too.

Baby need prayers, maybe if I pray for baby, baby will gain strength and do things.

I'm a Christian you know, and he weren't like this you know [the child had been functioning at a lower level]. I took him to the Throne of Grace, and I laid on him right here and I prayed on him day and night and I ask God to touch him because he used to run all over the place as though him mad ... but I entreated him to God and I laid on down on him and I pray and I say God touch him. I kept on asking the Lord to touch him, and I can see for *sure* him better.

The Kumina Queen says, 'You have to call to God before you do anything ... me deal with God direct ... me no deal with the duppy one [*obeah* man] ... me speak seven different languages and speak in tongues ... I can't make him [the child] talk, God have to give that.'

Table 26.2 Use of traditional healing practices

Practice	Yes	No
Use of olive oil	32	49
Use of medicinal food or drink	19	62
Use of special baths	17	64
Speaks to God	17	64
Visits an *obeah*	9	72
Other practices*	7	74

*Includes such things as eating from a calabash, burying the child in a hole to the waist for 1 hour, rubbing grapefruit juice and brandy on the 'mole' (brain), dressing the child in red, and not cutting the child's hair until he talks.

The frequency with which specific healing practices are used is seen in Table 26.2.

The use of non-prescription home remedies was not statistically significantly related to the child's diagnosis or degree of disability or the caretaker's degree of faith. Also not significant was what the caretakers stated as their primary concern regarding the child's situation (i.e., the child's lack of fulfilling physical milestones versus other concerns such as the inability of the child to go to school).

However, there is a strong tendency for those who believe in the possibility of a supernatural cause of the disabling problem to also use traditional healing practices. More specifically, those who believe that the child's disability is possibly caused by a supernatural force are more likely to use olive oil on the body, to drink medicinal tea, and to 'speak' with God.

Two other variables are statistically associated with the use of non-prescription healing practices. First, there is a relationship between not using indigenous treatment techniques and a delay in seeking action related to treatment for the disabled child. Once the child had been diagnosed as having a problem, those who do not use indigenous treatment techniques were also delayed in registering at the 3D Project.

For this study population, the concept of intracultural diversity is supported by the range of variation of beliefs and behaviors with regard to disability and rehabilitation. Although there are significant relationships when trying to discover variables correlating with a particular dependent variable, there is no indication that any single independent variable is of particular significance in determining a family's beliefs or behaviors.

CONCLUSIONS

It is presumed that there are people with disabilities in every society and that there will be specific medical care systems and explanatory models that account for the beliefs about the disability and the cultural patterns of behaviors having to do with disability diagnosis and treatment. The presence of a particular system is undoubtedly related in part to societal attitudes toward disability, the degree to which people with a disability are stigmatized, the material realities of the environment, and the adaptation mechanisms that are available for any individual and their family. This study provides data that define the culture of disability for a particular population and allows for the development of an appropriate cultural response by the 3D Project in rural Jamaica.

REFERENCES

Brathwaite E 1978 The spirit of African survival in Jamaica: Kumina. Jamaican Journal 42: 45–63.

Campbell S 1974 Folk lore and food habits. Jamaican Journal 8 (2/3): 56–65

Cassidy F 1982 Jamaica talk. McMillian Caribbean, London

Fabrega H 1974 Disease and social behavior: an interdisciplinary perspective. MIT Press, Cambridge, MA

Fabrega H, Manning P K 1979 Illness episodes: illness severity and treatment options in a pluralistic setting. Social Science and Medicine 13B: 41–51

Foster G 1976 Disease etiologies in non-Western medical systems. American Anthropologist 78: 773–782

Gleaner Co 1985 Geography and history of Jamaica. Gleaner Co, Kingston, Jamaica

Kleinman A 1980 Patients and healers in the context of culture. University of California Press, Berkeley, CA

Leavitt R 1992 Disability and rehabilitation in rural Jamaica: an ethnographic study. Fairleigh Dickinson University Press, Rutherford, NJ

Lowe H 1972 Folk medicine in Jamaica. Jamaican Journal 6(2): 20–24

Morrish I 1982 Obeah, Christ and Rastaman: Jamaica and its religion. James Clarke, Cambridge

Paterson O 1982 Persistence, continuity and change in the Jamaican working class family. Journal of Family History 7(2): 135–161

Robertson D 1982 Jamaican herbs: nutritional and medicinal values. Typeart Services, Kingston

Thams S 1986 Jamaican folk tales. Peace Corps Publication, Kingston

UNICEF 1994 The state of the world's children. Oxford University Press, Oxford

Walker S 1986 Attitudes toward the disabled as reflected in social mores in Africa. In: Marfo K S, Walker S, Charles B (eds) Childhood disability in developing countries: issues in habilitation and special education. Praeger, New York

27

Barriers to successful community based rehabilitation in Jamaica

Marigold Thorburn

INTRODUCTION

Community based rehabilitation (CBR) has now accumulated a documented history of about 16 years. More and more programs are being established, although research on the many aspects of implementing it is only fairly recent. While there are wide differences in the concept of CBR (Thorburn 1996), most people seem to agree that it must include intervention of some type, whether by professionals, community workers, parents, people with disabilities (PWD), or volunteers.

Because successful CBR depends to a great extent on involvement and participation of family members and the community, several aspects of this core element of CBR and home-based early intervention have been researched. In Jamaica, an early stimulation project (ESP) began in 1975 (Thorburn et al 1979) and since 1985, there has been a more comprehensive CBR program known as the 3D Projects (Thorburn 1991). Our experience was that approximately 30% of children with disabilities (CWD) did not progress because of lack of parental participation.

This chapter will describe the results and conclusions drawn from a series of studies over the past years to elucidate barriers to the successful implementation of CBR. All these were carried out in Jamaica between 1988 and 1996 within 3D Projects (see Ch. 26).

In trying to clarify the process of developing CBR at the individual and service levels, a case management model, broadly stated in six main steps, is useful. These steps are:

1. Detection (or suspicion) of a disability
2. Identification of the type and severity of the disability
3. Assessment, usually by a professional
   a. a clinical/psychological measurement of impairment (e.g. visual acuity, audiological)
   b. a functional assessment (i.e. the ability to carry out tasks expected of the person according to age, sex, etc.)
4. Individual program planning, based on the assessment and individualized to the child/person's needs
5. Implementation of the program
6. Follow-up evaluation of progress.

An expanded model, incorporating the levels of personnel, screening and documentation instruments needed in Third World countries, was outlined by Thorburn (1990). This model has proven very useful in human resource planning and in training personnel to understand the approach of CBR. For example, understanding the disability process, the approach to programming, the roles of different workers, and the instruments needed can be confusing even for professionals. Task analysis which breaks a complex task down into component steps in the right sequence facilitates understanding of the whole intervention process during training.

In addition, this model makes it easier to determine where problems or barriers occur when a CBR program is trying to flourish. For example, during the 1980s, initial problems were recognized at stages 2 and 3 due to a lack of appropriate technology. Subsequent research to investigate and develop appropriate disability identification and assessment procedures solved the technical problems (Thorburn 1993, Thorburn et al 1993a).

The most tricky problems, however, seem to be those that occur at the stage of implementation; the programs devised for an individual's needs must be acceptable to, and put to work by, the family, the support person who provides or monitors the intervention, and the community. This aspect is the focus of this chapter.

DISABILITY AND REHABILITATION IN JAMAICA

Jamaica is a small, mountainous, sub-tropical island in the Caribbean. English is the official language, but a creole version is the main vernacular. The population is 2.5 million, with a demographic structure that is typical of Third World countries: approximately 45% of people are under 15 years of age.

With regard to rehabilitation services, Jamaica is no exception to most developing countries. The services for PWD are mostly confined to the capital city, Kingston, and there are few rehabilitation professionals. During the past 20 years, however, community based projects have been set up and they now serve 11 of the 14 parishes (the equivalent of counties in the USA).

In the International Epidemiological Study of Childhood Disability (IESCD) (Durkin et al 1990) of children 2–9 years of age in the parish of Clarendon, it was found that 16% had disability symptoms by screening positive on the Ten Questions (see Ch. 12) (Thorburn et al 1992a). Mild, moderate, and severe disabilities were found in 9.4% of the children (Paul et al 1992). Prevalence rates for adult PWD, available only from a small study (Thorburn 1982), showed an increase with age, going from 1% in the 19–45 year age group to 4.4% in the 45–60 year age group.

In 1994, a situational analysis of disabilities and rehabilitation in the English-speaking Caribbean (PAHO 1994) reported that the childhood group most neglected was the large percentage of mildly disabled and that there was also a serious deficiency in services for the older person with a disability. The priority needs for CWD and their families identified by self-advocacy groups of PWD and parents were transportation, income-generating projects, social benefits and respite care. For adolescents and adults, the needs were expressed for job placement, supportive and mobility aids, and also self-advocacy organizations (PAHO 1994). No need was expressed for early intervention or CBR.

3D Projects was established in 1985 as the first CBR program in Jamaica. It is based in the parish of St Catherine and has a network of rural community groups including parents of CWD, and adolescents and adults with disability. Services are provided in the parishes of St Catherine, St Thomas, Manchester, and St Mary.

The 3D services (Thorburn 1991) include a home visiting program, clinics, a stroke rehabilitation program, training for staff, parents, and human service personnel in the community, an adolescent/adult program, integrated special education, parent activities, research, and documentation. The staff structure is based on the Canadian manpower model (National Institute on Mental Retardation 1971). Local people, who are mostly mothers of CWD, are trained as community rehabilitation workers (CRWs). 3D Projects is also involved in raising the public awareness of the needs and capabilities of PWD. This has been greatly enhanced by the efforts of parents in educating new parents of CWD and through drama and social activities.

Family profiles

The IESCD in Jamaica (Thorburn and Desai 1989) yielded the main background information on demographics, health statistics, and family and community profiles for CWD in Jamaica, while a study by Leavitt (1992) of health beliefs in 3D Projects' clients provided the foundation for further work on attitudes of families. The following is data from the IESCD about family and household structure which is probably fairly typical for rural Jamaica at that time (Thorburn 1997).

About half the heads of household claimed to have middle-class or skilled occupations; however, 21% were unemployed, and the rest had low-income occupations. More than half (60%) owned their houses, 42% had electricity, 44%

owned a TV, and 80% had a radio. About a quarter (26%) of the families were living two to three persons to a room and 40% were in homes with over 3 people per room; 55% had only one or two rooms; and only 19% had four or more rooms. Only 13% had water piped to the house.

Of the children in the survey, 23% were not living with their mothers, a recurring factor found by Desai et al (1970), Leavitt (1992), and Thorburn et al (1993b). Although disability symptoms were more common in children whose mothers were absent (17.5% as opposed to 15%), the difference was not significant.

According to Leavitt (1992), the majority of caregivers of CWD (almost 60%) reported or showed no evidence of stigma attached to the child, a finding subsequently confirmed by Bischoff et al (1996); a large minority said that they had heard others make negative comments. There was some association of these different responses with whether the caregiver would consider long-term institutional placement (even though this was not an option), the absence of adult males in the household, and socioeconomic status (negative comments were associated with poorer status).

Two-thirds of the children could go outside the home like non-disabled children in the family. For those who could not, it was said to be because the child was too big or because he or she was 'rude' (naughty). Seventy percent of the respondents in the study said they would not consider placing their child in an institution, and fewer than half felt that the child had changed their lives. These views were associated with the presence of males in the house, the lack of negative comments by others, and very strong religious faith. These responses were not related to the type or severity of the disability.

Evaluation of CBR intervention

After the completion of the IESCD, which helped to elucidate and validate the first five steps of the case management model outlined above, evaluation was the next task. This has turned out to be a difficult challenge (Thorburn 1992). An evaluation of the early stimulation project (ESP) in 1978 (Thorburn et al 1979) had focused only on the effectiveness of the program as shown by the developmental progress of the child. After 10 years it seemed more important to know the wider impact of the CBR program on the family.

Two surveys, one in St Catherine in 1989 and one in Clarendon in 1990 (Thorburn 1992), interviewed all the clients. Parents' views about the home visits and the community workers were sought, as were changes in knowledge, attitudes and practices, and their opinion about the program.

Generally the results were very positive and almost identical in the two areas. Almost 75% said their knowledge about disability issues had increased; 56% claimed that their attitudes had changed and that the program had positively affected their relationship with their child. Between 80 and 85% enjoyed the home visits by the CRWs and felt good about them but 55 to 60% said they still needed more information, especially about schooling, behavior, and speech. The accuracy of their knowledge about their child's disability was better than that of a group of families interviewed in the IESCD in Clarendon who had not received any intervention (Thorburn et al 1992b).

While 93% said they would recommend the program to another parent, only 47% said they had attended parent training and meetings. It appears that the home visiting aspect of the program was regarded as most beneficial since the caregiver did not have to go anywhere, whereas the training and the meetings with other parents, on which 3D laid great importance, demanded leaving the home. It was this rather disappointing finding that led to further research looking more carefully at what factors had an effect on parent involvement in the program.

In recent years, increasing efforts have been made to evaluate CBR, as shown by the numbers of reports appearing in the very useful newsletter *ActionAid Disability News* from India. A major constraint has been the complexity of CBR itself, with a wide variety of variables affecting progress and the high technology/academic content and process of evaluation procedures. Jonsson (1994) has made a commendable effort to de-mystify this process with 'Operations Monitoring and Analysis of Results' (OMAR), a manual and simple computer program. In 1995 and 1996, 3D attempted to use OMAR to evaluate 3D and two other community-based services, but a number of methodological constraints and errors made the results inconclusive. The problems encountered included the need to use qualitative rather than quantitative studies, difficulties in communicating with respondents, the retrieving of files, follow-up of mobile clients, and analyzing results (unpublished reports). The experience was very useful but there is still not a meaningful, user-friendly evaluation protocol. Because of the difficulties in evaluating CBR projects *per se*, it has been essential to continue the quest for information regarding the impact of particular human variables on home based early intervention (HBEI) and community based rehabilitation (CBR). Much of the research at 3D Projects is doing just that.

HUMAN BARRIERS TO HOME BASED EARLY INTERVENTION AND COMMUNITY BASED REHABILITATION

The following describes some of the research conducted, mostly under the auspices of the 3D Projects, by Thorburn and others that helps to elucidate the human barriers to HBEI and CBR. These results can provide a better understanding of how to improve the effectiveness and impact of CBR.

The burden of having a child with a disability

It is generally presumed that a CWD adds a burden to the family. Terwindt (1992) conducted a study in 3D in the parish of St Thomas to clarify some of the reasons why parents may not always participate in HBEI programs to the

It seems that parents with positive attitudes towards their child and the disability had better experiences with health services. Also parents with a child with a mild disability had better experiences than parents of children with moderate or severe disabilities.

Seminars are now being held with medical and nursing staff to try and rectify this situation, but doctors tend to be hyper-sensitive regarding these issues.

The impact of community attitudes toward disability and rehabilitation

A survey carried out in 1993 in St Catherine and St Mary parishes sought to further explore the question of attitudes toward disability within the general community (Thorburn 1995). A stratified sample of different age, sex, and occupational groups was questioned on supernatural beliefs, misconceptions about disability, awareness of rights of PWD, knowledge of services, and willingness to offer assistance to PWD.

A minority of the sample (18%) held supernatural beliefs, such as that the disability was due to an evil spirit, punishment for a sin, or occurred because the mother had seen a disabled person when she was pregnant. However, these beliefs were less prevalent than the idea that disabled children are 'sent by God' (40%), supporting Leavitt's findings (1992). In contrast to Leavitt, this study found that the higher frequencies of supernatural beliefs were significantly associated with the lower-income-earning occupations and with people 50 years of age and older. It should be noted, however, that Leavitt's sample was almost exclusively from the lower income groups.

The need for training of CWD was accepted, but people were unaware that PWD can get adequate training and rehabilitation in their own homes; they assumed that special schools and homes are the best place. This has substantial implications for home based training. Furthermore, only 50% of the respondents recognized the equal rights of PWD with respect to job opportunities.

The declared willingness of over 90% of respondents to help a neighbor or to volunteer in a program was encouraging, but has to be tempered by the recognition of socioculturally defined limits as to what would be acceptable (Bischoff et al 1996). The notion that community volunteers in CBR may, at times, be a realistic strategy might be feasible even though this has not been so regarded in the past in Jamaica.

The impact of the role of relatives and neighbors

Many mothers on occasion – some for a lot of time – experience the need for care outside the family. In rural areas of Jamaica this falls on the extended family; in the city there are back yard 'nurseries', a very common form of day care. Unfortunately, because of the stigma accompanying disabilities and the extra attention required, children with the severest disabilities are less likely to be accommodated.

Terwindt (1992) concluded that the role of relatives and neighbors in helping families varies. While many caregivers relied on close family to help out, they placed very little reliance on people outside the family. Caregivers expected little assistance from others although contact with other parents of CWD (through 3D) was a notable positive influence.

Following on the above, Bischoff (1994) conducted a more in-depth investigation of the role of neighbors of families with CWD in an area that then lacked services. This showed that half of the caregivers drew on neighbors for short periods of time, but most caregivers did not want to overburden them. It seemed that the parents who expressed an ability to cope were more likely to request help from neighbors. According to Bischoff et al (1996): 'Many caregivers showed an impressive ability to cope. They obviously succeeded in breaking down an overall task, posed by their child's disability, into manageable bits and pieces which enabled them to get their neighbors involved: one can only ask for help if one can first define for oneself tasks of culturally appropriate size for which then to muster support' (Bischoff et al 1996).

In contrast, the people who were not coping neither requested help nor received any. At least 20–25% of the parents could be considered 'non-copers', who need more help in changing attitudes and practices (Thorburn 1992). Recognizing that the negative responses expressing unmet needs could be linked to such factors as severity of disability, poverty, or other domestic problems, Bischoff et al (1996) point to the need for other options such as assistance from neighbors or a CBR project, to relieve burdens for the 'non-coper', especially when children are severely disabled. The CRW should be aware of these factors and should share her own experiences and coping methods as examples to support the non-coping parent.

All these points endorse Miles's (1990) criticism that 'it is inappropriate for WHO to estimate that 98% of disabled people are "totally neglected in developing countries" (Helander et al 1983)' (Miles 1990).

STRATEGIES TO MINIMIZE THE HUMAN BARRIERS TO CBR IMPLEMENTATION

The effectiveness of CBR at the family and community level depends, in large part, on the acceptance of and participation in home based training by family members. This, in turn, affects the credibility of home and community based intervention as opposed to traditional, 'professional' rehabilitation. The following summarizes where efforts have been made and where there needs to be continued focus to foster success.

Facilitating parent activities and acquisition of information and skills

Parent activities have been an important part of the 3D program since its outset. Parent training and parent-to-parent counseling has been effective in mobilizing parent involvement and changing negative attitudes and practices. 3D Projects has also deliberately involved parents as resources in training, services and workshops for community personnel – professionals and community workers. A corps of parent trainers can now run training courses almost independently.

Frequent discussions with groups of parents about their reactions to having a CWD have made it clear that the distress, confusion, isolation, guilt, and shame experienced to varying degrees by many parents is considerably alleviated both by visits from 'parent counselors' and by involvement in parent groups that discuss awareness, accurate information, and rights, and give support. To this end, 3D Projects has produced video manual productions called 'Parent-to-Parent Counseling' and 'Parent Training'.

During the past 5 years, there have also been specific training courses on behavior management for parents of CWD. These courses have been greatly appreciated, and many people express the view that all parents should have this training. This is a strategy worth developing and is also the subject of a video manual production called 'Child Rearing Skills' that 3D has produced for community leaders. This video has been shortened and adapted for a parent training manual called 'Pathways to Parenting' produced in Jamaica by Parenting Partners (1994).

More recently, in a series of 16 parent orientation courses of 3 days duration in different parts of the Caribbean, 9 post-course and follow-up evaluations were analyzed (Thorburn 1996) to determine the effectiveness of the courses. Parents' main goals in coming to the courses were 'to be a better parent', 'to learn more about my child', and 'how to cope/help the child better'. Parents prioritized better understanding of disability, improved coping, meeting other parents, and improved self-esteem and confidence as the major benefits of the courses. In three countries, many of the parents had never received an adequate diagnosis or explanation of their child's problem at all. Clearly, information and networking are desperately needed.

CRWs are also an important asset for parents' groups. They should be sensitized towards their own achievements as parents of CWD without any rehabilitation help 'of which they rightly can be proud so as to make them aware of what to look for in the life stories of their clients' families'. This is obviously desirable. 'The self-esteem caregivers can derive from knowing that professional rehabilitators acknowledge their achievements would seem a good basis for imparting more in-depth knowledge and educational skills' (Bischoff et al 1996).

Changing attitudes and knowledge about disability

While superstitions and misconceptions that might prevent participation by family members (and by PWD) exist, Thorburn (1995) found a willingness on the part of a large majority of individuals to assist PWD. It seems likely that an emphasis on positive attitudes, knowledge about disability, and the rights of PWD will help with this process. In the experience of 3D Projects, community orientation workshops have proven to be very helpful in mobilizing interest and participation in CBR programs.

Improving communication with health services

Communication barriers between health care workers and parents are a detrimental factor. Clearly, health staff in all aspects of the services where PWD are encountered need more training in knowledge, management, and communication skills to give parents a better understanding of their children. Ideally, all health care and counseling needed by families for CWD could be given in the regular health care services, thus effecting the goal of 'Health Care for All' *and* equality of access for PWD. The main barrier is the overburdened and under-financed state of the public health services.

Sensitization to negative child-rearing practices

This is a delicate subject because it implies criticism of deep cultural traditions and practices. However, there is increasing concern at the present time about the practices described earlier, particularly in relation to the continuing upsurge of violence in the community and child abuse in particular in the Caribbean. While this issue is being hotly debated, consideration has to be given at least to sensitizing people about their behaviors and what the likely consequences of these behaviors are on their children. In the case of CWD, the negative effects are particularly powerful given the extra disadvantages of CWD compared with their peers.

Reinforcement of 'natural' interventions

Even though PWD and parents do not prioritize this need (PAHO 1994), early detection and intervention are considered to be essential services for all CWD. Bischoff's observations (1994) about the importance of identifying the initiatives of parents to solve problems of their own accord suggest that a closer look should be taken at other indigenous rehabilitative practices that could be reinforced. For example, in Jamaica, a specific cultural practice that seems to have an appreciable effect on physical and motor development was described by Hopkins and Westra (1988) as a 'formal infant handling routine'. This comprises a series of consecutive actions or exercises carried out by the caregiver daily following the infant's bath. This starts at birth and continues to about 10 to 12 months of age, depending on when the infant starts to walk.

A recent study by van der Putten carried out in 3D Projects in a district of the parish of Manchester on 28 children with and 24 without disabilities showed that the routine was still practiced by many mothers and caregivers (van der Putten & Finkenflügel 1996). Although no formal studies have measured its therapeutic effect, one of the exercises, stretching, is similar to range-of-motion exercises.

If the parents have found their own ways of aiding or increasing improvement in their child, and it is approved of by CBR and professional workers, this will make intervention even more satisfying. This needs to be emphasized more in dealing with parents. For example, the following is part of the story of a mother of a child with Down syndrome, recorded by Bischoff (1994):

(Others) are trying to tell me that him will soon grow out of it . . . and I heard that you cannot grow out Down Syndrome. They just see him and they say maybe he will talk and you must keep him out of this and you must give him this and that . . . and you must go cut underneath the tongue and him will talk. But me don't do any of those things to him . . . just leave him and sit and eventually talk with him, *sit and talk with him and so he improve.* (Bischoff's emphasis)

This supports the idea that much of so-called intervention can be looking for sensible, spontaneous efforts that families are already making and reassuring them that they are doing the right thing and very little other 'rehabilitation' is needed.

FUTURE RESEARCH

Future research will be essential for CBR if one believes that CBR is the main strategy for Third World (and other?) countries to provide rehabilitation services to reach more people.

A number of barriers must still be overcome, mainly in convincing people that it is worth-while to spend time assisting families in their main areas of need. Cost and sustainability are major concerns and the point raised by Terwindt (1992) about the need to strike a balance between the more costly, individualized attention and programming and general, but not necessarily very child-specific, support to families needs to be examined more carefully. This combined with the role of the community and how much can be realistically expected of community members in the way of financial and/or participatory support needs to be elucidated.

Research on these areas is very challenging. It is not simply biological or even educational or behavioral, but rather complex and multidimensional. It has to look at people's goals for themselves, the barriers to achieving them, their personal strengths and resources and the strategies they can or have developed to reach them, as well as ways of mobilizing people in the community, hopefully reducing their negative and counter-productive attitudes and practices by providing appropriate and humanitarian knowledge and skills.

REFERENCES

Bischoff R 1994 Caring for disabled children in Jamaica: what is their neighbour's role? MSc thesis, University of Heidelberg, Institute for Tropical Medicine and Public Health

Bischoff R, Thorburn M J, Reitmaier P 1996 Neighbourhood support to families with a disabled child: observations on a coping strategy of caregivers in a Jamaican community-based rehabilitation programme. Child: Care Health and Development 22: 397–410

Campbell H C 1977 An evaluation of the effectiveness of the Portage Guide to Early Education for young hearing impaired children. BEd thesis, University of the West Indies

Desai P, Standard K L, Miall W E 1970 Socio-economic and cultural influences on child growth in rural Jamaica. Journal of Biosocial Sciences 2: 133–143

Durkin M S, Davidson L L, Hasan M, Khan N, Thorburn M J, Zaman S 1990 Screening for childhood disabilities in community settings. In: Thorburn M J, Marfo K (eds) Practical approaches to childhood disability in developing countries. 3D Projects, 14 Monk Street, Spanish Town, Jamaica, pp. 179–198

Helander E, Mendis P, Nelson G, Goerdt A 1983 Training for people with disabilities in the community, 3rd edn. RHL 83. WHO, Geneva

Hopkins B, Westra T 1988 Maternal handling and motor development: an intracultural study. Genetic Social and General Psychology Monographs 114: 377–408

Jonsson T 1994 OMAR in rehabilitation: a guide on operations monitoring and analysis of results. UNDP Interregional Programme for Disabled People. United Nations Development Programme, Geneva

Leavitt R 1992 Disability and rehabilitation in rural Jamaica: an ethnographic study. Fairleigh Dickenson University Press, Rutherford NJ

Miles M 1990 The 'community base' in rehabilitation planning: key or gimmick? In: Thorburn M J, Marfo K (eds) Practical approaches to childhood disability in developing countries. 3D Projects, 14 Monk Street, Spanish Town, Jamaica, pp. 287–302

National Institute on Mental Retardation, Canada 1971 A national mental retardation manpower model. Roeher Institute, Toronto

Op-Heij J, Dik M, Thorburn M J 1997 Experiences of parents of children with disabilities with the health services in Jamaica. West Indian Medical Journal 46: 83–87

O'Toole B 1988 The relevance of parental involvement programmes in developing countries. Child: Care Health and Development 15: 329–342

PAHO 1994 Situation analysis of disability and rehabilitation in the English-speaking Caribbean RHB 93 Pan American Health Organization, Barbados

Parenting Partners 1994 Pathways to parenting. (Available from the Caribbean Child Development Centre, University of the West Indies, Kingston 7, Jamaica.)

Paul T J, Desai P, Thorburn M J 1992 The prevalence of childhood disability and related medical diagnoses in Clarendon, Jamaica. West Indian Medical Journal 41: 8–11

Shearer M, Shearer D 1972 The Portage Project: a model for early childhood education. Exceptional Children 36: 210–219

Sobo E J 1993 One blood: the Jamaican body. State University of New York Press, Albany, USA

Terwindt F 1992 Caregiver involvement in the rehabilitation of disabled children in Jamaica. MSc thesis, University of Heidelberg Institute for Tropical Medicine and Public Health, Germany

Thorburn M J 1982 Preliminary results from a study of disability in the Lucea area of Hanover. PATH newsletter 10: 1

Thorburn M J 1990 Childhood disability in developing countries: basic issues. In: Thorburn M J, Marfo K (eds) Practical approaches to childhood disability in developing countries. 3D Projects, 14 Monk Street, Spanish Town, Jamaica, pp. 15–46

Thorburn M J 1991 A community approach to helping disabled children in Jamaica. International Journal of Mental Health 20: 61–76

Thorburn M J 1992 Parent evaluation of a community based rehabilitation programme in Jamaica. International Journal of Rehabilitation Research 15: 170–176

Thorburn M J 1993 Recent developments in low cost screening and assessment of childhood disabilities in Jamaica. Part 1: Screening. West Indian Medical Journal 42: 10–12

Thorburn M J 1995 Attitudes towards childhood disability in Jamaica. Paper presented at the 21st International Conference of the Paediatric Association of Jamaica, Kingston

Thorburn M J 1996 Roles and relationships of CBR in the community. In: Brown Roy I, Baine D and Neufeldt A H (eds) Beyond basic care: special education and community rehabilitation in low income countries. Captus Press, York University Campus, Ontario, Canada

Thorburn M J 1997 Raising children with disabilities in the Caribbean. In: Roopnarine J L, Brown J (eds) Caribbean families: diversity among ethnic groups. Advances in Applied Developmental Psychology 14. ABLEX Publishing, Greenwich, Conn., pp. 177–204

Thorburn M J, Desai P 1989 Low cost methods for rapid identification and assessment of childhood disability in Jamaica. Final Report. Department of Community Medicine and Psychiatry, University of the West Indies, Kingston 7, Jamaica

Thorburn M J, Brown J M, Bell C 1979 Early stimulation of handicapped children using community workers. Paper presented at the Fifth Congress of the International Association on the Scientific Study of Mental Deficiency, Jerusalem

Thorburn M J, Desai P, Paul T J, Malcolm L M, Durkin M, Davidson L L 1992a Identification of childhood disability in Jamaica: evaluation of the Ten Question screen. Ibid 262–270

Thorburn M J, Desai P, Paul T J 1992b Service needs of disabled children in Jamaica. International Journal of Rehabilitation Research 150: 31–38

Thorburn M J, Paul T J, Malcolm L M 1993a Recent developments in low cost screening and assessment of childhood disabilities in Jamaica. Part 2: Assessment. West Indian Medical Journal 42: 46–52

Thorburn M J, Paul T J, Desai P, Malcolm L M 1993b Development of an impact questionnaire to measure the burden of care of a disabled child. Paper given at the Twentieth International Conference of the Paediatric Association of Jamaica, Kingston, Jamaica

Van der Putten A A J, Finkenflügel H J M 1996 Formal handling routines: child rearing practices in Jamaica. West Indian Medical Journal 45(Supplement 2): 13–14

28

Impact of the Harare parents' groups for children with a disability and their parents: are caregivers satisfied with the service?

Jennifer Jelsma
Maude Zhanje

INTRODUCTION

David Teager, president of the World Confederation of Physical Therapy, has pointed out that throughout the world the rich are getting richer and the poor are getting sicker (Teager 1995). This is particularly true in developing countries and any agency wishing to provide rehabilitation services to most of the people in need will likely be overwhelmed by the task. Rehabilitation management of young children provides a special challenge in most developing countries because of the proportionally larger number of children to adults. In Zimbabwe, for example, half of the population is under 14 years of age (Central Statistics Office 1988) (see Ch. 25 for more information on Zimbabwe). How can therapists maximize the impact of meager health resources? How can the greatest number be helped without compromising the quality of services?

These questions confronted the health providers of a newly independent Zimbabwe in 1981. One response to the need for accessible and affordable rehabilitation was the initiation of a 2-year training for rehabilitation technicians to enlarge the pool of rehabilitation workers (Hanekom 1984, Finkenflügel 1991). Another strategy adopted was the establishment of a centralized Children's Rehabilitation Unit (CRU) in Harare, capital city of Zimbabwe. The CRU then initiated and supported community based parents' groups (PGs) for the caregivers of children with disabilities (CWDs). (Author

Jennifer Jelsma was actively involved in both the above programs.)

Strategies like the PGs have grown out of the need of many parents, and particularly parents of CWDs, to depend on expertise and help from professionals in the care of their children. The quality of this interaction can influence the extent to which families can adapt to having such a child. The literature has noted an increasing concern about the different perceptions of caregivers and professionals with regard to issues related to the child's therapy. Rosenbaum & King (1990) found little concurrence between the order of priority in which caregivers and professionals listed the most valuable components of care. Cunningham (1985), however, defines the new role of the caregiver as a co-therapist and teacher, while others caution against overburdening parents by expecting unrealistic levels of involvement in home programs (von Wendt et al 1984). To a certain extent, the issue of parental needs and perception of services has been addressed in the developed world (Bax 1985, Haylock et al 1993, Hinojosa 1991), but it is less understood in the developing world. In each context, it is important to find out the perceptions of the parents within the programs that professional rehabilitation workers offer.

In quantitative terms, the success of the PG approach in Zimbabwe has been documented and since 1993, approximately 500 children have been in contact with these groups (Jelsma et al 1995). However, the impact of the PGs has not been measured in qualitative terms. This chapter, through presenting research data, explores the family relationships between the CWD and his parents and siblings, the qualitative impact of PG attendance on caregivers, their satisfaction with the services that they have been receiving and their preferences regarding different forms of intervention. Do the caregivers prefer the decentralized but less specialized services provided in the PGs or the supplementary visits to the central institution? Has PG attendance met the perceived needs of the caregivers and aided the family in accepting and caring for their CWD?

THE STUDY
Background

PGs were first formed in 1987. Recognizing that PGs can be an essential part in the establishment of CBR services, one of the authors (JJ) originally pioneered this approach from the central facility, the CRU. Aspects of different models of CBR, such as the use of neighborhood centers (Miles 1985), the use of local volunteers (O'Toole n.d., WHO 1982) and the provision of low-cost aids, were integrated in an eclectic approach to CBR. Subsequently PGs were established in the high-density areas close to the neighborhoods in which the children lived. In time, other institutions in Harare dealing with the rehabilitation of children helped in establishing and servicing PGs in many of the city's high-density areas. This was done in collaboration with the CRU, and the programs were very similar to the original. One of these institutions was the Jairos Jiri Children's Centre (JJCC).

The PGs meet two to four times a month at decentralized locations, such as local municipal clinics and pre-schools. They are run by rehabilitation technicians (RT), who have had a 2-year generalized training in basic techniques of rehabilitation. Most of the children who attend the PGs have been seen and assessed by a physical therapist at JJCC before incorporation into the group. The progress of each child is intermittently monitored by a physical therapist, a communication therapist or an occupational therapist. The child may be referred back to the central facility to be further assessed and possibly given more specialized treatment by a therapist (or RT under more direct guidance of the therapist) whenever more intensive intervention is necessary.

PG sessions usually begin with a talk on some topic of interest. An outside speaker, such as a social worker or communication therapist, may be invited to address the group. This is followed by discussion and questions. There is also an exercise class during which some aspect of function such as head control or feeding is taught to the entire group. Finally each child individually sees the RT for a brief review of the specific handling techniques suggested by the therapists. Aids and appliances are also provided to PG attenders if necessary; these include wheelchairs, prone boards, corner seats, crutches and calipers.

The aims of the original model of PG participation (Hanekom 1988) included the following:

1. To educate parents on the causes, prognosis and management of their children's disability.
2. To encourage the growth of group autonomy and action independent of professional participation.
3. To encourage the growth of friendship and support among the parents.
4. To monitor the progress of the children, assist the parents in carrying out the prescribed treatment programs and as necessary, modify the treatment programs.
5. To refer back to the central facility for specialist attention as necessary.
6. To ensure follow-up of all CWDs in these areas through the assistance of volunteers.

The PGs differ from the mothers' groups in Bath, Britain, described by Stallard & Dickinson (1994) in providing not only counseling and emotional support but also physical therapy in a group setting.

Methodology

This study was carried out with the cooperation of the JJCC. Caregivers in five different groups supported by the centre were interviewed. Because cerebral palsy (CP) accounts for the greatest number of CWDs in the groups (Sifana 1994), interviews were conducted with the caregivers of children with this diagnosis. The second author (MZ), a Zimbabwean graduate physical therapist presently working at the CRU, gathered the data, questioning 50 caregivers about their attitude toward the PGs. All data were gathered through structured interviews in the vernacular, Shona. In addition to demographic information, the caregivers were asked about different aspects of participation in the PGs. Some questions were open-ended. The

responses to others were marked on a five-point scale ranging from 'strongly agree' to 'strongly disagree'. To distance herself from the rehabilitation team, the researcher did not wear a uniform and made it clear that the information gained was entirely confidential and would not prejudice the child in any way. Caregivers had the option of not participating but, in fact, all agreed to take part. Constant comparative analysis (Hinojosa 1991) of interview data was used to identify emergent themes expressed by the caregivers. The PGs were held at the local municipal clinic and all the caregivers walked to the place where their PGs met; only two had to come more than 5 km.

Results

Characteristics of the children and their families

All children had been diagnosed as having CP by a pediatrician and were 12 months of age or older. The median age of the children was 37 months, with a range from 15 months to almost 9 years. There were 23 males (46%) and 27 females (54%).

The caregiver, defined as any person spending up to 7 hours each day with the child, was female in every case. She was the principal person engaging in the child's home program and assisting with most activities of daily living. Over 90% of the caregivers were the mothers of the children; the other caregivers were maternal grandmothers, aunts, siblings or domestic helpers. All the caregivers lived in the high-density areas and as such were in a low-income group. Their mean number of years of education was 9 (*i.e.* up to 2 years of secondary school education).

Only 5 caregivers had a full-time job; an additional 13 were involved in some income-generating employment such as selling vegetables or crocheting; 23 were unemployed apart from caring for the child.

Thirteen (26%) of the caregivers reported a breakdown in their marriages as a result of having a disabled child. Reasons cited by the caregivers included: the husband could not accept that he could conceive a disabled child; problems within the extended family, particularly with the in-laws encouraging their son to remarry; and the belief that witchcraft had caused the child's disability. Most of those whose marital status remained unchanged had 2 or more older children, and this might have had a stabilizing influence on the marriage. All the respondents reported that having a CWD strained family relations, particularly with the extended family.

PG attendance

Approximately 30 PG sessions took place in the 12 months preceding the interviews and the median number of meetings each person attended was 7, with a range of 3–26. Each caregiver was therefore present for approximately 30% of the meetings. The reasons the caregivers gave for not attending a meeting included work commitments, household chores and the need to visit rural areas.

In addition to attending the PGs, 21 caregivers had also attended the JJCC for supplementary individual therapy. This happened when the RTs or the parents felt that the child needed more specialized therapy. The mean distance to the JJCC was 12.3 km and most parents used public transport to get to the centre. The median number of visits to the JJCC was 1, with a range of 1–17. Most of these caregivers reported that they would attend individual therapy more often if they could afford transport.

What did the caregivers know about cerebral palsy?

It is particularly important to understand what the caregivers know about CP in the light of the traditional belief system in Zimbabwe regarding the cause of disability (McAlister 1989, Mariga 1989). For example Mariga (1989) reports that some rural mothers whose children are disabled believe it is so because they took contraceptives at one time. In other instances the CWD may be seen as a reflection of something wrong with the mother. Often, the disability is seen as an act of a witch (*muroyi*) (Mariga 1989). A *muroyi* can

bewitch a person and only traditional healers (*n'angas*) are in a position to identify the witch and disperse the spell. The *n'anga* is the traditional healer who is believed to be able to diagnose the social causes of an illness. He is in contact with the ancestral spirits and is able to identify which spirits are displeased and need appeasement. He also dispenses herbal medicine. A study commissioned by the rehabilitation unit of the Ministry of Health (1990) found that 35% of respondents attributed epilepsy to supernatural causes (i.e. ancestral intervention, evil spirits or witchcraft).

In this study, 24 of the caregivers reported that the major cause of CP was congenital or, to use their own words, 'the brain did not form properly at birth'. Another 17 believed that their child's disability had been caused by someone or some supernatural being and 8 of these blamed members of the extended family. One-quarter (13) specifically mentioned witchcraft or the evil influence of another as the cause. Interesting responses included:

My husband's sister has no children of her own and she was jealous.

I had my child immunized and perhaps the ancestral spirits were displeased.

My parents-in-law did not want their son to marry me.

Fifteen did not know whether any of their other children would also have CP, and 22 reported that they did not know if a cure for CP existed. A religious sect, the Vapostori or Apostolic faith, is strong in Harare, and 5 caregivers who were members believed that CP could be cured by faith healing and prayer or appeasing the spirits. Only 1 felt that continuous exercises for the legs would cure her child.

Thirty-nine caregivers identified the RT or therapist as the person from whom they had learned the most concerning their child's condition. Three reported that another caregiver within their group had taught them the most about CP. Other sources of information were books or pamphlets, other family members and, in 3 cases, the *n'anga*.

How satisfied were the caregivers with different aspects of group attendance?

Generally a high level of satisfaction with their own understanding of CP was indicated. Caregivers also felt that their families and therapists/RT were helpful with the home program and that they enjoyed meeting with other caregivers at the groups. However, those who attended both individual therapy at the central institution and the PG preferred this to only attending the PGs. Although all felt they had benefited from the PGs, the majority wanted the rehabilitation worker to spend more time treating their children rather than talking and answering questions.

There was no consensus about whether the groups should spend more time during the meetings on other activities such as sewing or handcrafts: 19 felt a definite need for engaging in productive activities but 21 strongly disagreed. A summary of the responses is given in Table 28.1.

Not all caregivers could identify three useful strategies that they had learnt from attending the groups. The majority (26) felt that various handling skills were the most important gains. Others listed knowledge and acceptance of their children's condition as important. Only 1 caregiver reported learning nothing from the groups, and her child had been receiving individual therapy at a central institution regularly.

When asked to identify three key factors that could improve the quality of service, 42 caregivers (84%) suggested more therapy, in the PG setting, as the most useful. Institutionalizing their children was mentioned as a desirable option by 19 caregivers. Several organizations in Zimbabwe provide residential care in addition to education or training, and these are generally well regarded. The JJCC, for example, has one pre-school residential center and one primary school with boarding facilities for children with physical disabilities. Institutionalization may be the one chance that the child will get to receive a structured education.

One caregiver opted for periodic respite care. The rest showed strong reluctance to leave the

Table 28.1 Summary of caregivers' satisfaction with the parents' groups

Question	Number of responses (N=50)				
	Strongly agree			Strongly disagree	
	1	2	3	4	5
I understand my child's condition and how he/she became disabled	16	17	10	3	4
I feel able to competently carry out the home program I was taught	12	14	11	12	1
The rest of the family helps to carry out the home program	20	9	10	6	5
I feel the rehabilitation worker helps us cope with our child's problems	11	21	19	8	1
I feel able to ask questions about my child's condition	9	14	13	11	3
I really enjoy meeting other caregivers at outreach clinics	13	19	16	2	0
Answering questions is more useful than treatment demonstrations	7	9	3	24	7
Individual treatment at JJCC is more useful than PG attendance (N=21)	20	1	0	0	0
We caregivers should spend more time on other activities during PG sessions	19	7	3	13	8
Both the child and I have benefited from attending the groups	26	18	6	0	0

care of their children to anyone else; they did not feel anyone else could cope with the demands of caring for the child. Financial support and aids and appliances were mentioned by 20 as likely to improve care. In fact, 66 aids and appliances were reported to have been lent to the children. These included 16 wheelchairs, prone boards, corner seats, crutches, splints and calipers.

Discussion

Family relationships

Clearly, having a CWD in the family changes intra-family relationships. The family is likely to go through various stages of acceptance from shock, denial, sadness and, hopefully, to adaptation and finally reconstruction (Bax 1985). In practice, this study showed that the family is often unable to withstand having a CWD as a member. Virtually all the relationships experienced a period of conflict and eventually one-quarter of the marriages broke down (68% of caregivers resided with the father of the child, compared to 86% prior to the birth of the child). This situation is similar to that described by Bean (1994), who says that often the woman is blamed for the disability and left alone to care for the child.

The effect of the extended family appears to be ambivalent. A study on the stress levels of 33 mothers of children with CP in equivalent PGs in Harare (M'Kumbuzi 1995) reported relatively low levels of stress. Only 2 mothers showed moderately severe symptoms of non-psychotic mental illness. M'Kumbuzi (1995) attributed the low incidence to the fact that in 73% of the cases another relative lived with the nuclear family. She postulated that having someone else within the family other than the parents or caregiver provided opportunities for relief from care and reduced the isolation of the caregiver from life outside the family. Her conclusion was that 'the Zimbabwean cultural practice of encompassing the extended family within a close knit unit may be positively helping to maintain the mental health of the caregivers of children with CP' (M'Kumbuzi 1995).

In the present study, the parents often seem to perceive the extended family as either the cause of the disability or as a factor contributing to the breakdown of marriage. On the other hand, those caregivers who did have a supportive family, particularly maternal grandparents, seemed to be the most confident of their ability to care for their children. Whatever the role of the extended family may be, PG attendance may help the participants deal with family conflicts. In addition, education regarding the causes of CP may enable the caregivers to better defend themselves against blame by other family members.

In this group of lower-income women, low stress levels were noted and caregivers expressed surprise that they should not be expected to cope with the management of their children. The severe psychological and emotional stress reported by well-educated, majority Caucasian parents caring for young disabled adults in the San Francisco Bay area by Hallum & Krumboltz (1993) was not evident. The fact that all the children in this study were still young and the severity of their disability might not yet be evident may be a factor contributing to this difference.

Caregivers' knowledge of CP

Ross & Thompson (1993) interviewed parents of children with CP and living in inner London. They reported perceived low levels of understanding of their children's condition, with almost half reporting having little or none. In contrast, in the Harare groups only 14% said that they felt their knowledge to be insufficient. In reality, the caregivers entertained several misconceptions: the majority were not sure whether their other children would get CP, some thought that CP was a progressive disease, and one quarter were sure that there was a cure. Witchcraft was cited as a cause of CP by 26% of mothers, a proportion similar to the 27% noted in other PGs by Sifana (1994).

The central institutions distribute pamphlets in the vernacular to the caregivers when their children are first diagnosed as having CP. The statements designed to test caregivers' knowledge were based on these pamphlets. The value of the printed information is obviously questionable under these circumstances; only 6% reported that they had learned important information from books or pamphlets. This would support Miles (1987) in his contention that printed information is not an effective mode of transmitting information in societies where few people can read and fewer still seek knowledge from written texts. The role of rehabilitation workers in informing parents of the diagnosis and prognosis of their children is very important particularly since no caregiver reported that a medical practitioner had taught her most about her child.

Hinojosa (1991) reported that mothers of pre-school children with CP in New York, some of whom were economically disadvantaged, expressed a need for the therapists to spend more time talking to them and explaining the rehabilitation process. Similarly, only 2 of the 21 mothers of children with CP in inner London interviewed by Ross & Thompson (1993) agreed with the statement, 'I wish the physiotherapist would spend less time chatting to us and more time treating our child'. This was not true of the group under study. The caregivers did not seem to perceive a need for more discussion, and the majority felt that time spent answering questions was of less use than demonstrations of treatment.

Caregiver's role as co-therapist

As mentioned above, there has been much emphasis in recent years on maximizing the involvement of the family in the management of CWDs. The traditional model of therapy, in which the therapist plays the dominant role, has been criticized as 'wrongly assuming that the professional is in control and the parent is then encouraged to take part, when it is the parent's life, child and future' (Ross & Thompson 1993). One aim of the establishment of the PGs was to foster the autonomy of the caregivers and reduce dependence on professionals (Hanekom 1988). What is the reality? In the developing

world, much is expected of parents, particularly of mothers. The mother is already overburdened with the roles of wife, full-time mother, homemaker, and, in some cases, the breadwinner as well (Hamblin 1987). The rehabilitation worker's advice regarding handling and treatment may make further demands on her time and lead to frustration and possibly guilt if she is unable to carry out the suggestions. The mother may not wish to take on the role of co-therapist as described by Cunningham (1985) and may prefer that professionals shoulder the responsibility for treatment.

In this study, the caregivers strongly expressed the need for more individual treatment sessions. To cope with primary responsibility for therapy, the parents, like those described by Thorburn (1989), expressed the need for continuous support from both support groups and professionals. All the mothers who were attending individual therapy at the JJCC felt that these sessions were more beneficial than treatment in the group setting. The primary reason for this preference was that the physical therapists had more time to attend to the treatment than the RT who were running the PGs. The children would also benefit from specialized equipment and toys. They did not see the rehabilitation enterprise as primarily being 'an information system' (Miles 1987). As reported in parents of children with motor disabilities in Oxford, UK, by Haylock et al (1993), Zimbabwean caregivers wanted more professional, 'traditional Western' hands-on treatment. Over one third of the interviewees in this study suggested that institutionalization would be an acceptable option for their children.

Are these findings an indication of a growing dependency of caregivers upon professionals? Or do they perhaps confirm that caregivers are rejecting their roles as co-therapists and would rather spend their time playing and interacting with their children as opposed to teaching them how to sit, walk or talk (Hinojosa 1991)? The desire to institutionalize their children may be a function of the very active role that the JJCC has had in providing high quality schooling for CWD. It is possible that the caregivers would perceive such schooling as preferable to that offered by the local education authority.

CONCLUSIONS

Have the PGs met the aims articulated by the rehabilitation workers who established the groups? The mothers perceived that the aim of education had been met, although in reality there were still several with misconceptions regarding their child's condition. Friendships between the mothers have sprung up, and all caregivers reported having benefited from attending the group. The majority showed a high level of satisfaction with the rehabilitation worker's ability to help them with specific problems, but the problem of inadequate 'hands-on' treatment time was a cause of dissatisfaction. The caregivers universally wanted more individual therapy for their children.

This expressed desire for additional 'traditional Western' therapy and institutionalization poses problems for the progressive rehabilitation worker. The concept of empowerment of parents appears excellent, but do parents wish to be empowered? Do they wish to remain uninvolved, silent and dependent on others to speak for them and provide services (Thorburn 1989)? Is it possible that the rehabilitation worker imposes a greater burden on the caregivers, who do not wish to be considered as a 'ready made team for all-day rehabilitation' (Levitt 1986)? These mothers definitely wanted therapists to do the therapy, possibly so that they could perform the parenting. Von Wendt et al (1984) have cautioned against overburdening parents by expecting unrealistic and inappropriate levels of involvement in the management of their children. Although M'Kumbuzi (1995) found a low rate of non-psychotic mental illness related to stress, over half of her subjects responded affirmatively to the statement that 'there were moments when I felt life was so tough that I cried or wanted to cry'. There may well be a conflict of interest between the need for the child to receive good therapy and the caregiver to fulfill responsibilities to others and herself.

However much the rehabilitation worker may wish for the community to take responsibility and for the family to take an active role in rehabilitation, there must be a commitment by both the community and the family to CBR and home based care. Concerned workers cannot impose a community based philosophy on a society that still has a conventional understanding of the provision of medical and rehabilitation care. The expectations of the community and rehabilitation workers should develop at the same pace, and both groups should ultimately opt for the same model of service provision. Evidently the PGs have met certain of the aims of their founders, although not in the field of therapy provision. It might be that the caregivers need to be weaned away from the articulated dependency on professionals. On the other hand, perhaps professionals should be accommodating the expressed need to provide more individualized therapy by restructuring the groups to allow for more handling by the rehabilitation worker within the context of the groups.

In conclusion, the rehabilitation worker has a dual responsibility – to the child and to the parents. A balance must be struck between the right of CWDs to reach their functional potential and the right of a caregiver to be a wife, mother to her other children, and person in her own right. The model of service provision in the form of PGs seems to be generally acceptable. However, this model needs to be further developed in any particular context to provide a rehabilitation service that meets the needs of caregivers for support and the needs of children for effective hands-on therapy. The biggest challenge of all is to provide an effective and acceptable service for caregivers and their CWDs, within the very real limits of the rehabilitation and medical budgets of developing countries.

Acknowledgments
To the mothers of Glen View, Highfield, Kambuzuma, Mbare and Mufakose, Vivienne M'Kumbuzi for assistance in preparation, Michael Bol and the rehabilitation technicians at Jairos Jiri Children's Centre.

REFERENCES

Bax M 1985 Meeting the parents' needs. Developmental Medicine & Child Neurology 6: 139–140

Bean G 1994 Women as carers. Community Based Rehabilitation News 17: 6

Central Statistical Office 1988 Demographic and health survey. Central Statistical Office, Ministry of Finance, Economic Planning and Development, Harare, Zimbabwe

Cunningham C 1985 Training and education approaches for parents of children with special needs. British Journal of Medical Psychology 58: 285–305

Finkenflügel H J M 1991 Help for the disabled – in hospital and at home. World Health Forum 12: 325–329

Hallum A, Krumboltz D 1993 Parents caring for young adults with severe physical stress: psychological issues. Developmental Medicine & Child Neurology 35: 24–32

Hamblin T 1987 A new dimension in management programmes for cerebral palsied children in India. Physiotherapy 73: 307–308

Hanekom J M 1984 Rehabilitation assistants – possible answer to rural disability in Zimbabwe? African Journal of Rehabilitation 2: 4

Hanekom J 1988 The Children's Rehabilitation Unit. African Journal of Rehabilitation 2: 11–13

Haylock C L, Johnson M A, Harpin M A 1993 Parents' views of community care for children with motor disabilities. Child Care, Health and Development 19: 209–220

Hinojosa J 1991 How mothers of preschool children with cerebral palsy perceive occupational and physical therapists and their influence on family life. Occupational Therapy Journal of Research 10: 144–162

Jelsma J M, Cortes-Meldrum D, Moyo A, Powell G 1995 The Children's Rehabilitation Unit, Harare: an integrated model of rehabilitation. Pediatric Physical Therapy 7: 140–142

Levitt S 1986 Handling the child with paediatric development disability. Physiotherapy 72: 161–164

McAlister M 1989 Community based rehabilitation in Zimbabwe. Physiotherapy 75: 432–433

Mariga F 1989 Attitudes towards disability. Paper presented at a Conference on Community Based Rehabilitation,

Harare 11–15 April, under the auspices of the Ministry of Health

Miles M 1985 Where there is no rehabilitation plan. Mental Health Centre, Peshawar, Pakistan

Miles M 1987 Handicapped children in Pakistan: targeting information needs. Health Policy and Planning 2: 347–351

Ministry of Health, Zimbabwe 1990 Survey of knowledge, attitudes and practice of the general population in Zimbabwe, with regard to disability. Rehabilitation Unit, Ministry of Health

M'Kumbuzi 1995 Impact of caring for child with cerebral palsy on the mental health of care givers, University of Zimbabwe, Harare, Zimbabwe BSc thesis

O'Toole B (n.d.) Involvement of volunteers, parents and community members with children with special needs. In: UNESCO Special education. UNESCO, France pp. 25–32

Rosenbaum P, King S 1990 Home or children's treatment centre; where should initial assessments of child with disabilities be done? Developmental Medicine & Child Neurology 31: 314–352

Ross K, Thompson D 1993 An evaluation of parents' involvement in the management of their cerebral palsied children. Physiotherapy 79: 561–565

Sifana 1994 Ages at which children we referred to the Children's Rehabilitation Unit, University of Zimbabwe, Harare, Zimbabwe BSc thesis

Stallard P, Dickinson F 1994 Groups for parents of preschool children with severe disabilities. Child: Care, Health and Development 20: 197–207

Teager D 1995 Address to the WCPT. World Confederation of Physical Therapists, Newsletter, December, 1995, p. 1

Thorburn M J 1989 Working with parents. CBR News 11: 46–48

von Wendt L, Ekenberg L, Dagis D, Janlert U 1984 A parent centred approach to physiotherapy for their handicapped children. Developmental Medicine & Child Neurology 26: 445–449

World Health Organization 1982 Community based rehabilitation. Report of a WHO Interregional Consultation, Colombo, Sri Lanka. (RHB/1R/82.1) WHO, Geneva

29

Cross-cultural parent education and early intervention: Cuban and African-American families in Miami, Florida, USA

Helen Masin

INTRODUCTION

According to predictions, Miami, Florida, as it is today, is representative of the urban community in the United States of America (USA) of the year 2050. According to the 1990 census in the USA, approximately 75% of the population at that date was Anglo/European American, 12% African American, 9% Hispanic American, and 3% Asian American. By the year 2050, White non-Hispanic Americans will represent approximately 53% of the total population, African Americans 15%, Hispanic Americans 24%, and Asian Americans and Pacific Islanders 9%. (US Department of Commerce 1996)

The rehabilitation professional in Miami, in Dade County, Florida, is in a unique position to become aware of the impact of cultural beliefs on the delivery of physical therapy services in the USA. According to the *Miami Herald* (Staff 1992), 'South Florida [has been] transformed by a decade of social and economic upheaval, into an international multilingual mix that changed more dramatically than anywhere else in the country.' Nearly half of all Dade County residents were born abroad. In Dade County, 57% of families speak a language besides English at home. Large-scale immigration to Dade County from Latin America began with the anti-Castro Cubans in the 1960s; Cubans continue to come today although the largest influx was in the early 1980s. In addition, during the 1980s, thousands of Haitians fled to Florida to escape economic deprivation and political instability. The civil war and Sandinista rule in Nicaragua brought 100 000 refugees to Florida. Similarly, Colombians, Peruvians, Hondurans and Guatemalans have immigrated secondary to problems in their respective homelands. Given this diversity of cultures among the families being served, the rehabilitation professional must recognize that different cultures may have different ways of dealing with health, illness, and disability.

As a physical therapist educated in New York City, New York, and Atlanta, Georgia, I was not prepared for the cultural differences experienced when moving to Miami in 1980. Although I had worked in a variety of pediatric settings in the USA and the UK, I was unaware of the issues unique to Miami that would affect the delivery of patient care. As the physical therapist for an early intervention program serving 80 infants, toddlers, and their families, from a variety of ethnic and cultural backgrounds, I immediately realized I had to increase my knowledge of my clients' way of life. Moreover, as a researcher, I wanted to understand the impact of ethnicity on the intervention. This chapter describes a study to investigate the maternal knowledge of and attitudes toward physical therapy during early intervention at the Debbie Institute of the University of Miami Mailman Center for Child Development in Miami. This research addresses the issue of 'culturally competent' service delivery.

LEGISLATION AND SERVICES IN THE USA

Early intervention legislation

In the USA, federal law mandates the delivery of physical therapy services for children with disabilities and their families in a 'culturally competent' manner. Culturally competent care is defined as a 'set of congruent behaviors, attitudes and policies that come together in a system, agency, or among professionals to work effectively in cross cultural situations' (Cross et al 1989, p. 13). Culturally competent care recognizes and incorporates the importance of culture, and of assessing cross-cultural relations,

understanding the dynamics of cultural differences, expanding cultural knowledge, and modifying services to meet culturally unique needs.

This federal legislation evolved over 2 decades in response to the demands of parents of children with disabilities. In 1975, Congress enacted Public Law (P. L.) 94-142, which stated that all children 6–21 years of age, regardless of their handicapping condition, were entitled to a free, appropriate education in the least restrictive environment. In 1986, P.L. 99-457 mandated that early intervention services be provided for children with disabilities from 3–5 years old and recommended services for children from birth to 3 years. Both laws have been re-authorized as P. L. 102-119, the Individuals with Disabilities Education Act of 1991.

EVOLUTION OF EARLY INTERVENTION SERVICES

The evolution of early intervention services has stemmed from the involvement of families of children with disabilities. These families lobbied the US Congress to authorize the funding necessary to provide services for their children. In the USA, the term early intervention describes a wide range of services for infants, toddlers, preschoolers, and their families that have been identified as having or being at risk for developmental delays. Physical therapy is one service utilized in early intervention programs. Others include special education, speech and language therapy, audiology, occupational therapy, psychology, social work, nursing, and nutrition.

The concept of early intervention is based on the premise that 'all children should have the opportunity to develop their maximum potential regardless of race, creed, economic status, or handicapping condition' (Effgen 1990, p. 97). This premise is based on six primary principles:

• the first years of life are a period of rapid growth and development that lays the foundation for later development
• infants have the capability to interact and form attachments
• infants are able to learn

- parents are responsible for nurturing and providing early learning experiences
- developmental outcomes are determined by the interactions between both biological and environmental factors
- structured programming can improve the abilities of children and their families (Effgen 1990).

Effgen stated that the goal of the physical therapists on an early intervention team is to 'specifically encourage sensorimotor function by enhancing perceptual and motor development, musculoskeletal status, neurobehavioral organization, cardiopulmonary status and effective environmental adaptation, and to provide support to the families in the care of their child with special needs' (Effgen 1990, p. 97). She identified five basic assumptions that form the basis for physical therapy practice in early intervention:

- the plasticity of the nervous system (in other words, the nervous system may be molded)
- young children are sensorimotor learners
- the acquisition of motor skills is a major component of early development
- intervention should start early to promote optimal outcome and prevent secondary disability
- physical therapy services must be family centered in order to provide maximum intervention (Effgen 1990).

REVIEW OF LITERATURE

Although physical therapy traditionally utilized a child-centered model of service delivery, the federal mandate requires the provision of early intervention services in a family centered model. Educational researchers (Sameroff 1982, Dunst 1988) note that families play a critical role in their children's development. Since culture shapes family beliefs about child-rearing and health, physical therapists must understand both family dynamics and culture in order to provide optimal therapy services. Trout & Foley

(1989), defining the family of the handicapped child as the child's ecological system that is essential to the child's optimal development, recommends that professionals must know the family if they want to know the child.

Christensen's (1992) research with clinical professionals indicated that the ability to work effectively with culturally diverse families requires professionals to acknowledge their own cultural background and develop a general understanding of specific cultures. Christensen stresses that cultural background can be a powerful force in the relationship between professionals and the families they serve. This understanding of the family and its culture is extremely important for rehabilitation professionals as the populations being served are becoming increasingly diverse.

Given the anticipated diversity of the US population in the 21st century, physical therapists must educate themselves to work with populations different than their own as well as to diversify membership in their own profession. Physical therapists and physical therapy students polled by the American Physical Therapy Association in 1994 were 82–86% Caucasian; African Americans, Asian Americans, Hispanic Americans, American Indians, and other ethnic groups represented less than 3% each (APTA 1994). Physical therapy strategies successful with more homogeneous populations may not succeed when the client's ethnic group differs from that of the physical therapist.

Resources which may assist physical therapists in becoming familiar with cultures different than their own include transcultural studies in medicine, medical anthropology, and nursing. Transcultural studies have shown that understanding cultural variables is critical to working effectively with different ethnic groups (Anderson 1989; DeSantis 1989; Harwood 1981). Jackson (1982) found that the amount of time spent with the client affects patient satisfaction with medical care among African Americans receiving treatment for hypertension. DeSantis (1989) found increased compliance regarding nursing interventions with Hispanic and

Haitian mothers when the professional explores and respects the client's belief system. Harwood (1981) found that ethnic differences appear to be important determinants of observed differences in health behavior. His data indicate that ethnicity is particularly relevant to an individual's beliefs and behavior with regard to the various health practices.

The explanatory model described by Kleinman (1976) explains the etiology, onset of symptoms, pathophysiology, course of sickness, and treatment for the particular problem being addressed. On the cultural level, differences between the explanatory model of the family and that of the professional can produce miscommunication. Respect for the explanatory model of the families can facilitate patient–professional communication. For healing to occur, there needs to be a 'fit' between the family and the professional regarding the expectations, beliefs, behaviors and evaluations of the outcome.

CULTURE AND LIFEWAYS

For the therapist to understand the interactions between the explanatory model and the cultural variables, one must understand the nature of culture itself.

Culture as defined by Anderson & Fenichel (1989) is the specific framework of meanings within which a population, individually and as a group, shapes its lifeways, including the ways parents and professionals interact with one another. Specific cultural issues which affect health professional services include family role definition, relationships and child-rearing techniques, beliefs about health, illness and disability, and communication and interactional styles (Anderson & Fenichel 1989; see also Chs 2, 4, 8, 26, 27 and 28).

Saunders (1954) elaborated on other aspects of culture and showed how it affects a person's daily life:

- culture is a complex whole with interrelated parts
- culture has a historical continuity that transcends generations

- culture has a strong influence on the individual's self-perception and relations with people and the non-human environment
- culture changes and can be changed
- culture is complex, and processes for transmitting it are rather inefficient, so no individual ever acquires the whole of a culture.

Saunders (1954) identified several characteristics of the Anglo/European culture that may affect the patient–practitioner relationship. For example, in the USA, the culture of medicine itself is enmeshed in:

- the government as seen in Medicare
- religion as seen in hospitals associated with a religious orientation
- education as seen in medical schools and schools of allied health and nursing
- the economy itself as seen in the debates in Congress regarding health care costs.

Because the health care system and US culture are enmeshed, utilization of the medical services may be confusing to immigrants raised in other cultures. The family seeking care may not understand the expectations of the practitioners and vice versa. There is a greater chance for satisfaction if professionals are willing and able to adapt their treatment regimes to make them fit the expectations of their clients. (Saunders 1954)

For professionals to modify their approach to their clients, they must first be aware of the culture in which they were raised and educated. A dramatic example of such awareness occurred when I first arrived in Miami. A toddler in the early intervention program was being followed by the neurology clinic for management of grand mal epileptic seizures. The toddler was having breakthrough seizures at school, and all the staff members were very concerned. Because the child's family was Creole-speaking from Haiti, an interpreter talked with the child's mother about the importance of giving her son the phenobarbital which the physician had prescribed. The interpreter found out that the mother was administering the medication regularly at the appropriate dosage. However, the

hild was still having seizures at school. To get
more information, a staff member asked the
mother to demonstrate how she was administer-
ng the phenobarbital. When she did this, it was
pparent that a cultural variable had not been
ddressed. The mother had been bathing the
hild in the phenobarbital, which was custom-
ry in the part of Haiti where she had lived. The
taff had been operating on the Western medical
model of oral administration of medicine; the
mother had been operating on her own cultural
model in which medicine was administered by
athing.

THE STUDY

Research methodology

The purpose of the pilot study was to determine
f factors related to ethnicity may affect early
ntervention services at the Debbie Institute. The
ilot study used a questionnaire to assess per-
eived parental understanding of physical ther-
py, parental perceptions of physical therapy
ffectiveness, and, using a Likert-type scale,
arental satisfaction with physical therapy.
Demographic data were gathered using multi-
le-choice or fill-in-the-blank questions. The
uestionnaire concluded with open-ended ques-
ions dealing with qualitative aspects of the per-
eived maternal knowledge and attitudes
oward physical therapy.

The results indicated that parents were gener-
lly satisfied with physical therapy effectiveness
nd had a moderate understanding of what
hysical therapy actually did for their child.
However, 20% of the respondents left questions
lank that related to their understanding of
hysical therapy. These blank questions raised
ome concerns about the parental understand-
ng of physical therapy.

Interviews with Cuban-American profession-
ls at the research site indicated that response
differences may have been influenced by a cul-
urally biased survey or a variety of cultural
ariables. The survey sample, including Cuban-
American, African-American, Haitian, and other
Central and South American ethnic groups, may

not have been adequately sensitive to intergroup differences.

Based on these preliminary findings, the
questionnaire was modified to control for ethnic
differences and only the two largest respondent
groups in the pilot study were compared. These
were Cuban Americans and African Americans.
To get a larger sample size, the study expanded
to include two other early intervention programs in Miami. These were the Easter Seal
Society of Dade County and United Cerebral
Palsy of Miami. Thus, the survey sample
increased to 170 families.

Using the modified questionnaire, this
research investigated three hypotheses:

1. There are no significant differences in
maternal attitudes toward physical therapy
effectiveness between Cuban Americans and
African Americans.

2. There are no significant differences in perceived maternal understanding of physical
therapy between Cuban Americans and African
Americans.

3. There are no significant differences in
maternal satisfaction with physical therapy
between Cuban Americans and African
Americans.

To control for gender, only mothers or maternal
guardians were identified as the respondents.

The revised questionnaire included four questions regarding maternal perception of physical
therapy effectiveness, nine questions regarding
perceived maternal understanding of physical
therapy, eight questions regarding maternal satisfaction with physical therapy, four open-ended
questions regarding maternal satisfaction with
physical therapy, and 12 demographic questions. The questions were designed to investigate each respondent's experiences in physical
therapy with their children.

Three experts in physical therapy reviewed
and modified the questionnaire for construct
validity. The written survey was analyzed using
descriptive statistics and a t-test for independent samples. The surveys were written in
English and in Spanish to optimize respondents'
understanding of the questions. Nine personal

interview questions were developed to gain additional insight into the respondents' beliefs, attitudes, and behaviors regarding their child's disability and the role of physical therapy for the child and the family. Twenty taped interviews were conducted with 10 Cuban-American and 10 African-American families. Using Bogdan and Biklen's (1982) techniques for analyzing qualitative data, the interviews were transcribed, organized, broken into manageable units, synthesized, and searched for patterns to discover what was important to the respondents. Based on these analyses, themes emerged from the interview data that gave insights into the maternal beliefs and attitudes toward physical therapy in Cuban-American and African-American families.

To gain increased understanding of the maternal knowledge and attitudes toward physical therapy in Cuban-American and African-American families in Miami, the larger study was developed to combine both quantitative and qualitative (interview) techniques to get more in depth information from these families. Surveys were sent to all 170 families in the study and were completed by 122 respondents. Ethnicity was noted to determine when 30 surveys had been received from the Cuban American and African American families in order to meet the statistical requirements for the t-test.

Among these 122 responses, 31 were Cuban Americans and 33 were African Americans. Analyses were not made for the remaining 64 respondents or for the 48 nonrespondents although their ethnicity was documented. The 31 Cuban Americans identified themselves as such and the 33 African Americans identified themselves as such on the written survey. The survey was designed so that repondents identified themselves according to their own perception of their ethnicity. This proved to be an important feature of the research design because the respondents were more diverse than had been expected. All participants were advised that they did not need to complete or return the survey if they did not wish to do so. They were also advised that their responses would be used in summary form and that no one would be identified individually.

The bus drivers who transported the children to the Debbie Institute and the other two centers in the study delivered the surveys to the families. This proved to be a very effective way to engage the families in the research process because they already had a good relationship with the drivers. Families also returned the completed surveys via the bus drivers. The surveys returned to the research sites were logged on a master survey file.

Follow-up phone calls were made to 10 respondent Cuban-American and 10 respondent African-American families to determine their willingness to be interviewed after having completed the questionnaire. Of the 20 randomly selected mothers who were interviewed following the survey, only five chose to have face-to-face interviews. The remaining 15 mothers or guardians were interviewed by telephone.

The questions used in the interviews were adapted from Kleinman (1976) to elicit the families' explanatory model. The questions used family-oriented, jargon-free terminology. The interview questions related to all three hypotheses. In addition, the interview questions were designed to elicit maternal attitudes related to cultural norms. The questions were as follows:

1. What do you think has caused your child's situation (developmental delay)?
2. Why do you think it started when it did?
3. What does the (developmental) delay do to your child? What is its impact on your child?
4. What does your child's (developmental) delay do to you? What is its impact on you?
5. What kind of physical therapy would you like to have for your child?
6. What are the most important results for your child which you hope to get from physical therapy treatment?
7. What are the chief problems which your child's delay has caused you?
8. What is the worst thing that could happen because of your child's situation?

. Do you have any questions about the survey or these interview questions? Do you have any questions about physical therapy in general?

Results

Four questions were analyzed to assess maternal perception of effectiveness of physical therapy (hypothesis 1=H1). There were no significant differences between Cuban Americans and African Americans (see Table 29.1). Table 29.1 indicates that both groups felt that physical therapy services were effective for their children.

Nine questions were analyzed to assess perceived maternal understanding of physical therapy between Cuban Americans and African Americans (hypothesis 2=H2). The t-test revealed statistically significant differences in perceived maternal understanding of the purpose of physical therapy, the physical therapy treatment in school, and the use of adaptive equipment at school and at home.

Table 29.2 indicates that Cuban Americans and African Americans differed significantly on four questions. These differences indicated that Cuban Americans' better understanding of the physical therapy services may relate to the finding that more Cuban Americans reported attending physical therapy treatments, individual education plan (IEP) meetings, and home exercise training programs than did African Americans. Through attending these meetings, Cuban Americans may have learned more about the purpose of therapy (Q6), the type of physical therapy treatment (Q10), and the use of adaptive equipment at school (Q13) and at home (Q14).

Eight questions were asked to assess maternal satisfaction with physical therapy (hypothesis 3=H3). Statistical differences were found in relation to maternal feelings about control in planning physical therapy and in relation to satisfaction with the physical therapist's response to maternal suggestions (see Table 29.3). Table 29.3 indicates that African Americans were more satisfied with the physical therapists' responses to their suggestions than were Cuban Americans (Q18). However, Cuban Americans felt that they could exert more control (Q16) over their child's physical therapy services. This may have been due to better attendance of Cuban Americans at physical therapy treatments, IEP meetings, and home training sessions.

Demographic findings were tabulated and included parental participation in therapy activities such as evaluation, treatment, and program planning. Information regarding maternal age, education and ethnicity was included for both

Table 29.1   T-test for significant differences between Cuban Americans and African Americans regarding maternal perception of physical therapy effectiveness (H1) for Q24–Q27

	CA Mean	CA St dev	AA Mean	AA St dev	T-value	St sig
Q24	1.47	0.82	1.33	0.85	−0.67	−
Q25	1.53	1.04	1.61	1.03	0.31	−
Q26	1.53	1.04	1.67	0.92	0.56	−
Q27	1.63	1.16	1.76	1.0	0.47	−

Key
CA = Cuban American
AA = African American
St dev = standard deviation
Q24 = Do you think physical therapy has improved your child's ability to move?
Q25 = Do you think physical therapy has helped you to better understand your child?
Q26 = Do you think physical therapy has given you support as a parent?
Q27 = Do you think physical therapy training has helped increase your skills in working with your child's movement skills?

Table 29.2 T-test for significant differences between Cuban Americans and African Americans regarding perceived maternal understanding of physical therapy (H2) for Q6–Q14

	CA Mean	CA St dev	AA Mean	AA St dev	T-value	St sig
Q6	1.45	0.62	1.82	1.01	1.77	<0.05
Q7	2.23	1.12	1.12	2.12	−0.39	–
Q8	1.68	0.7	1.7	0.95	0.09	–
Q9	1.87	0.96	1.85	1.03	−0.08	–
Q10	1.39	0.76	1.67	0.92	1.33	<0.05
Q11	1.97	0.05	1.97	1.31	0	–
Q12	2.27	1.34	2.21	1.54	0.16	–
Q13	1.6	0.81	2.0	1.3	1.48	<0.05
Q14	1.14	0.73	2.76	1.46	3.21	<0.05

Key
CA   = Cuban American
AA   = African American
St dev = Standard deviation
Q6   = How well do you understand the purpose of your child's physical therapy treatment?
Q7   = How well do you understand physical therapy terminology?
Q8   = How well do you understand your child's physical therapy goals?
Q9   = How well do you understand your child's physical therapy evaluation?
Q10   = How well do you understand the physical therapy treatment that your child receives in school?
Q11   = How well do you understand the type of activities your child does in physical therapy?
Q12   = How well do you understand the physical therapy training that your family received for doing a home exercise program?
Q13   = How well do you understand the use of adaptive equipment (walkers, standers, braces, or toys) at *school*?
Q14   = How well do you understand the use of adaptive equipment (walkers, standers, braces, or toys) at *home*?

groups. No demographic information was obtained regarding income levels. The greatest variability in responses was found in the ethnic distribution of all the respondents other than Cuban Americans and African Americans. Demographic data were also collected for frequency and duration of physical therapy services for the two groups and sources of referral to therapy.

Open-ended questions were asked, and the mothers or grandmothers were encouraged to speak about the strengths and weaknesses of the physical therapy program, any changes that the family would recommend, and anything else they wanted to say about their child's physical therapy services.

Although both groups focused on the positive aspects of therapy, the Cuban Americans were much more likely to comment on the relationship between the therapist, the child, and the family. One Cuban-American mother summarized the importance of this relationship by stating:

I think the attitude, her giving of herself and the love of caring shown by the physical therapist and the desire of her to make my son better. The human aspect is the most important and special with these children.

Her comments were congruent with cultural beliefs of Cuban Americans that emphasize the importance of *personalismo* in dealing with professionals. For the Cuban Americans, the relationship with the professional was as important as what the professional did (Gomez 1991).

For the African-American mothers, their praise was different. It expressed their appreciation, but only one commented on a relationship

Table 29.3 T-test for significant differences between Cuban Americans and African Americans regarding perceived maternal understanding of physical therapy (H3) for Q1–Q5 and Q15–Q18

	CA Mean	CA St dev	AA Mean	AA St dev	T-value	St sig
Q1	1.19	0.54	1.3	0.59	0.77	–
Q2	1.42	0.67	1.33	0.69	−0.52	–
Q3	2.23	1.12	2.12	1.11	−0.39	–
Q4	1.73	1.14	1.88	1.32	−0.48	–
Q5	1.50	0.82	1.36	0.74	0.71	–
Q15	1.37	0.85	1.48	0.87	0.51	–
Q16	1.63	1.00	2.18	0.92	2.28	<0.05
Q17	3.53	1.33	3.85	1.37	0.94	–
Q18	2.10	1.58	1.30	1.38	−2.15	<0.05

Key
CA   = Cuban American
AA   = African American
St dev = Standard deviation
Q1   = How satisfied do you feel with the physical therapy in general?
Q2   = How satisfied are you regarding the effectiveness of the physical therapy staff with your child?
Q3   = How satisfied are you with the frequency of your child's contact with the physical therapist?
Q4   = How satisfied are you with the educational materials your child's physical therapist has given to you?
Q5   = How satisfied are you with your child's progress in physical therapy?
Q15   = How important (necessary) do you feel your family is in carrying out physical therapy activities?
Q16   = How much control (input that matters) do you feel you should have in planning your child's physical therapy goals?
Q17   = How often do you make suggestions to your child's physical therapist?
Q18   = How satisfied (pleased) are you with the physical therapist's response to your suggestions?

with the physical therapist. This mother stated her feelings as follows:

I am grateful for the service my daughter has received and I am pleased with her progress.

Implications

Cuban American interview findings and their implications

The findings from the interview data and the open-ended questions on the survey indicate that Cuban-American cultural beliefs do affect maternal perceptions of physical therapy. For example, the cultural concept of *personalismo* appears to play an important role in the success of the therapy intervention. Mothers focused on the impact on their lives and the lives of their

families of having a child with a developmental delay. Although the mothers acknowledged the support received from their extended family, they reported feeling depressed, sad, and frustrated by their children's delays.

Several mothers mentioned the economic strain of seeing so many medical professionals. Perhaps the Cuban cultural concept of the professional as 'all knowing' made the mothers feel that these multiple visits were in their children's best interest. Many families did not understand their role as co-partners in planning for a child's therapy services. The process of speaking up and telling professionals what they wanted was difficult for many of the Cuban American mothers. The interviews also indicated that Cuban Americans relied heavily on the extended family for support and guidance. Even if the professional felt they had much to offer the child, suggestions would not be followed through at home if the family did not value the input.

The importance of having the therapist develop a relationship with the child and the family is clear from the mothers' comments regarding their close relationship with the physical therapist. One mother stated:

The relationship between the physical therapist and the parent is also very important. I find it very comforting knowing that it does not matter what questions or concerns I may have, my child's therapist is always there to listen and help.

By taking the time to talk informally with the family prior to beginning the formal evaluation, the therapist will be laying the foundation for the development of *personalismo* that may improve the patient–professional communication, thereby enhancing patient compliance.

African-American interview findings and their implications

The interview findings indicate that the cultural beliefs of African-American families do affect their satisfaction, understanding, and perceptions of physical therapy. African-American families have a greater interest in physical therapy as it relates to improvements in their children's motor development. Mothers mentioned that it hurt them to see that a child with a disability could not play like his or her siblings. Because play is an important aspect of learning in African American culture, this statement seems to convey the sense of grief these mothers experience. African-American culture emphasizes a strong 'kinetic' component that includes nonverbal as well as verbal communication as important variables.

Several African-American mothers expressed an interest in having a parent training program for their children's physical therapy activities. African-American culture may emphasize more interactional and auditory learning as compared to the introspective learning of the Anglo/European cultures.

The interviews also provided insight into the African-Americans' beliefs about religion and disability. Several mothers mentioned that the outcome for their children was with 'the Man upstairs', or they thanked God for the school services. For these religiously-oriented families, the therapist may suggest that they access the support system of their church and its outreach programs to assist them in obtaining services and in purchasing equipment for children with special needs.

A third area of focus was the importance of the kinship family taking responsibility for the child if the parents were absent. Out of the 10 families interviewed, two of the children were in the care of a grandmother or aunt because the natural mother was unable to care for the children.

Because early independence is valued for children in African-American culture, the physical therapist is in a better position to promote this independence. It has been postulated that the African-American culture developed this desire for early independence because slave families were often separated and children needed to be independent to survive. Because play is also valued in African-American culture, the therapist can suggest therapeutic uses of play to help achieve therapy goals. The awareness of the closeness of the kinship network can assist the therapist when planning home based treatment. The physical therapist may ask other family members to attend therapy sessions to learn how to implement positioning, handling, and other therapeutic play activities. Since the kinetic component is an important source of communication, the therapist may emphasize demonstration, modeling, and verbal discussion of motor skills for the families in addition to the written home program.

Similarities in Cuban-American and African-American findings and implications for professionals

Several mothers from both groups expressed concerns about doing enough for their children. These findings are extremely important in that therapists can be very supportive to families by reassuring them that they are doing the correct things to help their children. Hopefully, these mothers' reassurances can help reduce the mother's anxieties.

Several mothers expressed confusion regarding their role as co-partners with the professionals serving their families. Therefore, therapists must educate parents in how to assume their roles as team members in planning physical therapy activities for their children. Both groups expressed praise and thankfulness for the services of the physical therapists. These findings indicate that mothers generally appreciate and value the therapists' support and input.

CONCLUSIONS

If professionals wish to provide culturally competent care, they must become aware of their own culture and the culture of Western medicine. This will enable them to appreciate the perceptual filters that may bias them when providing care for clients from other cultures. My experience with the superficial bathing for administration of phenobarbital for the child with grand mal seizures was a dramatic example of this.

Currently, most physical therapists in the USA come from an Anglo/European background. Anglo/European culture is characterized by a need for control over the environment, need for change, time dominance, human equality, individualism, privacy, self-help, competition, future orientation, action, openness/honesty, practicality/efficiency, and materialism (Shilling & Brannan 1989). In addition, Hall (1981) stated that 'what one pays attention to or does not attend to is largely a matter of context' (Hall 1981, p. 90).

Graham & Miller (1995) describe the characteristics that dominate most North American and northern European societies as low context: highly individualistic, assertive, dominating, results-oriented, independent, strong-willed, competitive, quick to make decisions, impatient, time-conscious, solution-oriented, control-seeking, well-organized and self-contained. The culture stresses the need for human equality, change, future orientation, action and self-help. Early intervention seeks to meet all these goals

as a way of dealing with a child born with disabilities. These elements are also incorporated in the philosophy of early intervention that states that all children are entitled to services to enable them to achieve their optimal potential.

However, many of the clients of early intervention programs come from cultures different from Anglo/European culture. For example, Cuban Americans and Hispanic Americans in general prefer a style in which human interaction dominates. They prefer immediate rewards rather than future rewards, live in the present, have strong family relationships that take precedence over the individual, and have a tendency toward dependency and an acceptance of fate (Saunders 1954, Shilling & Brannan 1989). Graham & Miller (1995) describe Hispanic culture as being high context: indirect, highly affiliative, team-oriented, systematic, steady, quiet, patient, loyal, dependable, informal, servicing, sharing, slow in making decisions, respectful, and listening. These individuals take longer to become acquainted with and trusting of one another. After trust is established, communication is fast. The culture values the past and is slow to change. Asian and African-American cultures are also often considered high context.

The concept of early intervention is perceived as very different by people of high-context cultures because their cultural values do not stress change, future orientation, or self-help. Given the differences in the beliefs of high- versus low-context cultures, the physical therapist must know how suggestions may impact on families coming from other cultures.

The results of this study indicate that differing perceptions of parental roles and parental understanding of physical therapy goals and activities may be linked to the differing cultural backgrounds of the therapists and their clients. Health professionals working with clients of cultures different from their own must take responsibility for learning about their own culture and the culture of medicine, learning about the culture of their client, and creating a bridge between the two cultures if they wish to enhance the patient–professional interaction for the common good.

REFERENCES

Anderson P, Fenichel E 1989 Serving culturally diverse families of infants and toddlers with disabilities. (Available from National Center for Clinical Infant Programs, 733 15th Street, N.W., Suite 912, Washington, D.C. 2005.)

APTA 1994 Physical therapy fact sheet. American Physical Therapy Association, Education Division Alexandria VA

Bogden R C, Biklen S R 1982 Qualitative research for education: and introduction to theory and methods. Allyn and Bacon, Boston

Christensen C 1992 Multi cultural competencies in early intervention: training professionals for a pluralistic society. Infants and Young Children, 4(3): 49–63

Cross J L, Bazron J Dennis K, Isaacs M 1989 Towards a culturally competent system of care. (Available from CAASP Technical Assistance Center, Georgetown University Child Development Center, 3800 Reservoir Road, NW, Washington, D.C. 20007.)

DeSantis L 1989 Health care orientations of Cuban and Haitian immigrant mothers: implications for health care professionals. Medical Anthropology 12: 69–89

Dunst C J, Trivette C M, Deal A G 1988 Enabling and empowering families – principles and guidelines for practice. Brookline Books, Cambridge, MA

Effgen J K 1990 Role of physical therapy in early intervention (Task Force on Early Intervention), Paediatric Physical Therapy, p. 97

Gomez M 1991 Culturally sensitive issues when working with Latino families. In Early Intervention: the family and you. Presentation at the Mailman Center for Child Development, Miami, FL

Graham M, Miller D. The 1995 Annual. Vol. 1 Training, San Diego, CA, Pfeiffer & Co.

Hall E T 1981 Beyond culture. Anchor Books, Doubleday, New York

Harwood A (ed) 1981 Ethnicity and medical care. Harvard University Press, Cambridge, MA

Jackson J 1982 Urban black Americans. In: Harwood A (ed) Ethnicity and medical care. Harvard University Press Cambridge, MA pp. 36–129

Kleinman A 1976 Concepts and a model for the comparison of medical systems as cultural systems. Social Science and Medicine 12: 85–93

Masin H L 1991 Parental attitudes toward physical therapy services at the Debbie School early intervention program Manuscript. University of Miami Department of Pediatrics, Miami, FL

Masin H L 1995 Perceived maternal knowledge and attitudes toward physical therapy during early intervention in Cuban-American and African-American families Pediatric Physical Therapy 7: 118–123

Sameroff A 1982 The environmental context of developmental disabilities. In: Bricker D (ed) Intervention with at risk and handicapped infants. University Park Press, Baltimore

Saunders L 1954 Cultural differences and medical care. Russell Sage Foundation, New York

Shilling B, Brannan E 1989 Cross cultural counseling: a guide for nutrition and health counselors. (Available from United States Department of Agriculture and United States Department of Health and Human Services Washington, DC.)

Staff (1992) Census data reveal area's vast changes. Miami Herald, 3 April 1992, p. 1

Trout M, Foley G 1989 Working with families of handicapped infants and toddlers. Topics in Language Disorders 10(1): 57–67

United States Department of Commerce 1996 Population projections of the United States by age, sex, race, and Hispanic origin, 1995 to 2050. Bureau of the Census, Feb 1996

30

Professional development, personality and self-esteem of Palestinian physical therapists

Lesley Dawson

INTRODUCTION

The name Palestine evokes different emotions depending on one's nationality, religion or political interests. Most of us can remember seeing Prime Minister Rabin of Israel and President Arafat shaking hands on the lawn of the White House in Washington or listening to Hanan Ashrawi articulating the needs of her countrymen and women. Less pleasant memories are the TV footage during the *Intifada*, the Palestinian uprising between 1987 and 1990 (Lockman & Beinin 1990), and the recent car and bus bombings in Tel Aviv and Jerusalem. For me Palestine is not just a piece of land but a people among whom I have lived and worked for 10 years.

The two areas making up the present Palestine, the West Bank and Gaza Strip, are separated from each other by 80 km of Israel. The larger West Bank is in excess of 5000 square km with a population of around a million people, 70% of whom live outside the urban areas in villages and refugee camps. The topography of the West Bank varies from the lush oasis of Jericho in the east to more barren hills in the west. Many Palestinians live and work in East Jerusalem, which, although reunified with West Jerusalem since 1967, has geographical, religious and cultural links to both the West Bank and Gaza Strip. Gaza seems to be one continuous stream of humanity with almost a million people living in an area of 365 square km bordered on the west by the sea. Both areas resound with the voices of children and young people as half

Table 30.1 Health status comparisons between Israel and Palestine*

	Israel	Palestine
Infant mortality rate	7.9/1000	40/1000
Life expectancy	76 years	61 years
Doctors/population	1:340	1:1000
Nurses/population	1:198	1:800
Nurses/hospital bed	5.25	1.12
Hospital beds/population	0.96/1000	0.70/1000
Primary health clinics	1:2090	1:4184

* These statistics are based on Swersky et al 1992 and SAAR 1993.

the population are below the age of 25 (Qleibo 1992).

The health challenges of Palestine combine those of developing and developed worlds. Table 30.1 shows some health related statistics comparing Israelis and Palestinians. The major provider of health care is now the Palestine Health Authority, which has taken over responsibility for government hospitals that were administered by the Israeli Civil Administration since 1967. The United Nations Relief and Works Agency also provides health care, especially in Gaza where three-quarters of the residents have refugee status (Palestinian Health Council 1994, Gaza Health Services Research Centre 1995).

Physical therapists are relative newcomers to the health care team in the Middle East. Earliest practitioners were expatriates working as volunteers in charitable organizations for people with disabilities (PWD). As the importance of the profession was realized, Palestinians were sent abroad to Jordan, Egypt or Eastern Europe to train (Bithell & Lumley 1987). Local training for assistant physical therapists began in the 1970s and accelerated during the *Intifada* because of the injuries sustained during confrontations between the *shabab* (young men) and the Israeli Defence Force (Giacaman et al 1989). However, supply and demand for physical therapy is not equal because of the lack of finances to pay

salaries. Professional development was boosted by the patient needs and physical therapy shortcomings experienced during the *Intifada*. In 1989 a physical therapy program was developed at Bethlehem University (BU) to begin to meet the need for appropriate undergraduate and continuing education for physical therapists. There are a few occupational therapists and one or two speech and language therapists practicing in Palestine. Occupational therapy education began at BU in 1996 and it is hoped that other rehabilitation professions will develop in the future.

There are about 300 physical therapists and physical therapy assistants registered as members of the Palestinian Physiotherapy Associations. All those who work in East Jerusalem, the West Bank and Gaza Strip are eligible for membership, provided they have had an educational program of at least 2 years, recognized by the Palestinian Health Ministry.

The findings given here refer to a group of 164 Palestinian physical therapists and physical therapy assistants who participated in a study in 1995 (Dawson 1997). The purpose of the study was to ascertain the relevance of an innovative physical therapy curriculum to Palestine and whether that curriculum would produce a more forward-looking practitioner than traditional curricula. This was done by means of questionnaires regarding the relationship between personality, self-esteem and professional development. Personal characteristics influence a person's selection of a profession and success within that profession, and self-attitudes affect self and significant others' perceptions of professionalism and personal professional development (Rovezzi-Carroll & Leavitt 1984). The Palestinian group was compared with 53 Irish physical therapists. This comparison represents a contrast between groups of Arabs and Europeans who share many similarities in their history.

PROFESSIONAL DEVELOPMENT

The level of development of a profession depends on a variety of influences. Models of health care, infrastructure of health services, history of the profession and the political situation are some of the external constraints. Alongside these issues are professional attitudes and values and the characteristics of the individuals themselves. A biographical questionnaire was included in order to elicit therapists' feelings, interests and attitudes to their professional education and practice (see Table 30.2).

The Palestinian group is young by comparison with groups in other studies (O'Neill 1976, Dawson 1982, Wagstaff 1987), with a mean age

Table 30.2   LESQ Phi coefficient and Mann Whitney results for Palestine and Irish physical therapists

	Palestinians	Irish	Phi/MW
	%	%	
Sex M/F	58/42	17/83	0.00001
Age (20–29)	72	34	0.00001
Married	59	46	0.0001
Children	38	36	NS
Entered HE after 1980	100	44	0.00001
Type of school	65 government	46 church	NS
Four year program	32	39	NS
Graduated after 1980	100	51	0.00001
Degree	32	41	0.034
Satisfied	80	86	NS
Working	70	95	0.01
Working 5 or more years	21	57	0.0001
Satisfied	80	87	NS
Prefer pediatrics	42	32	NS
Prefer orthopedics	73	70	NS
Prefer neurology	41	37	NS
Prefer cardiovascular	5	25	0.0002
Prefer obs/gynae	6	17	0.02
Prefer exercise	82	86	NS
Prefer electrotherapy	20	41	0.0016
Prefer manipulation	56	46	NS
Prefer massage	17	23	NS
Both sex patients	82	97	0.008
Preparation for work	80	49	0.00001
Decide treatment	49	91	0.00001
Health education role	50	88	0.00001
Teach caretakers	64	29	0.00001
Doctors' knowledge of PT	80 very well/well enough	62 quite well	0.03
Nurses' knowledge of PT	85 very well/well enough	58 quite well	0.0001
Social workers' knowledge of PT	85 very well/ well enough	39 quite well	0.00001
Organize workshops	16	41	0.0001
Lecture at workshops	21	45	0.00008
Patient education materials	39	45	NS
Teacher most responsible for learning	33	7	0.001
Self most responsible for learning	69	95	0.0002
Employer most responsible for learning	10	0	NS
Differences in practice	62	89	0.0022

of 28 years, 72% of whom were between 20 and 29 years of age. The sample is representative of the Palestinian physical therapy population and indicates the youth of a profession which began about 25 years ago. The sex ratio of 59% males to 41% females is different from most European countries.

Unlike Europe, where social mobility is common, the majority of Palestinian physical therapists have stayed close to home for their education and employment (Cossali & Robson 1986). This is particularly true for the women in the group, as it is not acceptable for Muslim women to travel far from their families to study. Muslim fathers want to know that their daughters are living and working in a respectable place and the closer to home the better. Another reason for the lack of educational mobility is the level of the university entrance examination (*Tawjihi*), which prevents acceptance outside the Arab world. The *Tawjihi* level is lower than the British 'A' level and Israeli *Bagrout* examinations, although some American colleges and universities accept Palestinian students.

Two-thirds of practicing Palestinian physical therapists studied to diploma level, that being the only possibility for physical therapy education inside the country until 1989. Until recently, the only Arab country open to Palestinians that offered a degree in physical therapy was Egypt. Gazan students were able to take this opportunity while West Bankers went to Jordan, which offered a 3-year diploma. Less than a quarter (21%) of the sample were graduates from the first 4-year degree program or the 3-year part-time program to degree level offered at BU (open to physical therapy diplomates and assistants). Wherever they studied, 80% of the sample were reasonably satisfied with their education.

The working situation for physical therapists is sometimes primitive and scope of practice is limited. Physical therapy departments are often small, dark and inaccessible, with little concern for patient or therapist comfort. Scope of practice, until recently, was limited to orthopedic conditions and passive forms of therapy. However, in an area with high unemployment

and limited financial resources, 78% are employed, mainly in outpatient clinics in urban areas. Most health institutions are located in the south and central areas of the West Bank and around Gaza town in the Gaza Strip making it necessary for both staff and patients to travel some distance for work or treatment. When there are road blocks, curfews and closures, hospitals and clinics may be severely understaffed. The prohibition on Palestinians entering Jerusalem has left the hospitals there without staff coverage. It also deprives non-Jerusalemites of the services of the best hospital to which they have access, the Makassad Islamic Hospital in East Jerusalem. Some Palestinians, who can afford to pay the higher costs of health care in West Jerusalem, use the Hadassah Hospital when they are able to gain access. Despite the limited opportunities and lack of choice of places to work, 80% of the group were quite well satisfied with their work.

Patient and modality preference show the limited scope of professional practice. There are 2.5% of the Palestinian population in need of rehabilitation compared to the world figure of 1.5%, most of whom are children with cerebral palsy (Fig. 30.1) and adults with permanent neurological impairment requiring physical therapy (Giacaman et al 1989). Yet, 73% of thera-

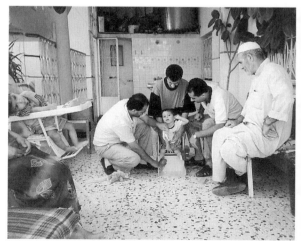

Fig. 30.1 Three physical therapy students fitting a child for a chair they have made for him at his home in Jericho.

pists prefer to deal with orthopedic cases. The orthopedic model of physical therapy originates from the education of the physical therapists themselves and that of doctors with whom they work. The fact that only 42% of the sample enjoyed working with children and 41% with patients with neurological problems supports observations made by Bithell & Lumley (1987) that Palestinian physical therapists are not trained to deal with children with cerebral palsy or adults with neurological damage. Neither cardiothoracic nor obstetric physiotherapy is common in Palestine (Al Khdour & Maas 1995). Treatment modality preference showed 82% preferred exercise, 56% manipulation and 20% electrotherapy. (See Table 30.2 for statistical significance when Palestinians are compared to Irish physical therapists.)

The expressed preference for hands-on therapy is surprising. When one visits physical therapy departments and clinics, one is shown, with great pride, the latest electrotherapy equipment (Bithell & Lumley 1987). Therapists will tell you that therapeutic modality use is patient driven, so electrotherapy equipment must be available. The technician approach of most physical therapists suggests that electrotherapy is often used inappropriately with little clinical reasoning to determine the best use of modalities or available equipment.

Physical therapy examination requires that one palpate the patient for signs of tissue abnormality. Islam prohibits physical touch between a male and female unless they are closely related (Ahmed 1988). In other Arab countries the prohibition on opposite sex therapist/patient physical contact is total (Roberts-Warrior 1995) but within Palestine only 18% of therapists prefer not to treat opposite sex patients. Western influences, especially among Christian Palestinians, tend to engender more liberal practices in patient/therapist relationships. Still many clinics have separate sections for male and female patients, each staffed by same-sex therapists.

Two-thirds of the sample recognized that there were differences between the practice of physical therapy in Palestine and other countries. Major differences itemized were available resources, public knowledge about physical therapy and preferred treatment modalities; 37% believed that the present political situation and Arabic culture limited the scope of practice in Palestine; and 33% attributed differences to Palestinian society's lack of knowledge of what physical therapists can offer, particularly in the field of neurological rehabilitation. Others felt that limitations on practice came from poor-quality education and clinical training.

Identification of the role of the physical therapist within the health care team is only now being discussed by health care planners. Almost half of the sample felt that deciding the treatment plan for individual patients was always the responsibility of the therapist 'because they are trained to do this.' Members of the profession are able to defend their own rights as independent practitioners, but not willing to share their skills with non-professionals.

Therapists' perceptions of other team members' knowledge of physical therapy is good. Most respondents thought doctors, nurses and social workers were quite well informed about physical therapy. While this attitude may reflect progress over the last 10 years, and, perhaps, cultural politeness, it does not support reality when compared with standards in Europe (Al Khdour & Maas 1995).

Perceptions of their own health education role and participation in teaching skills to PWD and their caretakers were less certain. Half (50%) of the respondents felt they had a role as health educator and 64% were concerned about sharing their skills effectively. The major topic for health education was back care (42%) and the most popular teaching topic was therapeutic exercise.

Public health education materials in Arabic have been developed by doctors and nurses on such topics as breast feeding, contraception, smoking and diet. One hospital in East Jerusalem has recently produced materials with written instructions and drawings to demonstrate exercises to be done at home by patients after laminectomy and joint replacement surgery. The sample showed that 39% had prepared patient materials for home exercise programs.

Continuing education for health care personnel has only recently been initiated as previously it was considered that a practitioner had the necessary knowledge, skills and attitudes at graduation for a lifetime of professional practice (SAAR 1993). Upgrading professionals to meet today's needs is only necessary when perceptions of those needs change. The presence of many international staff and the intervention of foreign non-governmental organizations during the *Intifada* are among the factors changing patient and staff perceptions. Prior to 1989 most continuing education (CE) in the profession was provided by foreign physical therapists who perhaps knew more about their own needs for CE than those of Palestinian physical therapists. Local physical therapists relied on outside support partly because it was offered, because of limited opportunities to go abroad and as a result of the dependency engendered by years of occupation.

Within the scope of the physical therapy program at BU, a CE committee was set up in 1992, funded by the European Union, to provide CE for the physical therapists of the West Bank and Gaza Strip. Because of traveling difficulties two committees developed, each of which was responsible for CE in its area: they planned, implemented and evaluated CE programs between 1992 and 1996. Over half of the sample had attended CE, 14% had been involved in the organization of CE and 11% had taught in CE courses. Major responsibility for learning was assumed by 69% of the respondents, while 33% gave the major responsibility to their teachers. The concepts of student-centered learning and life-long learning are not considered in primary and secondary education in Palestine, and even some college and university teachers find them strange ideas.

PERSONALITY

Personality profiles are available for professional groups in different countries (O'Neill 1976, Rovezzi-Carroll & Leavitt 1984, Wagstaff 1987) and can help to understand characteristic

behavior of successful practitioners. Certain aspects of a physical therapist's character may be considered universal because of the humanistic nature of the job and the caring and helping characteristics of the basic tasks involved. The influence of international networks and organizations, overseas scholarships and fellowships bring a global context to the profession but other qualities considered necessary for the practice of physical therapy are culturally based and differ between countries. If these qualities can be highlighted it may help therapists moving from their own to another culture for study or work opportunities to overcome the problems associated with culture shock and ethnocentrism.

In this study an inferential theory of personality is assumed in which there are universal traits that are shared, to a lesser or greater extent, by all human beings. Each trait is considered to have a bi-polar quality with all respondents displaying tendencies somewhere along a continuum. Characteristics inferred from an individual's self-report answers in a questionnaire are seen as indications of the person's underlying personality. The Cattell 16PF questionnaire reduces personality data to 16 personality factors.

Questionnaire B of the 16PF was used for Irish respondents and was translated into Arabic for use with the Palestinian sample. Table 30.3 shows a summary of the personality profiles of the two groups. Sten score tables assume that the raw score mean of the population will be between 4.5 and 5.5. Scores above or below this band indicate group differences.

Different scores were found for a number of factors. Palestinian physical therapists exhibit warmth (A+), lack emotional stability (C–), are bold (H+), suspicious (L+) and shrewd (N+) and show self discipline (Q3+). Irish physiotherapists show a profile of high intelligence (B+), emotional stability (C+), sensitivity (I+), radicalism (Q1+), and self-discipline (Q3+).

The two groups share high scores for self-discipline. Self-discipline is seen in terms of personal aspirations and the ability to work in conditions in which it seems difficult to main-

Table 30.3   Cattell 16PF results for Palestinian and Irish physical therapists

Factor	Dimension	Palestinians	Irish	Difference	Significance
A	Warmth	5.7	4.5	High	0.0001
B	Intelligence	5.2	6.7	Low	0.0001
C	Emotional stability	4.2	5.9	Low	0.0001
E	Dominance	5.6	4.7	High	0.002
F	Impulsivity	5.5	5.7	–	NS
G	Conformity	4.9	5.6	Low	0.009
H	Boldness	6.5	5.8	High	0.0001
I	Sensitivity	4.5	6.2	Low	0.0001
L	Suspicion	6.0	5.2	High	0.005
M	Imagination	5.6	5.2	–	NS
N	Shrewdness	6.9	5.4	High	0.0001
O	Insecurity	5.7	5.3	–	NS
Q1	Radicalism	5.7	6.2	–	NS
Q2	Self-sufficiency	4.8	5.1	–	NS
Q3	Self-discipline	6.7	6.5	–	NS
Q4	Tension	5.4	5.3	–	NS

 ain good standards. Is it the education of physical therapists that produces people who are self-disciplined, does the working environment influence the development of this trait or are those who pursue physical therapy self-disciplined by nature? Physical therapy students complain that they have to work much harder, assimilate more information and attend more classes than the average student. The ability to assist patients and clients solve individual problems requires clear, logical thinking and skills concerned with sifting through data to arrive at appropriate objectives and to evaluate the efficacy of treatment interventions. Such processes are made easier by self-discipline. Palestinian diplomate physical therapists who complete the 'Top up' program at BU after a gap of many years between their initial diploma and upgrading to a degree, deserve respect as they manage to juggle job and family and study in a culture where part-time study is not common and mature people do not admit to needing further training.

The Irish group shows higher intelligence than Palestinians. Higher intelligence is to be expected in groups who have participated in higher education. Palestinians have been described as among the most intelligent people in the world (Glubb 1969, Findlay 1994) and yet their 16PF profile shows average intelligence. Some writers have suggested that perceptions and demonstrations of intelligence are culturally determined (Karson & O'Dell 1976, Cattell 1989). Questions translated from English to Arabic may express sentiments that are unimportant in the Middle East.

The Irish group shows greater emotional stability than Palestinians. Emotional stability is a necessary trait for a group that deals with the physical and psychological problems of individuals with impairment, disability and handicap. Physical therapists need empathy while being able to keep their own emotional needs from interfering with their ability to help. This quality is perceived as a prerequisite in Western society for dealing with other people but not in the Middle East. Emotionalism is a valued quality for those who say they want to help people in Palestinian society, particularly since the *Intifada* (Lockman & Beinin 1990). It is seen as a sign of patriotism to show emotion toward the young people injured during this time who are regarded as heroic freedom fighters. The political situation itself contributes to the lack of emotional stability of a group of people who have, until recently, had little control over their own destiny (Di Giovanni 1993, FAFO 1993). Lack of emotional stability may mean that not all patients are given equal attention. Those who engage one's sympathies most and improve quicker are likely to receive better treatment than those whose problem is chronic and who cause too many problems. Physical therapists' emotional instability may be associated with feeling that their education was inadequate and is often expressed as defensiveness about their treatment standards (Bithell & Lumley 1987, Giacaman et al 1989).

Warmth (A+) is a phenomenon of Arabic society dating back to the desert life style of the Bedouin (Hourani et al 1993). Arabs cannot understand why Westerners do not invite visitors to their homes so readily. In the Middle East one of the first phrases one learns to understand is *ahlan wasahlan* meaning (welcome). You may have just met a person and they immediately invite you to their shop or home. Once inside, the minimum hospitality you will receive is a cup of tea or coffee. Palestinian friends tell me that the welcome is always genuine, although hosts do not expect you to visit each time you are invited. You may be invited to eat with a family by the husband without consulting his wife, in which case you sit and make polite conversation while the women and children of the family scurry around buying and cooking food (Qleibo 1992, Pryce-Jones 1990, Rantisi & Beebe 1990). Warmth has been described as both a local and international characteristic of physical therapists (O'Neill 1976, Dawson 1982, Wagstaff 1987). Physical therapists with human warmth find that patients confide in them and appreciate the chance to ask the questions they did not dare ask their doctor.

Boldness reflects the extended family life of Middle Eastern culture. In a society where extended families share living quarters, eat meals together and discuss everything of importance to any individual member, everyone is used to expressing their opinions. Foreigners living among Arabs will be asked very personal questions very early in the relationship. Locals will want to know if you are married, how old you are and how much money you earn. If you answer to the first question is yes, they will ask how many sons you have. If you answer no they will want to know why you are not married. Westerners, who may speak of personal or money matters with reluctance, initially find it difficult to parry such questions. The trait of boldness is stronger among males than females. From an early age girls are encouraged to be more submissive than boys, so as to have a good reputation in order to marry well (White 1992). Palestinian physical therapists show boldness in their willingness to challenge ideas and speak in public on any subject. Europeans might be embarrassed to speak if unprepared but Palestinians do not consider lack of preparation or poor speaking skills reasons for keeping silence (Pryce-Jones 1990).

Suspicion reflects the history of the Palestinian people. Their perceptions of promises made by the Western powers after the First and Second World Wars and in recent years, and inability to gain control of their own lives may have contributed to this factor. The increasing popularity of Islamic fundamentalism is a response to the perceived effects of Western materialism and permissiveness on young Muslims. Hamas (the militant Islamic group against the Olso Accords) began to encourage a return to the roots of Islam and is seen by many Palestinians as an alternative to progressive Westernization.

Physical therapists' suspiciousness is seen in their unwillingness to share ideas and resources with colleagues in case someone should claim their ideas. Arab society is hierarchical and everyone aims to be near the top of the pyramid. Knowledge brings power, which is not to be shared with others (Hamada 1990). A Palestinian physical therapist, especially a man, does not take kindly to criticism by others which makes it difficult for peer learning to take place.

Shrewdness is seen in the ability to keep negotiating when a Westerner would have given up. The shrewdness of Palestinians has been experienced by anyone who has tried to bargain with a shopkeeper in the *suk* in the Old City in Jerusalem. No transaction is simple very shopping expedition takes longer than anticipated. Bargaining is part of the fun of shopping in the Middle East, and if you do not bargain you deprive both yourself and the shopkeeper of an enjoyable aspect of business.

SELF-ESTEEM

Self and others' perceptions affect the way we behave. The persona we portray is influenced by our self-esteem and in turn affects how we deal with others. Self-esteem refers to 'the evaluation that the individual makes and customarily maintains with regard to himself' (Coopersmith 1967). Burns (1991) calls it the worth a person feels about himself 'respecting himself for what he is, not condemning himself for what he is not.'

The Taiser Self-Esteem Questionnaire (TSQ) was used to compare students in England and Saudi Arabia (Abdallah 1989). As it was shown to be reliable and valid for use with cross-cultural groups and was already translated into Arabic it was used to compare Irish and Palestinian physical therapists. The TSQ is a four-point Likert scale requiring responses ranging from strongly agree to strongly disagree. Questions are posed in both positive and negative fashions and refer to both self-attitudes and imputed attitudes of others to self. It was assumed that most respondents would answer positively to those questions couched in positive terms and negatively to those written in negative terms. Abdallah (1989) categorized responses under the heading of physical appearance, positive self-worth, negative self-image and trustworthiness. Table 30.4 summarizes the results.

Palestinian physical therapists showed similarities to their European colleagues in being self-satisfied and seeing themselves as honest, attractive, successful and reliable. They would say others saw them as confident, successful and likeable. It is difficult to see oneself as honest or reliable unless one were satisfied with oneself. This picture is one of positive self-worth. Is this a characteristic of physical thera-

pists? Physical therapists with a positive view of themselves and life in general will likely better motivate patients, clients and carers toward an optimistic view of their own or their relative's chances of good recovery from injury or coping with disability (Egan 1994, Dunkel Schatter et al 1992). If you do not believe in yourself and what you are doing, it is quickly noticed by those you try to help.

Positive self-worth is likely to influence practitioners' roles as confident professionals. Palestinian physical therapists are aware that their therapist role makes them special and brings added status in their community. Perceptions of self-worth can contribute to competence but there may be a mismatch between ideal and real self (Burns 1984). Fantasizing that the two aspects of self are congruent is a way of coping with deficiencies in practice (Coopersmith 1967, Hamada 1990). A Palestinian physical therapist is reluctant to admit to not knowing the answer to questions or problems posed by patients and wants to give the impression of knowing all the answers.

It is not an Arabic trait to be particularly introspective. Few Palestinians can view themselves without reference to their occupation or family connections. They find it difficult to describe themselves to someone else or analyze mistakes or weakness in their performance. In school someone else will determine your level. Who you are in the Arab world is determined by which family and clan you belong to. Children are the heart of the family and grow up believing that everything they do is good. That belief is constantly reinforced by their extended family members (Pryce-Jones 1990). If a teacher or employer finds fault with a student or employee, the individual being censured will blame it on someone else as he is not able to look at his own performance objectively (Abdallah 1989).

Palestinian physical therapists are keen to be judged competent and want to have skills and knowledge comparable with Western professionals. Particularly among the men, there is a great interest in electrotherapy and high-technology approaches to physical therapy. This

Table 3.4 TSQ results for Palestinian and Irish physical therapists

Attribute	Palestinian	Irish	Significance
Positive self-attitude	1.53	1.78	0.001
Feel valued by others	1.72	1.80	NS
Wish for more self respect	2.16	2.95	0.0001
Sometimes feel useless	2.96	2.62	0.003
Honest person	1.43	1.40	NS
Able to do things well	1.59	1.73	NS
Do not inspire confidence	3.60	3.62	NS
Not satisfied with self	3.35	3.34	NS
Worthwhile person	1.75	1.55	0.027
Would like to change	2.56	2.96	0.0001
Self-confident	1.51	1.95	0.0001
Mixed up	2.97	3.43	0.0001
Want to be someone else	3.31	3.48	NS
Low self-opinion	3.62	3.45	NS
Blame myself	2.47	2.68	NS
Attractive personality	2.02	2.04	NS
Worry what others think	2.96	2.57	0.001
Others see me as failure	3.18	3.16	NS
Take good care of myself	1.74	1.98	0.008
Feeling of well-being	1.84	1.87	NS
Satisfied with appearance	1.74	2.18	0.0001
Can't do things well	3.00	2.91	NS
Sensitive person	1.74	1.84	NS
I like myself	1.93	1.55	0.0001
I am happy	2.00	1.71	0.001
My friends trust me	1.66	1.57	NS
I feel a failure	3.42	3.43	NS
I can't trust people	2.62	2.53	NS
I am satisfied with friends	1.82	1.77	NS
Other people like me	1.94	1.91	NS
My family rely on me	1.58	1.32	0.001
I am a friendly person	1.73	1.55	0.032
I am satisfied with family	1.64	1.61	NS
I have good qualities	1.71	1.69	NS
I am a decent person	1.55	1.59	NS

may result from the Islamic prohibition on touching between the sexes, even in a therapeutic context. With machines it is possible to treat both sexes at a distance. The greater importance of theoretical knowledge and low emphasis on psychomotor skills in physical therapy education and practice affects therapists' perceptions of treatment modalities. Using one's hands is seen as a manual job. A person does not study

in higher education to use manual skills but to use his brain. Practicing a skill until one has reached an acknowledged level of performance is not clearly understood, and physical therapists are judged to be able to do something either because they read about it or saw someone demonstrate it.

The aspect in which Palestinians were more positive than the Irish group was that of satis-

action with personal appearance. Personal appearance is considered very important as Palestinians often judge others on first impressions. In the hospital or clinic physical therapists like to look like doctors and enjoy being mistaken for medical practitioners. Palestinian students will make a greater effort than their European peers to look smart and attractive in the university. Part of the reason may be that this is one of the few places where men and women can mix freely and single young people have to make the most of such opportunities. The dress code for university teachers is as formal as in the business world.

For a number of responses the Palestinians indicated a more negative self-image than the Irish group. Palestinians wished they had more self-respect, would like to change many things in their lives, feel mixed up and that they cannot trust others. It would not be surprising to find negative self-attitudes in a population who have been limited geographically and politically for so long. It may be hard to have self-respect when you feel that the world has forgotten you. Nor is it unusual to want to change when your life seems to be controlled by larger political circumstances. Having just achieved a measure of autonomy, yet finding that their aspirations were unrealistic and will take many years to achieve is a good reason for feeling mixed up. It is hard to trust people when among the promises made by numerous leaders and agencies over the years, few have come to fruition.

Negative self-image can stem from the Palestinians' transitional situation as a society. They cannot be truly described as part of the developing world because of their educational level, health patterns and social systems (Barghouthi & Daibes 1991). Neither are they yet part of the developed world, however much they may aspire to that situation. In an attempt to find a place in the world the Palestinians have substituted education for land (Cossali & Robson 1986). In the Middle East land is still the basis of personhood and evidence of wealth and status. Loss of land brings negative self-image through refugee status. For refugee families, education has become the vehicle for social

advancement, bringing better prospects for job, home and life partner.

Emphasis on status makes it difficult to encourage the concept of cooperation between therapist and patient in the rehabilitation process. In Palestinian society the therapist is still the expert and the patient has a more passive role. Recent adoption of the community based rehabilitation (CBR) model of health care delivery has not been received wholeheartedly by physical therapists, who see CBR workers as competitors for patients and lowering the standards of rehabilitation services (Coleridge 1994).

CONCLUSION

Considering the enormous upheavals experienced by Palestinians over the last 50 years it is amazing what they have achieved. Present day and future autonomy brings with it increasing opportunities to develop and change but also responsibilities that previously were not shouldered. It is helpful that many countries are assisting the Palestinians to build up their health infrastructure, but one drawback to the plethora of assistance can be confusion. Each group advocates its own approach to health problems and systems, but few are concerned to discover what is culturally appropriate (Deegan 1993).

Palestinian health personnel and planners need to develop their own model of health care and a unique vision of health in their country. This model is slowly emerging and the vision is becoming clearer. Palestinian physical therapists, in company with the rest of their health care colleagues, have the personal and professional characteristics to participate in that vision and make it come true. Boldness will give courage for new ideas, self-discipline will encourage perseverance, human warmth will foster policies which take into account the needs of PWD and positive self-worth will give one confidence in having the ability to solve problems. Professional development of physical therapy in Palestine over the last 25 years in terms of teamwork, continuing education and health education augurs well for development in the future.

REFERENCES

Abdallah T 1989 A cross-cultural study of self-esteem and locus of control. Doctoral thesis, University of York

Ahmed A S 1988 Discovering Islam: making sense of Muslim history and society. Routledge, London

Al Khdour Z, Maas L M 1995 Physiotherapy in obstetrics and gynaecology in Palestine. World Confederation of Physical Therapy, Washington, DC

Barghouthi M, Daibes I 1991 Infrastructure of health services in the West Bank and Gaza Strip for health care planning: the West Bank rural PHC survey. Health Development Information Project, Ramallah

Bithell C, Lumley C 1987 Physiotherapy in the West Bank and Gaza Strip: a discussion paper. British Council, Jerusalem

Burns R B 1984 The self concept: theory measurement and behavior. Longman, London

Burns R B 1991 The self concept: theory, measurement and behavior, 2nd edn. Longman, London

Cattell H B 1989 The 16PF: personality in depth. Institute for Personality and Ability Testing, Champaign, Illinois

Coleridge P 1994 Disability training in the community: a needs assessment: West Bank and Gaza Strip. Health Development Information Project, Ramallah, West Bank

Coopersmith S, cited in: Burns R B 1984 The self concept: theory, measurement and behavior. Longman, London

Cossali P, Robson C 1986 Stateless in Gaza. Zed Books, London

Dawson V L 1982 A personality profile of the physiotherapy student. Master's dissertation, University of Bradford

Dawson V L 1997 Cultural implications for physiotherapy education: the Bethlehem experience, Doctoral Thesis, Loughborough University of Technology

Deegan H 1993 The Middle East and problems of democracy. Open University Press, Milton Keynes, UK

Di Giovanni J 1993 Against the stranger: lives in occupied territory. Viking, London

Dunkel Schatter C, Blasband D E, Feinstein, L G, Herbert T B 1992 Elements of supportive interactions: when are attempts to help effective? In: Spacapan S, Oskamp S (eds) Helping and being helped: naturalistic studies. Sage Publications, London

Egan G 1994 The skilled helper: a systematic approach to effective helping, 5th edn. Brooks/Cole, Pacific Grove, California

FAFO 1993 Palestinian society in Gaza, West Bank and Arab Jerusalem: summary of a survey of living conditions. Center for International Studies, Oslo, Norway

Findlay A M 1994 The Arab world. Routledge, London

Gaza Health Services Research Center 1995 Health status of population: annual report Gaza Strip 1990–1994. Pales-tinian Health Council/Benevolent Society of the Gaza Stri

Giacaman R, Daibes I, Nammari R, Waller S C 1989 Toward the formulation of a rehabilitation policy: disability in th West Bank. Birzeit Community Health Departmen Ramallah

Glubb J B 1969 A short history of the Arab people. Hodde and Stoughton, London

Hamada L B 1990 Understanding the Arab world. Thoma Nelson, Nashville Tennessee

Hourani A, Khoury P S, Wilson M C 1993 The moder Middle East. I B Taurus, Jerusalem, Israel

Karson S, O'Dell J W 1976 A guide to the clinical use of th 16PF. Institute for Personality and Ability Testing Champaign, Illinois

Lockman Z, Beinin J (eds) 1990 Intifada: the Palestinia uprising against Isreali occupation. I B Taurus, London

O'Neill E 1976 An occupational profile of the physiothera pist. Master's dissertation, University of Bradford

Palestinian Health Council 1994 National health plan for th Palestine people, Palestine Health Council, Jerusalem

Pryce-Jones D 1990 The closed circle: an interpretation of th Arabs. Paladin, London

Qleibo A H 1992 Before the mountains disappear: an ethno graphic chronicle of the modern Palestinian. Al Ahran Press, Cairo, Egypt

Rantisi A G, Beebe R K 1990 Blessed are the peacemakers: Palestinian Christian in the Occupied West Bank Zondervan Books, Grand Rapids, Michigan

Roberts-Warrior D 1995 Cultural differences in therapy experiences in a Saudi Arabian hospital teaches one thera pist that therapy is more than physical. WCPT Daily News June 17, 1 and 4

Rovezzi-Carroll S, Leavitt R 1984 Personality characteristic and expressed career choice of graduating physical ther apy students. Physical Therapy 64(10): 1549–1552

SAAR 1993 Needs for training and continuing education ir health, engineering and agriculture in the Occupied Palestinian Territories. Society for Austro-Arab Relations Jerusalem

Swersky B, Kanaaneh H, Avgar A, Schonbrun M 1992 The Israeli equality monitor, issue number 2: health care ir Israel. Advar Center, Tel Aviv, Israel

Wagstaff P S 1987 A study of the personality, motivation and attitudes of finalist physiotherapy students in four mem ber states of the European Economic Community (the Republic of Ireland, the United Kingdom, the Netherlands and Greece). Physiotherapy 66(5): 691–696

White P 1992 Mourning in Bethlehem: the impact of the Gulf War on Palestinian society. Gracewing, Leominster, UK

The practice of cultural competence in the 21st century

The two chapters in Section 5, 'The Practice of Cultural Competence in the 21st Century', summarize the most salient points presented in the preceding sections and suggests specific ideas and approaches to facilitate cultural competence.

'Towards a public health perspective on rehabilitation', by Huib Cornielje, argues that rehabilitation professionals must work within the public health paradigm. This demands a consideration of the social and cultural determinants of health and ill-health and vigilance toward promoting health not only at the individual level but for the aggregate population as well. Public health implies a collective action toward health, in this case collective action by rehabilitation professionals.

Cornielje describes how public health practice and policies are both similar and different when comparing the developed and the less developed world, and how both the north and south have something to offer each other. He argues that given the primary health care perspective that has been galvanized by the World Health Organization (WHO), rehabilitation, in all countries, no matter their level of socioeconomic development, should embody key elements of a public health philosophy. That is, 'rehabilitation must be integrated into a multidisciplinary process in which participation and empowerment are at the core of an endeavor towards equity and full integration of the person with a disability (PWD) in the community'.

Cornielje calls for rehabilitationists to fully understand that 'therapy' alone is not the equivalent of rehabilitation. In fact that concept is confining. Instead, he urges therapists to be proactive and recognize, for example, that mobilizing PWD to become active in the disability rights movement or working in health promotion and disability prevention, might have a far greater impact on the life of the PWD. Like Neufeldt (Ch. 3), Cornielje suggests that both the PWD and rehabilitation professional work collaboratively and become open to change. They both must become aware of the social, political, and cultural aspects of rehabilitation, i.e. components stressed by public health professionals.

'Moving rehabilitation professionals toward cultural competence: strategies for change' provides practical approaches to encourage the development of a culturally competent professional through changes in the educational curricula and professional practice patterns. Ronnie Leavitt reiterates that each individual in a professional–consumer interaction is a unique 'cultural entity' with his or her own worldview and that we are still seeking theories and models for training that will prepare the professional to serve a culturally diverse society. Nevertheless, a set of core curriculum guidelines on culturally sensitive and competent health care is recommended. Leavitt also proposes that there needs to be greater focus on the development of culturally valid standardized screening instruments and culture-specific functional outcome measures.

The final chapter in *Cross-cultural Rehabilitation* recognizes that not all rehabilitation professionals are suited to work cross-culturally. For those who do decide to embark on this professional path, Leavitt offers suggestions to help prepare for immersion in a cross-cultural setting. Self-reflection, advance preparation, and realistic expectations are key. Professionals are told to expect culture shock, an occupational hazard of cross-cultural immersion. In spite of that, Leavitt proposes that the frustrations and challenges associated with a cross-cultural encounter are likely to be outweighed by the rewards of personal growth and development, the knowledge that PWD have benefited from your expertise, and the gratitude you receive from the people you work with.

Lastly, Leavitt summarizes some of the lessons to be learned from *Cross-cultural Rehabilitation: An International Perspective*. Prominent is the theme that all human experiences, including the experience of disability, are grounded in culture. By defining the culture of disability and rehabilitation for specific sub-cultures, the authors contribute to the understanding of the culture-specific explanatory models of PWD, supporting the notion of inter-cultural and intra-cultural diversity.

The development of an ideal model by which to provide rehabilitation has remained elusive, but clearly any such model must be culture-specific and not merely attentive to biomedical intervention. Leavitt suggests that rehabilitation be part of a broader commitment to community development and that rehabilitationists adjust to a paradigm shift whereby they become co-participants or partners with PWD in the rehabilitation effort. Leavitt closes by challenging the rehabilitation professional to embrace diversity and difference, reshape practice protocols, redefine research priorities, and develop the most appropriate service models and public policy to benefit PWD.

31

Towards a public health perspective on rehabilitation

Huib Cornielje

INTRODUCTION

Public health is the science and art of preventing disease, prolonging life and promoting mental and physical health through organized community efforts (WHO 1961). Public health, by definition, aims to promote people's health at an aggregate level, through collective efforts to combat or remove factors that threaten the health of a population. The emphasis is on community or collective efforts and responsibilities and not on the health interests of individuals. In such a paradigm, health professionals need to continually consider the social and cultural determinants of health and ill-health as vital factors which can to a large extent influence rehabilitation processes. Even more explicitly, rehabilitation professionals should be aware of different culturally determined attitudes and behavior towards health, ill-health and healing processes and be competent to deal both at an individual and at an aggregate level with those differences.

Public health in so-called developed countries is largely shaped by financial, economic, cultural and political factors (McKeown 1979). For example: 'Targeted child health programs can substantially reduce mortality, but long-term reduction in mortality will require continuing social change, increased economic security and political commitment to health and welfare in the context of a relatively stable political environment' (Ewbank 1993).

The practice of public health in Western countries is largely a matter of public policy since there are often excellent social health insurance systems and such basic services as clean water and sanitation. Presently there is an emphasis on preventive, promotive and protective tasks in a collective perspective.

Recently there has been a global, so-called 'new public health' movement which on one hand focuses on the 'old' 19th-century issues such as sewerage, water purification systems, improvement of housing and working conditions, but on the other hand pays attention to community based and oriented health care with a great emphasis on health-related behavior and lifestyle.

The declaration of Alma Ata (WHO 1978) and the 'Health for All' strategy of the World Health Organization (WHO) (WHO 1982) make clear that with all the similarities and differences that exist at national and regional levels, public health issues should be viewed in an international perspective. The backbone of public health is to a large extent formed by social reform with the ultimate goal of improving the health of the population.

Primary health care (PHC) was introduced by the member states of the WHO in the late 1970s as a response to – and assumed cheap solution for – the inadequate health care systems worldwide. In order to achieve health for all, community based care systems needed to be developed with an adequate distribution of resources devoted to services relevant to the needs of the individual, the family and the community at large. Furthermore, central to improving health is the idea that people should take greater responsibility for their health. Community participation and involvement in making decisions regarding health became one of the key elements of PHC. Care for and rehabilitation of people with disabilities (PWDs), elderly people and people with chronic diseases was recognized as being a part of a comprehensive PHC strategy. However, PHC programs were often confined to vertical programs focusing on either priority groups such as mothers and children or specific interventions such as polio eradication. Subsequently, rehabilitation of PWDs became largely ignored within PHC. The introduction of community based rehabilitation (CBR) was a logical development which concurrently took place with the formation of the worldwide disability rights movement. Rehabilitation and disability issues became part of the political agenda of national states and international bodies such as WHO and UNICEF.

In this chapter comparisons will be made between the public health developments in countries of the north and those of the south. The geographical meaning of 'north' and 'south' is but one of many contrasts. These contrasts will be used to search for similarities and differences to provide evidence that rehabilitation, both in the north and in the south, should embody key elements of a public health philosophy. Most notable is the philosophy that rehabilitation must be integrated into a multidisciplinary process in which participation and empowerment are at the core of an endeavor towards equity and full integration of the PWD in the community. These lessons will be directed both to developed and less developed countries.

Historically, the north (the developed countries) has been prescribing what would be good for the south (the less developed countries). Development principles such as community participation, which is regarded as a pillar of primary health care, far too often evolve into forms of manipulation; empowerment is often embodied in charity at best, and in oppression at worst; a search for equitable services often results only in a maintenance of the *status quo* of inequality and partiality.

TOWARDS A PUBLIC HEALTH PERSPECTIVE ON REHABILITATION

Rehabilitation disciplines need to take stock of how new insights into the role of public health and predicted changes in demography, epidemiology and health care policy influence their present and future role in the health care system.

The conventional role of rehabilitation professionals is reactive. This is in contrast with the pro-active efforts of public health. For rehabilitation to be required, there is an underlying assumption that there is an impairment, disability or handicap resulting from an illness, injury or congenital malformation. Rehabilitation is focused on individual needs depending on the level of impairment and/or disability and is usually given only in response to specific needs. Therefore, rehabilitation is primarily individually oriented and hence seems of little importance to public health. However, reviewing rehabilitation practice in both the north and the south, one can identify a number of exciting developments in the sphere of rehabilitation that are potentially of great importance for the public health sector.

Lessons from the south

Having had the privilege of working for 10 years in South Africa as a physical therapist in a number of rural and urban CBR programs, my position changed with regard to the significance of physical therapy in the lives of PWDs. One of the great lessons was that a restricted view of rehabilitation, focused only on the physical aspects of therapy, severely hampers any long-lasting effect of therapies given. A professional, Western, biomedical, scientific approach, which tends to narrow rehabilitation to therapeutic interventions, becomes an obstacle in the delivery of appropriate and effective rehabilitation services. Only after becoming frustrated by the confinements of the therapy room and visiting the health ward, the villages, the homesteads and the places where PWDs live, did an awareness emerge that therapy is not equivalent to rehabilitation.

Rehabilitation is a far more comprehensive philosophy. For instance, the concept of adapting the environment to the needs and demands of PWDs by means of improving the accessibility of a hut, or mobilizing PWDs to become active in disability rights movements must be included in an overall plan and not be neglected by professionals. In fact, these activities may make the greatest impact! Rehabilitation being confined to therapy: how often do professionals fall into this trap? Therapists continually work on training mothers in inhibition and facilitation techniques for children with cerebral palsy. Simultaneously it is forgotten that the very same mothers have five other children at home to take care of, have to collect water 3 km from home, have to work in the fields, may be in the role of both mother and father, and often are just trying to survive.

This awareness of a limited view of rehabilitation led to a process of transformation; not only do PWDs need rehabilitation, but professionals have to adjust and change to become aware of the social, political and cultural aspects of rehabilitation. Rehabilitation becomes a mutual developmental process in which both the PWDs and rehabilitation professional become open to change.

CBR was introduced at the beginning of the 1980s and was seen as the solution to problems of PWDs in the south. The WHO, governments and other international donor organizations recognized and realized that conventional Western rehabilitation had little to offer to the thousands of PWDs in the south. CBR was presented as the best solution for the many and complex difficulties of PWDs. CBR would improve the accessibility to rehabilitation and it was thought to be the best method to reach as many people as possible at the least possible price (Helander 1984).

Worldwide, several CBR models were initiated and developed. Some of these programs concentrate solely on the delivery of outreach services (Guillen 1995) and home based therapy (Loveday 1990) and therefore are primarily focused on individual therapeutic intervention, often following Western models of therapy. In contrast, there are developmental models (Philpott 1993) and sociopolitical programs focusing on empowerment, in which terminology such as 'liberation of the oppressed' and 'the struggle for disability rights' are practically demonstrated in the formation of disability self-help groups and disability rights movements (Cornielje 1993). In the latter context, CBR would develop into a program of empowerment with a focus on social integration and equal opportunities for PWDs. With rehabilitation recognized as an integral part of a broader community development approach, CBR is thus in sharp contrast to the medically oriented approach of conventional rehabilitation programs (Cornielje 1992).

Even those models that seem to be reduced to therapy at home or outreach services only, have potentially, something to offer to the north. The home based and outreach programs show many similarities with existing outreach programs in the north. As a physical therapist working in the early 1980s in a wealthy village in the Netherlands, very young people, people with severe disabilities, and elderly people were visited at their homes. Some would consider this CBR, but was it? Certainly, it was a means of improving accessibility of care, but was it part of an intentional philosophy and system advocating for the equalization of opportunities? How great were the concerns with, for instance, the social consequences of disability? Within the 20–30 minutes of treatment there was not much opportunity to give sufficient attention to the psychological status of clients, let alone pay attention to physical, social and cultural barriers.

Further, even if such interventions are affordable to the north, do such services need to be offered to large numbers of people by highly paid professionals? Long term institutional care is considered to be very expensive, but not enough evidence exists to prove that individual based home care (provided by professional therapists in the north and in the south by different categories of community rehabilitation workers) is more efficient *per se*. A growing awareness certainly exists that cost-effectiveness is fundamental to the furtherance of home based therapy (van Woerden & van Wiggen 1996).

While not yet enough evidence exists from the north with regard to the efficiency of home care, the situation in the south differs dramatically. For instance, the vast distances in rural areas, inadequate transport systems, poor infrastructure, absent referral systems and unsatisfactory working habits combined with insufficient supervision and support systems are serious hindrances in the management of efficient home based programs.

Recently a number of evaluation studies of pilot non-professional, primarily home based CBR programs in South Africa have been carried out (Cornielje et al 1995). These studies show that home based therapy is expensive, even if auxiliaries are involved. Therefore, home based CBR cannot unconditionally be considered the best model for a national rehabilitation paradigm. In the south, minimal budgets for rehabilitation, the absence of consumer movements and a lack of professionalized rehabilitation systems require, by definition, a public health approach.

Besides the individually oriented home based programs, one can increasingly observe efforts in the direction of more comprehensive CBR-like programs in the north. Diminishing national health budgets in the north seem to have provided an impetus to critically evaluate the effectiveness of numerous therapeutic interventions (Haas M 1993, van Woerden & van Wiggen 1996).

Lessons from the north

In some northern countries, developments can be observed for a more pronounced role of the therapeutic professions in the direction of public health (Ritchie 1989). In Europe, therapists have traditionally rendered a number of public health services such as teaching elementary physical education in school health services and providing pre- and postnatal exercise programs. The more recent involvement of physical therapists in health promotion and prevention activities in such fields as cardiac rehabilitation and support groups of patients with chronic diseases (such as ankylosing spondylitis) is new.

Original Scandinavian techniques such as massage and medical gymnastics were seen as preventive measures to avoid secondary complications of the disease and injury processes, reducing recovery time, improving the quality of the end result and helping patients back to normality (Hayne 1994).

Physical and occupational therapists have shown considerable interest in the development of their disciplines as part of occupational health services in the past decade. For quite some time, therapists have acted as trainers in the area of lifting and handling, and have recently assumed the roles of adviser, trainer and assessor. Within the occupational health services, trained professionals now provide health education and implementation of preventive measures based on ergonomic principles (Nagy 1994). However, preventive measures are still most commonly adopted only as a response when something has gone wrong.

Most recent developments in the Netherlands are focused on the area of fitness. Increasing numbers of Dutch people in all age groups dislike the culture of sport schools and fitness clubs and prefer to exercise under the guidance and supervision of a physical therapist. Potential target groups of the latest 'PhysioSport' and 'Pre-Sport' movement are: healthy persons, people with latent health problems, chronically ill people, the elderly, and employees in the context of occupational health (Visser 1995). One very recent development in this field is an initiative of the Netherlands Society of Psychosocial Therapy which launched a program for schools in Amsterdam called *de Klas Beweegt*, meaning 'the classroom moves'. This program is aimed at young students and tries to stimulate a consciousness among pupils about safe and healthy lifestyles, to create a basis for a more self-assured society, and to promote a better coping mechanism for youngsters in a society in which they will be confronted with stress. This is achieved through training sessions in the classrooms (training in maintaining and/or improving good posture, movement and relaxation (Geul-Klaren & In't Veld 1996).

Occupational therapists, particularly in the Scandinavian countries and the UK, have also shown an interest in preventive activities at the workplace. Their role in research in occupational health, for example, is well recognized. Occupational therapists in Portugal, under the auspices of a program funded by the WHO, are involved in preventive activities in mental health care and care for the elderly (H van Bruggen, personal communication, 1995).

The public health role of the occupational therapist in the Netherlands is not very impres-

sive in terms of the number of professionals involved. However, interesting experiments are taking place. For instance, the housing department of Amsterdam employs a number of occupational therapists who advise on housing policy. This advisory function should not be underestimated in terms of its public health impact. The primary focus is on individual advice regarding needs for appropriate aids, appliances and adaptations for people with chronic illnesses and disabilities. However, research provides evidence that the more successful municipal health services (in terms of administering this law) employ occupational therapists as case managers who have been placed in such positions so that they will be able to influence policy-making (Brancerapport Paramedische Zog 1996).

Recently, occupational therapists in the Netherlands have been granted increased opportunities to work in the primary care setting. As a result, they will be able to direct their work towards community based activities and expand their home based rehabilitation activities. Experiences in the primary care setting demonstrate that the 'products' of occupational therapy in the home setting surpass the conventional individual orientation of interventions (van Woerden & van Wiggen 1996). A more public health role becomes evident: that is, promotion and training activities at group levels. Examples of such public health interventions are conducting courses in 'Back Care', 'Care of the Chronic Sick at Home' and the 'Elderly and Health' program, which have been initiated by the Amsterdam White Cross Association in alliance with the Amsterdam Rehabilitation Center.

The practical role of rehabilitation professionals in public health is well accepted. However, their contribution towards a role in the area of policy development and management of the provision, control and supervision of care and rehabilitation is limited. Furthermore, the areas of epidemiological research, health promotion and education, and prevention do not receive adequate attention during basic training and professional practice. Therapists may argue that they spend enough time and effort in these areas of health care delivery. However, the type and quality of health promotion and prevention activities given is often insufficient, often on an *ad hoc* basis, and focused on secondary and tertiary prevention only.

Not all described public health interventions would be of equal importance in all contexts. Some are certainly of no interest – at the moment – for many countries in the south. However, larger gains in the quality of life of people living in the north and in the south could be achieved through some concerted and focused intervention efforts. Notwithstanding the degree of development of a country, a reorientation of rehabilitation policies and practices is needed towards reaching all in need, instead of focusing on expensive, specialist therapy for the very few who can afford highly technological care. This subsequently requires a change of attitude among all rehabilitation professionals, health planners and the public at large.

Quality of life: the great public health challenge for both the south and the north

For a long time the focus of public health interventions has been on the eradication and reduction of disease and death. Such a focus was to a large extent related to the existing philosophies regarding health and ill-health. Health was previously regarded as merely the absence of disease. With the change in the definition of health to include physical, social, and mental well-being, it has become apparent that it is not feasible to realize a state of absence of disease. The observed transition from acute infectious diseases towards more chronic diseases supports the more recent definition of health. The current emphasis of health interventions is on improving the quality of life and achieving an optimum well-being, rather than, as in the past, simply adding years to life.

This is certainly true for the north where the epidemiological transition resulting in increased survival into older ages has resulted in a greater concern for the provision of therapeutic and rehabilitative services. However, the delayed demographic transition in many countries in the south, where the necessary cultural changes with regard to fertility control do not occur automatically with development, will also mean an acceleration of the growth of the elderly population. Subsequently a rise of 'degenerative' and 'human-made' diseases and disabilities can be predicted. This will require an expansion of rehabilitation interventions (Hermans 1995). More severe disabilities will also result in an increase in handicaps and place a greater burden on society. A UK-based survey of older people living at home showed that disability affecting activities of daily living was a greater influence on perceptions of health than the presence of an active disease or condition (Partridge et al 1991).

This notion pleads for an approach that focuses on ecological, social and cultural variables. Within such a conceptual model interventions should not only be purely medical or therapeutic and individually oriented but also directed at the prevention of handicaps and action at the community level. Added to the commonly recognized determinants of the disease process should be those that particularly influence the disablement process which in turn leads to handicaps. These determinants are formed by the ecological, social and cultural obstacles such as physical barriers, lack of legislation with regard to the rights of PWDs and prevailing attitudes. The disablement process in such a paradigm is not seen as simply an individual problem.

Historically, it has been the rehabilitation disciplines that have played an important but insufficiently recognized role towards improving the quality of life of people with chronic diseases, subsequent disabilities and handicaps. Whereas a number of these interventions are palliative in character, a substantial number of measures/therapies focus on the enhancement of function and minimizing of disabilities. Further research should be focused on the effects of therapeutic interventions and the future role of rehabilitation disciplines in a public health paradigm, in order to meet the needs of the growing population.

The development of a public health paradigm

Since the 1980s, a worldwide emancipation movement of PWDs is increasingly challenging the effects of national and global rehabilitation policies. This movement, in the north known as the Independent Living Movement, and in the south emerging as the CBR movement, has exposed and will continue to expose the shortcomings of professionalized and elaborated systems of rehabilitation. Supposed beneficiaries who continue to be deprived of sufficient health, welfare and rehabilitation services will rightfully question the justification of rehabilitation policies and programs. Besides, inequalities in health and welfare standards continue. An escalation of inequality in health can be expected in view of the changing demography, restraints in social security systems and changes in the financing of health care. Particularly vulnerable groups, such as elderly people, people with chronic diseases, and PWDs will be confronted with the consequences of neo-liberal policies.

The current, more topical PHC elements (such as accountability, decentralization, efficiency, sustainability and quality assurance) specific to Western ways of thinking seem to be a logical result of changing political tides worldwide and rising global neo-liberalistic trends. Consequently, there is a risk that the needs of those who are caught in a culture of poverty will not be addressed appropriately, since it is usually far more uncomplicated and efficient to invest in the middle class. Besides, there is the risk that these trends will stimulate a further move into a cult of the healthy, the young, and the financially successful and independent citizen.

While these developments will continue within the 21st century, the intrinsic, but increasingly neglected values of the original PHC philosophy (such as equity, democracy, justice and solidarity) will provide solutions to the needs of the world's population. The dialogue within the disability movement, both at the national and international level, reflects the concerns of PWDs with regard to the emerging setbacks in the area of equalization of opportunities.

Historically, the role of rehabilitation disciplines in the area of public health has been marginal. However, an appropriate combination of the 'old' PHC ideology in which therapists ensure that mechanisms will be put in place to advocate and work for equalization of opportunities, and attention to 'modern' PHC topics could form the cornerstone of a developing rehabilitation policy in a universal public health perspective. Innovative thinking is required to guarantee the well-being of all, both in the north and in the south. Critical to an expansion of the public health role of rehabilitation disciplines is:

1. A more pro-active approach focusing on education of patients/clients, promotion of healthy lifestyles and prevention of handicaps. A group-oriented approach will not only be cost-effective, but vitally important to the effectiveness of interventions for a variety of chronic conditions since the motivation of patients will be raised significantly in comparison to individual interventions (Hidding 1993; Schaardenburg 1994; Taal 1995).

2. A shift of focus from an individual's normalization of function towards a more social approach of rehabilitation in which the ultimate goal is the integration of the PWDS into society and in which there is an equalization of opportunities.

3. A change from being the manager of the person with a chronic disease or disability to that of being a resource, thus enabling the client to better cope in reaching his own goals (Coleridge 1993).

4. Stronger political representation of the rehabilitation professions via patient lobby groups and disability rights movements. However, there is a risk that such collaborative initiatives will result in too strong a power-base for the professional bodies. Joint provider-consumer bodies could, as long as consumers have at least an equal stake in such a body, form powerful alliances in advocating for development of accessible, affordable and equal rehabilitation to all.

5. Health promotion and education in general but also more specifically geared towards, for instance, the areas of geriatrics and mental health.

6. An expansion of the consultancy role of rehabilitation disciplines in occupational and geriatric health.

7. An increased involvement of rehabilitation professionals in community based care. In the north this might be achieved through home care organizations. These organizations lack specific knowledge, for example, in the field of giving advice regarding assistive devices. Rehabilitation professionals could become consultants and trainers for such organizations. In the south the CBR model should be further promoted and developed.

The majority of PWDs in both the south and to a lesser extent in the north still do not have access to appropriate rehabilitation services. The dramatic demographic changes worldwide and limited health budgets require action from politicians, health planners, consumer groups and, last but not least, rehabilitation professionals. The response of rehabilitation professionals seems evident: develop a system of care which can provide solutions to the demands and the socially and culturally acceptable values and norms of rapidly increasing numbers of PWDs.

Rehabilitation professionals will find themselves increasingly working in a rapidly changing environment. This will require a consciousness among rehabilitation professionals concerning their own limitations in terms of cultural norms and values. It also requires a sensitivity towards other (indigenous) paradigms regarding health, illness, disability and rehabilitation.

Under these circumstances, rehabilitation systems are required which primarily focus on both the delivery of a package of essential rehabilitation and on culturally appropriate interventions. As much as the aggregate (public health) level of rehabilitation policy should come to the fore, the cultural relevance of interventions needs to be expressed in the execution of rehabilitation programs.

REFERENCES

Brancherapport Paramedische Zorg 1996 Netherlands Institute for Research in Primary Health Care (NIVEL), Utrecht, the Netherlands

Coleridge P 1993 Disability, liberation and development. Oxfam, Oxford, pp. 73–79

Cornielje H 1992 Transforming physiotherapy training: some thoughts. PhysioForum 7:15

Cornielje H 1993 A local disability movement as part of a CBR programme. In: Finkenflügel H (ed) The handicapped community. VU University Press, Amsterdam, pp.17–21

Cornielje H, Ferrinho P, Fernando A 1995 An evaluation of the CBR training programme of the Institute of Urban Primary Health Care, Alexandra, South Africa. Internal Report

Ewbank D C 1993 Impact of health programs on child mortality in Africa: evidence from Zaire and Liberia. International Journal of Epidemiology 22 (Suppl.1): 64–72

Geul-Klaren T, In't Veld H 1996 Oefentherapie centraal in de psychosomatische fysiotherapie. FysioPraxis 6: 9

Guillen C 1995 Rehabilitacion integral en la communidad. Proyecto RIC, Intern Document Cochabamha, Bolivia

Haas M 1993 Evaluation of physiotherapy using cost-utility analysis. Australian Journal of Physiotherapy 39(3): 211–216

Hayne C R 1994 From prevention into risk management. Physiotherapy 35(2): 101–107

Helander E 1984 Rehabilitation for all: a guide to the management of rehabilitation in developing countries. RHB/84.1. WHO, Geneva

Hermans J 1995 Veel aandacht voor thuiszorg in Europees Jaar van de Ouderen. FysioPraxis 5: 2–3

Hidding A 1993 Group physical therapy in ankylosing spondylitis. Dissertation. Krips Repro, Meppel

Loveday M 1990 Is CBR a second rate service? In: Finkenflügel H (ed) The handicapped community. VU University Press, Amsterdam, pp. 95–98

McKeown T H 1979 The role of medicine: dream, miracle or nemesis? Blackwell, Oxford

Nagy J A 1994 Bedrijfsfysiotherapie: een nieuwe wending aan preventie. FysioPraxis 13: 16–18

Partridge C J, Johnstone M, Morris L 1991 Disability and health services: perceptions, beliefs and experiences of elderly people. Centre for Physiotherapy Research, King's College, London

Philpott S 1993 Disability as a developmental issue – the challenge for occupational therapists. Bi-annual Congress of the South African Association of Occupational Therapists, Pretoria, South Africa

Ritchie J E 1989 Keeping Australians healthy: the challenge to physiotherapy practice posed by the concept of the new public health. Australian Journal of Physiotherapy 35(2): 101–107

Schaardenburg D van 1994 Arthritis in the elderly with emphasis on rheumatoid arthritis. Dissertation Rijksuniversiteit Leiden, Leiden

Taal E 1995 Self-efficacy, self-management and patient edu-

cation in rheumatoid arthritis. Dissertation, Eburon, Delft

Visser P 1995 FysioSport: een nieuwe ontwikkeling. FysioPraxis 12: 4–7

van Woerden H M, van Wiggen C W M 1996 'Ergotherapie aan huis' vanuit het Verpleeghuis. Nederlands Tijdschrift voor Ergotherapie 24: 16–23

World Health Organization 1961 WHO draft policy document of the Netherlands School for Public Health of 1994. WHO, Geneva

World Health Organization 1978 Health for All Series, No. 1. Declaration of Alma-Ata, Primary health Care. WHO, Geneva

World Health Organization 1982 Health for All Series, No. 7. Plan of action for implementing the global strategy for Health for All and index to the 'Health for All' series. WHO, Geneva

32

Moving rehabilitation professionals toward cultural competence: strategies for change

Ronnie Leavitt

INTRODUCTION

As a new millennium begins, the recognition of the necessity of cross-cultural competence is expected to grow. Cultural competence depends upon continuing self-assessment regarding culture, acceptance and respect for difference, vigilance toward the dynamics of differences, ongoing expansion of cultural knowledge and resources, and adaptation of services to meet the needs of a particular group. Historically, the available models for the provision of care have generally relied on the values and belief systems of the 'majority' – i.e. the white, middle-class person living in an industrialized, Western nation. These models have been culturally insensitive by denying the realities of non-Western systems of thinking. Today, however, although it is recognized that biomedicine and its healers have a lot to offer, there is now an increased awareness of the limitations of biomedicine, of a system based solely on a biological understanding of the human being. There is now a greater understanding of the need to pay attention to the material and non-material sociocultural factors when providing care. In the pluralistic medical systems that exist throughout the world, there is the recognition of the presence and utility of a range of health care beliefs and behaviors, as well as of practitioners of care. Furthermore, interest is rising in the need to provide health care in a more effective and efficient way, to maximize limited resources and to meet an ever-expanding array of health concerns, including those having to do with disability and rehabilitation.

For all these reasons, the field of cross-cultural health care and the idea that cultural competence is desirable have begun to flourish. Yet, cross-cultural study of how an individual, family, or society reacts to an impairment – that is, the meaning of disability in a particular context and the role and possibilities associated with rehabilitation – is still in its early stages.

This chapter will suggest ways to foster the development of a culturally competent rehabilitation professional through changes in the educational curricula and professional practice patterns; recommend ways in which a rehabilitationist can prepare for immersion in a cross-cultural experience; and summarize some of the most compelling themes that have emerged from this book.

FOSTERING THE DEVELOPMENT OF A CULTURALLY COMPETENT REHABILITATION PROFESSIONAL

To achieve cultural competence and show a commitment to a global vision of health care, professionals, both in training and in the field, must be exposed to the process of both recognizing one's own cultural identity and worldview and learning about others' cultural value system. The assumption is that competency in recognizing bias, prejudice, and discrimination and our discomfort when faced with difference, using cultural resources, and overcoming cultural barriers can be learned. An understanding of sociocultural variables in the health care setting and an individual client's worldview is expected to lead to an improved clinical encounter with better functional outcomes for the patient and a more rewarding personal experience for the professional. As Ibrahim (1995) proposes: 'Each individual in a professional-consumer dyad [should] be viewed as a unique "cultural entity" with an emphasis on the individual's "subjective reality" or worldview.... [This] can lead to professional-consumer cultural matching' (Ibrahim 1995, pp. 194–195). Nonetheless, 'The helping professions are still seeking viable theories and mod-

els for training that would prepare servic providers to provide valid, effective, reliabl and ethical professional services in a culturall diverse society' (Ibrahim 1995, p. 190).

Historically, few practicing rehabilitation pro fessionals have been suitably educated on th issues associated with the delivery of cross-cu tural health care. Often, their education ha ignored the influence of socioeconomic statu religion, race, or ethnicity, as well as the pres ence of differing explanatory models or differ ing verbal and non-verbal communication o learning styles. Strategies to overcome potentia barriers resulting from misunderstandings hav been sorely lacking, and, few schools or trainin programs provide adequate instruction abou culture and health.

To foster change in this regard, the Society o Teachers of Family Medicine's task force o cross-cultural experiences, in the USA, has rec ommended a set of core curriculum guideline on culturally sensitive and competent healt care for all family medicine residents (doctors i clinical training after medical school). It stresse the themes of self-reflection about one's ow culture and biases and increased knowledg about other people's way of life (see Appendi A for the guidelines). These curriculum guide lines are adaptable for other professiona groups. Their use, in the same or modified form is strongly encouraged. Nevertheless, th authors caution users of the document to b aware of its potential limitations and to conside their development as an ongoing process (Lik et al 1996).

Ideally, practitioners should integrate materia to foster cultural competence into multipl didactic and experiential learning experience throughout training. Didactic learning migh include learning another language or specifi details about a particular cultural way of life Experiential learning would include working i teams with professionals from other rehabilita tion disciplines and from other sociocultura groups in real-life practice settings that expos learners to different ways of life. For example clinical experiences in a homeless shelter, a inner-city clinic, an American Indian reserva

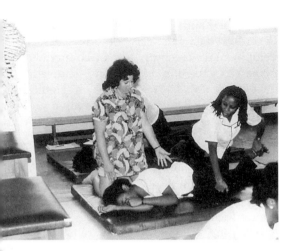

ig. 32.1 Teaching PNF at the University of West Indies, amaica, physical therapy school. Photo courtesy: Ronnie eavitt.

ion, or a foreign country can be especially educational (Fig. 32.1). A wide variety of specific multicultural training methods and exercises an assist in the preparation of such experinces. Appendix B offers a small sampling.

Likewise, a quest for cultural competence equires candid discussions regarding the need or better collaboration between the professional nd the client. The professional must strive to enter care around the client and the client's amily by taking on the role of facilitator or conultant. This, of course, is true for all patient–therapist interactions, but it especially pplies when two parties have the added limension of seeing the world from different ultural vantage points. Thus, for an encounter vith an individual patient, professionals might ecome knowledgeable about their clients' eliefs regarding family life or the causes of disbility. Furthermore, the professional might ctively attempt to formalize larger scale, politial change through legislative or political action y engaging in the process of advocating for nd developing disability rights groups. This uggests the need for practitioners to redefine heir role more broadly than they have in the ast.

Along similar lines, to be culturally compe-ent, a practitioner must have a global perspecive of care, that is, appreciate the need for

people involved in rehabilitation, with their differing customs, philosophies and ways of life, to come together to work for the common good. Helen Hislop, a pioneer physical therapist, used this theme as her focus during the plenary session of the World Confederation of Physical Therapy in June, 1995. She stated:

The value of diversity, individuality, and improvisation should be apparent to all of us. We are a group of independent clinicians, all playing the same game with the same objective, but each of us produces individual variations on the same basic theme, expressing individuality and talent that can combine to produce a unique effect, never twice the same, but powerful and beautiful. . . . You, individually and collectively, are the only means by which a change can overtake international physical therapy and give to it the preeminence it must earn You can force a change by acting in common cause that will result in a spurt of growth in the quality of our clinical services . . . that will take place in every corner of our round world. (Hislop 1995, p. 58)

Within the educational sphere, special attention should be paid to increasing the diversity of the student body, faculty, and staff. Not only does this mean encouraging more people of color to apply to academic programs, but the institutions must be prepared to facilitate successful completion of the program. The American Physical Therapy Association, for example, began formal initiatives to increase cultural diversity in physical therapy education in 1983. Some of its key initiatives are: the minority scholarship fund; Diversity 2000, an annual fund-raiser for the scholarship fund; public relations activities to recruit and retain students; a minority achievement award for academic programs that demonstrate ongoing success in recruitment and graduation of people of color; cultural diversity workshops; and more (Monahan 1997).

'Success', however, is elusive. Certainly the effort by individual educational programs is important, but it is vital for accrediting and licensing bodies to incorporate the practice of cultural competency in their standards, criteria, and requirements. Only then can these ideas become institutionalized within the educational sphere. Furthermore, institutions providing health and rehabilitative care must demonstrate organizational policies that support the recruitment and hiring of a diverse workforce and offer staff development that demonstrates a commitment to culturally competent care within the health care delivery system infrastructure.

The need for functional outcome assessment

In the quest for cultural competence, including the adaptation of services to meet unique cultural needs, the rehabilitation professional must have the tools by which to assess patient status and evaluate intervention results. To answer this need, the focus in health care assessment has shifted from impairment research to outcome research. Outcome measures evaluate disability status and indirectly evaluate patient expectations and perceptions regarding health and function rather than the presence of biological pathology (Testa & Simonson 1996). There is a growing awareness that decreasing an impairment does not necessarily lead to a commensurate decrease in disability status. The development of culturally valid standardized screening instruments and culture-specific functional outcome measures has to become an important goal for the rehabilitation professions.

Thus far, construct and content validity for some of the most common tests have been established only for individuals performing activities characteristic of the Euro-American culture. Yet, there is considerable variation across groups with regard to the kinds of functional activities that are essential for everyday life and also with regard to the age that children are expected to be able to perform these activities (Groce & Zola 1993). For example, the Euro-American standardized tests do not ask questions regarding the ability to move in and out of squatting or to use hands or chopsticks to eat. Tests appropriate to an Asian country would need these types of questions. Also, mothers in some cultures spoon-feed children until the age of 2 years or more. On a Euro-American test a child not yet manipulating utensils or independently eating some food

with their hands might be considered delayed. Recently, data analysis of the Denver Developmental Screening Test (a commonly used pediatric screening instrument) showed some developmental skills emerged at significantly different ages between the normative group of white, middle-class children in the USA and Alaska Native children (Kerfeld et al 1997). In a second study, Gannoti used the Pediatric Evaluation Disability Inventory (P.E.D.I). and also found differences between the normative group and a population of children living in Puerto Rico. (Gannoti 1998)

With the recognition that rehabilitationists will serve a diverse body of people, and the paucity of cross-cultural disability and rehabilitation research, culture-specific valid and reliable functional assessment tools and patient satisfaction scales need to be developed. Merely translating an assessment tool or research instrument like a survey into another language is not sufficient. Determining norms for concrete, specific functional activities that are appropriate for a population avoids culturally constructed concepts involving the measurement of such things as intelligence and language, gross motor, and fine motor skills. Instruments that are not culture-specific should be used with caution. At the very least, people using the assessment tool need to be sensitive to cultural needs and if possible, work with bicultural and bilingual colleagues. In addition, at the community level these tools will contribute to efforts to evaluate program outcomes; this seems particularly important in the coming years with the evaluation of additional community based rehabilitation (CBR) programs. Finally, these tools will provide useful information for cross-cultural comparisons in defining the social construction of disability and the most appropriate public policy.

PREPARING FOR IMMERSION IN A CROSS-CULTURAL SITUATION: PRACTICAL CONSIDERATIONS

What I consider exotic, charming, enchanting or captivating, you may consider annoying distasteful, offensive or even repugnant. What works for one does not work for another. For some people the opportunity to work in a cross-cultural setting is the chance of a lifetime. Others might find it a miserable experience. What personal characteristics are likely to foster a successful cross-cultural encounter? High on the list are a sense of humor, a sense of adventure, patience, flexibility, tolerance for ambiguity and difference, and cultural sensitivity. Being perceptive, empathic, innovative, organized and committed to sharing knowledge and skills are also very important. Working in a cross-cultural setting means being able to cope with the unexpected, and being prepared for situations never previously encountered. It is doubtful that anyone can be all of these things all of the time, but we can strive toward maintaining some of these attributes as often as possible. Ironically, every professional has some characteristics that are not conducive to a successful encounter. That is, we can be task-oriented, overachievers, and fearful of failure.

Not all rehabilitation professionals are suitable for working cross-culturally. That said, a practitioner who does decide to make the journey into another culture must aim for cultural competence. First and foremost, it is essential to understand and reflect upon the notion that each of us is immersed in our own culture, with its associated beliefs, attitudes, and behaviors that guide our personal and professional interactions. Our own culture is the framework that guides us in our everyday life. Furthermore, we need to take a hard look at both our tendency to stereotype as a means to simplify a complex world, and at the inherent biases we hold toward our own way of life and against that of those who are different. We need to acknowledge our tendency to understand life and draw conclusions based on superficial appearances rather than on well-founded knowledge.

In reality, we all tend to be ethnocentric, that is, believing that our own cultural way of life is the norm, the standard by which all others are judged. What we forget is that the next person, from another culture, is also ethnocentric. Thus, the ability to function effectively in another environment is no easy task; cultural competence is easy to espouse, yet very difficult to do. Do not underestimate the obstacles to achieving the goal of cultural competence. A lifetime of existence can not be so easily molded or manipulated to accept ways which can be very contrary to our own experiences and values.

At the same time, it is important to remember what cultural competence is not. It is not abandoning your own culture and becoming a member of another culture by taking on all of their attitudes, values and behaviors. It is not learning everything there is to know about another culture; that would be impossible.

Advance preparation is a critical component to a successful encounter. *Cross-cultural Rehabilitation: An International Perspective* provides an enormous amount of helpful theoretical and practical information, founded on the premise that useful information and ideas can be extrapolated from one culture and molded or manipulated to suit a different contextual environment. No two places or peoples are the same, yet principles and practices can be modified to become appropriate for a particular culture. What is essential is the need to consider a wide array of sociocultural variables and the principles of cross-cultural care.

At the same time, when working in a specific environment, within your own country or internationally, factual information about that particular environment is essential. Such things as geography, language (including verbal and non-verbal communication styles), political structure, economic and material resources, history, and cultural value orientations are all helpful, as are population characteristics such as ethnicity, religion, social structure and roles. Arguably, the most relevant variable is socioeconomic development. In much of the world, the norm is overwhelming poverty, particularly that classified as relative poverty whereby people can afford some basic necessities but cannot maintain a comfortable standard of living. The presence of poverty will assuredly influence what kind of rehabilitation is available. Knowledge of customs regarding such things as dress, food, greetings, forms of address, rites of passage, and common courtesies are also key. (See Appendix C for some resources published by governmental and private agencies that provide information about different nations and cultures and Appendix D for a sample of resources offering health-related culture-specific information.)

With regard to health, of utmost importance is a basic knowledge of infant mortality rates, life expectancy, disease and disability incidence and prevalence, health care delivery system structure (including the accessibility of hospitals, clinics, personnel, materials, etc.) and beliefs and behaviors associated with illness and disease or disability. Some cultures, for example, believe that disability is a form of punishment. A person may have sinned or violated a taboo, thereby causing the wrath of God or a source of wickedness. Alternative treatment practices, such as the Asian custom of using coin rubbing which results in raised red skin marks, to draw evil from the body, can be a source of misunderstanding. When using classic Western treatment procedures it is necessary to consider the appropriateness of that treatment within the context of the patient's culture. Elaborating on previously noted examples, in many Asian cultures people usually squat rather that sit for socializing, eating, and toileting. Thus, if a person has a fractured hip, a goal for the surgical procedure and rehabilitation process would be for a relatively greater range of motion than is typically sought in the West, even at the expense of stability. Also, eating with hands or chopsticks may require different movement patterns and range than is typically used by Westerners, thus necessitating different exercises and activities of emphasis.

In preparing for cross-cultural work, practitioners must also learn the goals and philosophy of the particular project or rehabilitation department. What is the background and rationale of the program? Particularly important is whether the program is primarily oriented to service, i.e. the actual implementation of treatment procedures, or to training and educating people who will take over responsibility for the program. Especially relevant to the therapist

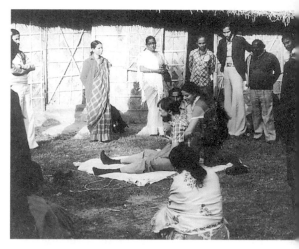

Fig. 32.2 Bangladesh. Demonstrating normal protective reactions to community health workers who are learning normal development.

who is expecting to educate is that methods of teaching and learning differ between cultures. Knowledge transmission in Western cultures, for example, often relies on taking notes and studying written texts, as well as intense discussions with a great deal of interaction between teacher and student. Other cultures rely more on a straight lecture format with few questions and little discussion. And other cultures rely almost entirely on oral training. A written list of exercises, even with diagrams, may not be as effective as demonstrating such exercises (Fig. 32.2). A dysjuncture between your goals and the program's goals may lead to disappointment.

When working in a cross-cultural environment, especially if resources are particularly limited, rehabilitation professionals may face a new twist on some familiar ethical dilemmas. Primary ethical principles of autonomy, beneficence, and distributive justice may need to be considered from new perspectives. Kay & Salzman (1994) enumerate several scenarios that might arise depending on the particular context. Let us assume that the situation involves a low-income nation with very limited resources, very few rehabilitationists and almost no facilities. The country depends upon external assistance and is pleased that expatriates are willing to work there.

Among the questions that are likely to arise are: What is the accepted scope of practice? In many instances, no laws will govern what you, or your counterpart can do, or even who can claim to be a physical, occupational, or speech therapist. Does the host country have different expectations of what you can or should do, knowing your educational and practice background, such as practicing without a physician's referral? Should you practice differently than the locals and create a double standard? Should you practice outside the scope of your usual practice, for example, by doing primary health care activities for which you have not been trained? What if you are asked to assist by giving injections, suturing, or educating about family planning or nutrition? What if these activities require most of your time and you are left without time to collaborate with PWD regarding their needs? What if, by upgrading the local professionals' knowledge and abilities, you help to enable one of the few qualified professionals to emigrate from their country, thereby leaving fewer professionals to work with PWD? No matter how you answer each question, in each case, the visiting clinician has an ethical responsibility to help inform the key individuals (such as physicians, government and non-governmental leaders) about what appropriately educated therapists are capable of doing. In the end, it must be up to the local people to determine how their system will work.

Another set of ethical questions concerns the use of technology and assistive devices (Fig. 32.3). For example, is it humanitarian, (or even useful), or is it impractical and fostering of dependence, to bring high technology or Western style equipment from a donor source, into an environment where that equipment is, with rare exception, not usable due to cultural or environmental constraints? What are the potential consequences of the donation? How much effort should you put forth to assist the privileged few with the procurement of high-tech, Western style assistive devices?

Culture shock

When working cross-culturally – whether in their own nation or in another country – rehabilitationists are likely to experience 'culture shock'. The term describes the more pronounced reactions to the psychological disorientation most people experience when immersed in a culture markedly different from their own. Some degree of culture shock is almost inevitable, and more often than not, it does not stem from any single event or series of events that you may easily confront. Rather, cumulative pressures develop from having your values constantly questioned. Your belief in your own culture and your ethnocentrism is threatened. You are cut off from familiar cultural cues and known patterns (Kohls 1979).

Culture shock is a cyclical phenomenon, involving four basic phases of adjustment. When you arrive in a new environment, and for a period of several weeks thereafter, you are likely to experience a sense of euphoria as you see and absorb new experiences. Later you will probably undergo a period of more pronounced, more unpleasant symptoms as you enter the second stage of culture shock. Differences that once seemed exciting or exotic become over-

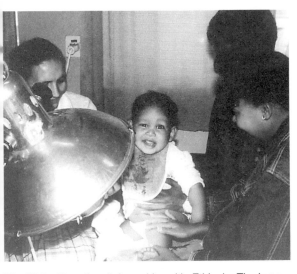

Fig. 32.3 Use of an 'infra red lamp' in Ethiopia. The lamp contains a regular bulb. Many patients receive this so that they think they are getting a 'modality'.

whelming and a source of anger. Differences associated with the non-material, less obvious value systems can especially affect how the visitor and host view the world from different vantage points. Perhaps the most difficult cultural differences to overcome psychologically, especially for North Americans and Europeans, relate to pace of life and notion of time. Westerners are action oriented and often unforgiving about such things as missed appointments, 'red tape', bureaucratic delays, and a sense that time is an unimportant concept. Combine this with the stresses of living and working under different physical conditions and an ambiguous situation, and culture shock becomes likely. Symptoms of this stage may include homesickness, withdrawal, irritability, stereotyping of and hostility toward the hosts, a lessened ability to work effectively, and physical ailments.

With time, there is a gradual adjustment and a level of appreciation for, and comfort with, the culture. With a general understanding of cultural value systems, for example a tendency toward collectivism (vs. individualism) or past orientation (vs. present or future orientation), this third stage leads to a better understanding of the logical reasons behind some of the behaviors that are most frustrating. If one remains for an extended period of time, you may adapt and likely become bi-cultural. However, do not underestimate how difficult it is to fully adapt to another culture.

Once back in a more familiar environment, you may experience a reverse culture shock. One is likely to undergo initial elation over being home again, but then, more quickly than you did while living in the other culture, you may experience depression and frustration and find difficulty adjusting. Back home, you expect things to be the same as before, but you are often changed by the cross-cultural experience. Many, for example, find Western lifestyles to be wasteful and lavish. Underlying value systems such as the expectation to be action oriented and time bound, no longer seem that important. Also, you may want to share your experiences with others, yet colleagues and friends are not

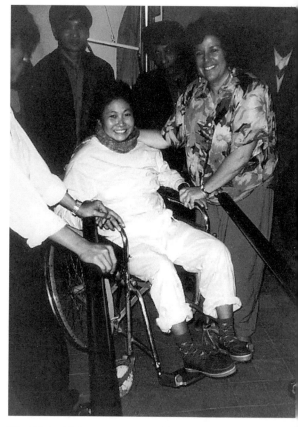

Fig. 32.4   Vietnamese woman left in bed for 3 months after traumatic head injury. Author Ronnie Leavitt assisted in fitting her for a wheelchair and standing her in parallel bars. Both women had tears of joy.

all that interested. Giving talks and presentations to interested groups can be a way of channeling your enthusiasm to those who share your interests. Again, being aware of this phenomenon, and seeking out others who have gone through a similar situation, is likely to be helpful.

In a sense, culture shock is an occupational hazard of cross-cultural immersion. There are no easy remedies but some things can help lessen its impact. Admitting to your ethnocentrism and understanding your own culture are the first steps. Learn more about yourself and your own culture through the eyes of your hosts. Also, continue to learn about the particular culture in which you are working. Ask questions and be astute in your observations. Have realistic expectations of yourself and others and remember that problems and challenges are inevitable. The more respect that you show for the people and culture, the more respect you are likely to command and the more effective a consultant/clinician you are. Additionally, be realistic about how much you can accomplish during a particular time period. It can be disheartening to leave a site with the realization that you have only made a dent and that many needs are left unmet. However, the gratitude you will receive from PWD and colleagues is likely to be one of the richest rewards of your life (Fig. 32.4). Many rehabilitationists return to their home setting feeling that they have gained more than they have given.

LESSONS TO BE LEARNED FROM *CROSS-CULTURAL REHABILITATION: AN INTERNATIONAL PERSPECTIVE*

Cross-cultural Rehabilitation: An International Perspective adds to the development of a relatively new area of study. Groce & Sheer (1990) and Ingstad & Whyte (1995) note the slow emergence of research regarding disability and culture and the need for a holistic conceptualization of PWD in their own cultural context. By way of cultural juxtaposition (chapters cover a range of cultures throughout the world and come from the perspective of differing academic disciplines to familiarize the reader with work being done by experts in a related field) there has been an attempt to provide an expansion of our own limited worldview perspective; to make us realize the limitations of seeing the world only through our own eyes and mind. Only through a greater understanding of different cultures, and an understanding of the different disciplines and their ability to contribute to the study of cross-cultural rehabilitation, can there be a dissolution of boundaries – both between cultures and between the disciplines. *Cross-cultural Rehabilitation: An International Perspective* provides an overview of a range of material that is likely new to many rehabilitation professionals. This resource aims to challenge the clinician, academician, and stu-

dent to work across cultures. It should be seen as a starting point from which to further study and discuss topics of particular interest. It should enable the rehabilitation professional to become more culturally competent.

Chapters range from providing a theoretical perspective to those describing case scenarios. From these, several compelling themes have emerged. The rehabilitation professional can extrapolate the information to their own cross-cultural situation and begin to explore ways to further cultural competence. For instance, to advance an understanding of disability cross-culturally, practitioners and researchers, in their attempt to improve functional outcomes, need to speak a universal language (using the terms impairment, disability, and handicap in the same way) and to understand the particular epidemiological considerations within an environment. There is a need to understand alternative cultural value systems and verbal and non-verbal communication styles, and the advantages of a collaborative teaching and learning environment, as well as to be cognizant of usable strategies to minimize existing barriers between people from different cultural contexts.

Themes

A prominent theme is that all human experiences, including the experience of disability, are grounded in culture. However, the perception of disability is not a universal phenomenon. Although PWD have existed through the ages, and in all societies, and there are predictors of how someone will fare in a community, the meaning and consequences of having a disability vary. Although the presence of negative attitudes toward, and discriminatory practices against, PWD is often the reality, there are exceptions. In part, variation is a result of the kinds of rehabilitation services available to that individual. By defining the culture of disability for particular sub-cultures, the authors contribute to the understanding of the culture-specific explanatory models of PWD (although, of course, the authors themselves are limited by their own cultural influences and experiences when reporting on any subject). The aim has been to draw attention to a variety of beliefs and behaviors associated with disability and rehabilitation in different locations and to variations within one place and in one time. The notion of inter-cultural and intra-cultural diversity has been supported.

A second dominant theme is that the development of an ideal model by which to provide rehabilitation has remained elusive, but clearly any such model must be culture-specific and not merely attentive to biomedical intervention. All models, both new and old, must be systematically scrutinized to determine which model works and is sustainable for a particular culture. This difficult task is further complicated by the fact that there is no universal agreement on what should be measured. Is a change in the developmental milestone of a child with a disability more or less important than a change in the effect that child will have on the life of the family? More research, especially from the point of view of the PWD, is critical.

Third, in most situations, and given the expectation of significant financial constraints, the chances for any model of rehabilitation to succeed will be enhanced if rehabilitation is an integral part of a commitment to broader community development, with input from multiple public and private sectors (such as those involved with education, or labor). Paramount would be the inclusion of PWD and/or their families, as well as local community leaders in the planning and implementation stages.

Fourth, it is also apparent that success will depend on professionals' recognizing the unique sociocultural circumstances and needs of the PWD. A case in point might be the need to acknowledge the importance of a range of cultural value orientations that might influence the kind of care that is deemed appropriate, the personal beliefs and behaviors associated with disability and rehabilitation, or the need to seek ways to make your goals and the patients' or families' goals compatible rather than conflictual. A family may become involved with an early intervention program, as in a Euro-American value system, but may refuse a surgi-

cal intervention for fear of destroying the child's spirituality. Strategies to maximize involvement of the families of PWD are often critical, but it may be unfair and unrealistic to expect family members to be involved with active rehabilitation. Each individual case must be assessed due to the transactional and situational nature of cultural identity, and mutual adaptation must be considered as a potential solution.

Fifth, rehabilitationists will need to adjust to a paradigm shift to become co-participants or partners with PWD and serve as collaborators or consultants rather than managers of rehabilitation activities. They may find it most productive to become more involved with a broader array of activities than heretofore seen as part of one's traditional professional responsibilities. As an example, the professional may become an advocate for the disability rights movement, keeping in mind the ultimate goal is for PWD to become empowered to have the freedom and equal opportunity to make their own choices in life. A focus on changing societal attitudes toward PWD might have a greater impact than an exercise regime. In essence, the 'culture of rehabilitation' needs to change and adapt in response to the environment and conditions present in a particular time and place. It must adapt to an increasingly diverse population thereby necessitating more cross-cultural interactions and a culturally appropriate intervention process.

CONCLUSION

In conclusion, persons with disabilities, almost half a billion strong, are often limited in their ability to fully integrate into society by physical or social barriers. From single individuals around the globe to multinational governmental and non-governmental organizations, there has been an upsurge in the effort to ensure human rights and full participation of PWD in all aspects of social and economic life. The formulation of the World Programme of Action Concerning Disabled Persons (1992) and the United Nations International Decade of Disabled Persons (1983–1992) are two examples of formalized attempts to facilitate change. Yet, change is typically very slow and arduous.

Constructive movement toward the future requires a vision. The vision can be obtained by pooling our ideas and resources and seeking a commitment from all those involved in the rehabilitation process. For rehabilitation professionals, there is a special moral and political imperative to facilitate the rehabilitation process whereby PWD can maximize their human potential by fulfilling their life's goals. Included in this obligation is the idea that all consumers of care, no matter what their specific identity, deserve the very best that a professional has to offer. To have the most impact on diminishing the disability status of a client, the rehabilitation professional must understand how disability is socially constructed for that particular individ-ual. That is, the disability and its consequences must be defined in the context of the person's sociocultural environment. This requires the professional to be culturally competent. The path of intercultural learning to cultural profi-ciency takes a long time and conscious effort.

In acknowledging the social construction of disability, rehabilitation professionals then face the challenge of embracing diversity and differ-ences, reshaping practice protocols, redefining research priorities, and developing the most appropriate service models and public policy to benefit PWD. The professional will feel greater satisfaction associated with providing care that is culturally competent and by improved out-comes for the PWD. The PWD is expected to gain the right to more personal choices and free-dom.

REFERENCES

Cross T L, Bazron B J, Dennis K W, Isaacs M R 1989 Towards a culturally competent system of care. Volume 1. National Technical Assistance Center for Children's Mental health, Georgetown University, Washington DC

Gannoti M 1998 PhD dissertation The validity and reliability of the paediatric evaluation of disability for children liv-ing in Puerto Rico. University of Connecticut

Groce N, Sheer J 1990 Introduction. Social Science and Medicine 30(8): v–vi

Groce N, Zola I 1993 Multiculturalism, chronic illness, and disability. Pediatrics **91**(5): 1048–1055

Hislop H 1995 In common cause. Presented at World Confederation of Physical Therapy, June 1995. PT Magazine (September): 56–61

Ibrahim F 1995 Multicultural influences on rehabilitation training and services: the shift to valuing nondominant cultures. In: Karan O, Greenspan S (eds) Community rehabilitation services for people with disabilities. Butterworth-Heinemann, Boston, pp. 187–205

Ingstad B, Whyte S 1995 Disability and culture. University of California Press, Berkeley

Kay E, Salzman A 1994 Volunteer PTs in developing nations. PT Magazine (October): 52–56

Kerfeld C, Guthrie M, Steward K 1997 Evaluation of the Denver II as applied to Alaska Native children. Pediatric Physical Therapy 9: 23–31

Kohls R 1979 Survival kit for overseas living. Intercultural Press, Chicago

Like R, Steiner R P, Rubel A 1996 Recommended core cur-riculum guidelines on culturally sensitive and competent health care. Family Medicine 28(4): 291–297

Monahan B 1997 The quest for diversity in the classroom. PT magazine (January) 72–77

Testa M, Simonson D 1996 Assessment of quality of life outcomes. New England Journal of Medicine 334(13): 835–840

Appendices to Chapter 32

Appendix A: Core-curriculum guidelines on culturally sensitive and competent health care*

ATTITUDES

Residents will develop attitudes that include:

1. Awareness of the impact of sociocultural factors on patients, practitioners, the clinical encounter, and interpersonal relationships
2. Acceptance of the physician's responsibility to understand the cultural dimensions of health and illness as a core clinical task in the care of all patients
3. Willingness to make their own clinical settings more accessible to patients by taking into consideration their residential location, means, and costs of transportation, working hours, language and communication needs, disability status, and other financial and environmental circumstances
4. Appreciation of the heterogeneity that exists within and across cultural groups and the need to avoid overgeneralization and negative stereotyping
5. Recognition of their own personal biases and reactions to persons from different minority, ethnic, and sociocultural backgrounds and the need to deal with cultural countertransference
6. Appreciation of how one's personal cultural values, assumptions, and beliefs influence the clinical care provided
7. Willingness to understand and explicate those values, assumptions. and beliefs and to examine how they affect the care provided to patients that share and do not share a similar perspective
8. Understanding of the limitations of cultural analysis and the role played by other historical, political, economic, technologic, and environmental forces in shaping the delivery of health care to individuals, families, and communities
9. Expressing respect and tolerance for cultural and social class differences and their value in a pluralistic society
10. A moral and ethical obligation to challenge racism, classism, ageism, sexism, homophobia, and other forms of bias, prejudice, and discrimination when they occur in health care settings and society in general.

---

* Reproduced with permission from Family Medicine, 1996.

KNOWLEDGE

Residents will develop an understanding of:
1. General sociocultural issues relating to health care
   A. Anthropologic concepts that are essential for the provision of culturally sensitive and competent health care
   B. How all cultural systems – including those of both patients and physicians – are sources of (congruent and incongruent) beliefs about health, communication about symptoms, and treatment
   C. The impact of culture on the recognition of symptoms and behaviors related to illness
   D. How diversity within a culture affects the provision and utilization of care
   E. How health care systems reflect the prevailing values of the culture(s) in which they exist
   F. Developmental models of ethnosensitivity (e.g. fear, denial, superiority, minimization, relativism, empathy, and integration) in relation to one's own ethnic and sociocultural background

2. Multiculturalism in the USA
   A. Selected minority, ethnic, and sociocultural groups (according to relevant local needs):
      1. Northern, Western, Southern, and Eastern European-American
      2. Black/African-Americans
      3. Asian/Pacific Island-Americans
      4. Latino/Hispanic-Americans
      5. Native Americans/American Indians/Inuit
      6. West Indian/Caribbean-Americans
      7. Middle and near Eastern-Americans
   B. Selected vulnerable or 'at-risk' groups
      1. Age-specific (infants, children, adolescents, adults, and older adults)
      2. Low income
      3. Homeless persons
      4. Immigrants/refugees
      5. Persons in specific occupations
      6. Migrant workers
      7. Gays and lesbians
      8. Persons with developmental disabilities
      9. Persons with physical disabilities
      10. Persons with mental disabilities
      11. Persons with addiction problems
      12. Persons who are incarcerated
      13. Other special populations
   C. The changing demographics of various population groups
      1. Historical experiences
      2. Sociocultural characteristics
      3. Economic characteristics
      4. Political characteristics
      5. Geographic characteristics
      6. Religious characteristics
      7. Linguistic characteristics

3. Cultural perspectives on medicine and public health
   A. The health-seeking process and illness behavior
      1. Sociocultural determinants of health and wellness
      2. The disease/illness distinction
      3. Personal/familial health and illness-related beliefs, values, attitudes, customs, rituals, and behaviors
      4. Sociocultural risk factors and interventions that can be used to modify these risk factors
      5. Kleinman's 'typology of health sectors'
         a. Use of the 'Professional Health Sector' (the organized regulated legally sanctioned health professions, such as modern Western biomedicine)
         b. Use of the 'Popular Health Sector' (the lay, nonprofessional, nonspecialist domain of society where ill health is first recognized and defined, and health care activities are initiated)
         c. Use of the 'Folk Health Sector' (nonprofessional, nonbureaucratic forms of healing that are either sacred, secular, or both)
         d. Interactions within and across the professional, popular, and folk sectors of care
         e. Outcomes of professional, popular, and folk healing
      6. Access issues and barriers/facilitators to care
   B. Cultural assumptions and their influence on the US health care system
      1. Basic value orientations (in relation to human nature, other people, activity, time, and the environment)
      2. Self-help/volunteerism/consumerism
      3. Advocacy/activism
      4. Populism/elitism
      5. Separatism/pluralism/integration
      6. Opportunity/optimism
      7. Efficacy/effectiveness/equity
      8. Prejudice/discrimination (eg. racism, classism, ageism, sexism, homophobia)
      9. Privilege/disadvantage
      10. Power/powerlessness/critical consciousness

4. The ethnosensitive (cultural) epidemiology of health and illness problems of diverse population groups
   A. Clinical problems relating to the nation's health promotion and disease prevention objectives
   B. Clinical problems having high mortality and morbidity rates
   C. Clinical problems relating to the stage of the individual and family life cycles and major life events (pregnancy, birth, marriage, death, etc.)
   D. Clinical problems that are linked to culture shock from migration, intergenerational value orientation conflicts, and acculturation/assimilation processes
   E. Clinical problems relating to 'folk illnesses' (e.g. 'high blood,' 'falling out,' 'evil eye,' ' susto,' 'ghost sickness,' 'koro')
   F. Clinical problems present in country or geographic area of origin

SKILLS

Residents will develop skills in the following areas:
1. Clinical practice
   A. Forming and maintaining a therapeutic alliance
   B. Recognizing and appropriately responding to verbal and nonverbal communication

C. Constructing a medical and psychosocial history and performing a physical examination in a culturally sensitive fashion

D. Using the biopsychosocial model in disease prevention/health promotion, the interpretation of clinical signs and symptoms, and illness-related problem solving

E. Prescribing treatment in a culturally sensitive manner

F. Using the negotiated approach to clinical care
  1. Berlin and Fowke's LEARN model
     (L) – Listening to the patient's perspective
     (E) – Explaining and sharing one's own perspective
     (A) – Acknowledging differences and similarities between these two perspectives
     (R) – Recommending a treatment plan
     (N) – Negotiating a mutually agreed-on treatment plan
  2. Explanatory model (EM) elicitation techniques
     Eliciting individual or family EMs: (i.e. 'ideas about the etiology, onset, pathophysiology, prognosis, and treatment of disease and illness')
  3. Illness prototype (IP) and patient request (PR) elicitation techniques
     Eliciting individual or family IPs: (i.e. 'ideas about sickness based on previous personal experiences, the experiences of significant others, or media-transmitted information')
     Eliciting individual or family PRs: (i.e. 'the type of help [clinical resource] the patient would like [hopes, wishes, wants] to receive from the practitioner')
  4. Pfifferling's cultural status exam

  5. Stuart and Lieberman's BATHE model – Background/Affect/Trouble/Handling/Empathy)
     Exploring the psychosocial context of the patient's visit to provide social support and as a basis for gaining insight

G. Using family members, community, gatekeepers, translators/interpreters, and other community resources and advocacy groups

H. Working collaboratively with other health care professionals in a culturally sensitive and competent manner

I. Working with alternative/complementary medicine practitioners and/or indigenous, lay, or folk healers when professionally, ethically, and legally appropriate

J. Identifying how one's cultural values, assumptions, and beliefs affect patient care and clinical decision making

2. Administrative practice
  A. Analyzing the sociocultural dimensions of one's own practice site and the implications for practice management
  B. Implementing a cultural sensitization training program for office/clinic staff
  C. Promoting cultural competence in health care organizations as part of total quality management and continuous quality improvement activities
  D. Using ethnographic and epidemiological techniques in developing a community-oriented family practice
  E. Influencing the cultures of health care organizations and professional groups (eg, managed care organizations, ambulatory care facilities, hospitals, nursing homes, specialty societies)

Appendix B: Resources for multicultural training exercises

Anti-defamation League of B'nai B'rith 1986 A world of difference. Boston, MA

BaFa' BaFa' 1977 Simulating training systems. Del Mar, CA

Brislin R, Yoshida T 1994 Improving multicultural interactions: modules for cross-cultural training programs. Sage, Newbury Park

Committee on Minority Health Affairs 1991 Racial and cultural bias in medicine: video and discussion guide. American Academy of Family Physicians, Kansas City

Dickerson-Jones T 1993 50 activities for managing cultural diversity. Human Resource Development Press, New York

Ibrahim F 1995 Multicultural influences on rehabilitation training and services: the shift to valuing nondominant cultures. In: Karan O, Greenspan S (eds) Community rehabilitation services for people with disabilities. Butterworth-Heinemann, Boston, MA, pp. 187–205

Kavanaugh K, Kennedy P 1992 Promoting cultural diversity: strategies for health care professionals. Sage, Newbury Park

Lambert J, Myers S 1994 50 activities for diversity training. Human Resource Development Press, New York

Locke D 1992 Increasing multicultural understanding: a comprehensive model. Sage, Newbury Park

Ponterotto J, Pedersen P 1993 Preventing prejudice: a guide for counselors and educators. Sage, Newbury Park

Teaching Tolerance. Biannual publication of the Southern Poverty Law Center, Montgomery, Ala

Weeks W H, Pedersen P B, Brislin R W (eds) 1979 A manual of structured experiences for cross cultural learning. Intercultural Press, Yarmouth

Appendix C:
Resources for additional information on culture

This list focuses primarily on resources produced in the USA. Other nations have similar resources.

1. *Background notes*. Published by the US State Department; 170 countries are covered. Between 6 and 10 pages long, they cover geography, people, history, government, political conditions, economy and foreign relations. Often with suggested reading. Available from the Superintendent of Documents, Government Printing Office, Washington, DC, 20402-9325. For information, call +1 (202) 647-6575.

2. *Bibliographic surveys*. These are annotated bibliographies. Ten volumes are available from the Superintendent of Documents, US Government Printing Office, Washington, DC, 20402-9325.

3. *Business customs and protocol*. This series is produced primarily for business people by the Stanford Research Institute. The series concentrates on how to get started, how to get things done and how to facilitate mutual understanding. Available from Stanford Research Institute International, 333 Ravenswood Avenue, Menlo Park, CA 94025.

4. *Country studies* (formerly called Area Handbooks). These valuable resources are updated regularly. They are prepared by the Foreign Area Studies Group at American University. These include 108 different countries covered to varying degrees of thoroughness. Also available from the Superintendent of Documents, US Government Printing Office, Washington, DC, 20402-9325. For information, call +1 (202) 647-6575.

5. *Country updates* summarize important information that the foreign resident might need. Available from Intercultural Press, Inc. PO Box 768, Yarmouth, ME 04096.

6. *Culturegrams* are published by Brigham Young University and cover 96 countries. The reports are brief, but cover customs and courtesies, the people, lifestyles and a small map. They contain information about local customs and there is an emphasis on practical tips on how to get along. Available from David M. Kennedy Center for International Studies, Publication Services, 280 HRCB, Provo, UT 84602, or call +1 (801) 378-6528.

7. *Encyclopedia of the Third World*. There are three volumes in the series, which can be consulted in the reference section of most libraries. Published by Facts on File, 460 Park Avenue South, New York, NY 10016.

8. *Human relations area file.* A tremendously valuable resource, but probably one that contains more information than the average person needs. It provides access to voluminous entries of an anthropological nature for many cultures and subcultures around the world. If you want to be thoroughly prepared, it is a goldmine of information. Many major university libraries house copies of the HRAF on microfiche. Information can be obtained from Human Relations Area File, 755 Prospect Street, New Haven, CT 06511.

9. *Professional organization special interest groups.* For example, the Cross-Cultural and International Special Interest Group (CCISIG) of the American Physical Therapy Association has additional resources and the names of individuals who have worked internationally.

10. *Other sources of information:*
    - Chamber of Commerce.
    - Church and missionary societies.
    - The embassy of the host country. Many also have Offices or Ministers of Tourism, which are frequently located in New York City, or the capital of your own country.
    - Universities and colleges in your area. The departments of anthropology and public health are likely to be the most useful.
    - Foreign exchange students.

Appendix D: Culture-specific health related resources

This list represents a sampling of some culture-specific health related resources.

Adams D L (ed) 1995 Health issues for women of color: a cultural diversity perspective. Sage, Thousand Oaks, CA

Braithwaite R L, Taylor S E (eds) 1992 Health issues in the black community. Jossey-Bass, San Francisco

Cross-cultural medicine. 1983 Western Journal of Medicine 139: (6)

Cross-cultural medicine – a decade later. 1992 Western Journal of Medicine 157(3)

Galanti G-A 1991 Caring for patients from different cultures: case studies from American hospitals. University of Pennsylvania Press, Philadelphia

Harwood A (ed) 1981 Ethnicity and medical care. Harvard University, Cambridge

Huff R M, Kline M V 1999 Promoting health in multicultural populations: a handbook for practitioners. Sage, Thousand Oaks, CA

Lynch E W, Hanson M J (eds) 1992 Developing cross-cultural competence: a guide for working with young children and their families. Paul H. Brooks, Baltimore, MD

Molina C W, Aquirre-Molina M 1995 Latino health in the US: a growing challenge. US Department of Health and Human Services, Public Health Services, Washington, DC

Office of Minority Health Resource Center 1995 Pocket guide to minority health resources. US Department of Health and Human Services, Public Health Services, Washington, DC

Pachter L M 1994 Culture and clinical care: folk illness beliefs and behaviors and their implications for health care delivery. Journal of American Medical Association 271: 690–694

Spector R 1991 Cultural diversity in health and illness. Appleton and Lange, Norwalk

Young T K 1994 The health of Native Americans; toward a biocultural epidemiology. Oxford University Press, New York

Zane N W S, Takeuchi D T, Young K N J (eds) 1994 Confronting critical health issues of Asian and Pacific Islander Americans. Sage, Newbury Park

Index